Rheumatic Fever in America and Britain

# Rheumatic Fever in America and Britain

## A Biological, Epidemiological, and Medical History

Peter C. English

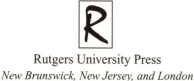

Rutgers University Press

*New Brunswick, New Jersey, and London*

**Library of Congress Cataloging-in-Publication Data**

English, Peter C.
    Rheumatic fever in America and Britain : a biological,
epidemiological, and medical history / Peter C. English.
       p.   cm.
    Includes bibliographical references and index.
    ISBN 0–8135–2710–4 (alk. paper)
    1. Rheumatic fever—America—History. 2. Rheumatic fever—Great
Britain—History. I. Title.
RC182.R4E54 1999
616.9'91'00941—dc21                                    99–14094
                                                           CIP

British Cataloging-in-Publication data for this book is available from the British Library

Manufactured in the United States of America

*To Sarah Warder English and the
three decades we have spent together*

# CONTENTS

# Illustrations, Figures, and Tables

# ACKNOWLEDGMENTS

This book has been a long time in coming. I am a medical historian who is convinced that each half of my career—primary care pediatrician and historian—enhances the other. Pursuing two careers does have a down side: time for historical investigation, especially away from my home base, Duke University, comes at a premium. Fortunately, generous grants have provided support for research. This project got under way with funds from the Josiah Macy, Jr. Foundation (1984–1986). It soon became clear to me that much of the pre-1900 history of rheumatic fever was a British story. In 1988 I spent a month at the Wellcome Library in London, supported by grants from the Josiah Charles Trent Memorial Foundation, the Burroughs-Wellcome Fund, the American Philosophical Society, and the National Institutes of Health/National Library of Medicine Extramural Programs. The NIH/NLM also provided partial salary support in 1988–89. Then came a five-year administrative interlude when I served as Chief of the Division of General Pediatrics and Director of the Pediatric Clinics at Duke. Although this was an exciting time to be on medicine's management "front lines," these duties took me completely away from rheumatic fever. When my tour of administrative duty ended, the managed care revolution was in full swing. As every practicing physician understands, this shift in the funding of American medicine has greatly eroded time dedicated to largely "unfunded activities," such as historical research. My work on this book proceeded only in the interstices between patients and teaching. In 1997, funds again from the Josiah Charles Trent Memorial Foundation and the Burroughs-Wellcome Fund, augmented by support from the Department of Pediatrics and the Dean of Arts and Sciences at Duke, permitted a sabbatical year which I spent at the Wellcome Institute for the History of Medicine. The manuscript was finished in London. My designation as the first Josiah Charles Trent Associate Professor of the History of Medicine at Duke University provided support for the final preparation of the manuscript for publication. I would like to express special thanks to Mary and Jim Semans and their generous family, benefactors of the Trent chair, who have encouraged me since my undergraduate days at Duke.

I would like to acknowledge the libraries and librarians who were particularly helpful to me over the years. Staffs at the Wellcome Library and at the Clinical Sciences Library and the Biological Sciences Library, both associated with University College, London, provided considerable assistance. At Duke University, Betsy Adams, Mary Ann Brown, and Susan Feinglos in the Medical Center Library and Barbara Busse, G.S.T. Cavanagh, Susan Smith Cavanagh, Gayle Elmore, and Suzanne Porter, in the Josiah Charles Trent Historical Collection provided years of assistance. In particular, I would like to thank Betsy Adams for checking the accuracy of every citation.

Along the way I have delivered papers at meetings, conferences, and workshops. Among the sponsoring institutions were the Johns Hopkins Institute for the History of Medicine (1983, 1991); Bradford Lectures in the History of Pediatrics, Children's Mercy Hospital, Kansas City, Missouri (1984); Hospital for Sick Children, Great Ormond Street, London (1985); College of Physicians of Philadelphia (1988); History of Medicine Society, University of Alabama–Birmingham (1988); University of Washington (1988); University of Kansas (Hixon Hour, 1991; Logan Clendening Lecture, 1995); University of Kansas–Wichita (1991); Triangle Workshop in the History of Science, Medicine, and Technology (1991); and the Wellcome Institute for the History of Medicine/University College, London (1998). I gained special insights in each of these presentations from conversations with one or more in the audience about the upheavals that rheumatic fever had wrought in their family lives. Some of these experiences have been included in this book.

Several colleagues read the complete manuscript: Jeffrey Paul Baker (Duke University), Ann G. Carmichael (Indiana University), Gerald Grob (for Rutgers University Press), Margaret Humphreys (Duke University), and Doris Zallen (Virginia Polytechnic Institute and State University). These historians added rich insights and blunt criticism. Baker, a pediatrician, and Humphreys, an internist, also read the manuscript with a clinical eye. Not all agreed with every aspect of my central argument. I am thankful to each. I take full responsibility, of course, for the final result.

The Wellcome Library and the Wellcome Institute for the History of Medicine hosted me twice. I want to pay special thanks to Sal Bragg, Bill Bynum, Chris Lawrence, Michael Neve, Vivian Nutton, and Roy Porter for their warm welcome. In London, I shared an office with Ian Dowbiggin and Doris Zallen. Many conversations with Ian and Doris added crucial perspective to this volume.

Dual careers are not possible without supportive colleagues. In the History Department, I have been blessed with a series of supportive chairs: Robert Durden, Anne Scott, Warren Lerner, William Chafe, and Alex Roland. Deans of Arts and Sciences, Richard White and William Chafe, provided needed assistance at key moments. In pediatrics, my division chiefs have always valued my work in history: Thomas Frothingham, Deborah Squire, and Dennis Clements. Martha Gagliano, Samuel Katz, Deborah Kredich, John Moses, Neil Prose, and Gordon Worley—all humanists and pediatricians—provided inspiration along the way. I am particularly grateful to the nurses and physicians in my pediatrics practice who cared for my patients while I was on sabbatical.

From Rutgers University Press, I received much needed critical comment and assistance from Doreen Valentine and Helen Hsu.

I have had the privilege of caring for several patients with rheumatic fever. One child, Adela V., stands out in my memory. Her infirmity rendered her an almost constant resident while I was in training at New York Hospital. I have thought of Adela often in the course of my writing.

Finally, my wife, Sarah, read and edited every word in this book (except these). One of my goals for this volume was to make it readable and as devoid of jargon as possible. Sarah's perceptive comments refined both prose and argument. It is to her and our marriage that this book is dedicated.

March 1999

# PREFACE

When I enrolled in medical school in 1969, intent on studying both diseases and their histories, rheumatic fever had largely vanished from the commonplace experience of physicians and their students. In 1970 rheumatic fever accounted for only 256 deaths in the United States, a startling decline from nearly 40,000 deaths in 1940.[1] While virtually a disease of history, like smallpox or the "English Sweate," rheumatic fever had not been forgotten. Indeed, encountering the memory of rheumatic fever was much like attending a traditional family gathering that continues on after the death of a loved one. Recollections and lore abounded; what remained of the disease produced fond recall among my medical school teachers of their formative clinical experiences. In truth, rheumatic fever had largely disappeared even from their medical youth. Physicians who had trained at Boston's House of the Good Samaritan, a hospital that specialized in the care of the sickest sufferers of rheumatic fever and where many of the innovations of the thirties and forties first saw light, remembered that some of the hospital's beds went empty during their training in the fifties.[2] Some of these same physicians remembered with persistent excitement their investigations into rheumatic fever a decade earlier during World War II, because the disease, long in decline, briefly enjoyed an epidemiological encore in barrack[3] and ship[4] life that crowded recruits into tight living spaces. Heightening these wartime experiences was the exhilaration of investigating the stunning efficiency of sulfonamide and, a few years later, penicillin in driving the nails into the coffin of a disease once so prevalent.[5] Antibiotics played a role, especially in prevention, but they were only a small part of the story. In fact, rheumatic fever had been in decline for a half century before the discovery of penicillin.

In 1970 there were still vestiges of rheumatic fever left visible for the newcomer to medicine. On rare occasions, a child came to the pediatric clinic with complaints so unusual that the question of rheumatic fever arose. In such instances we would seek out of necessity the "gray-hairs," because our regular teachers, pediatric house officers, had no first-hand experience with the disease. The elders would enter the examining room. If we had guessed correctly, great ceremony would be made in gathering together as many students and residents as possible for a demonstration and discussion of this fascinating disease. Dramatic physical findings formed the core of these rare sessions. Afflicted children had painfully swollen joints, usually wrists, ankles, or knees. In marked contrast to patients with other forms of arthritis, the suffering of these children demonstrated that this peculiar form of arthritis actually moved from joint to joint. Even more striking, these swollen joints in time would heal completely without leaving the child with a crippling handicap. Careful auscultation of the heart then followed, for no diagnosis of rheumatic fever could be made without some evidence of recent acquisition of heart disease. This part of the demonstration was often futile, because in 1970 proving cardiac injury often required a close reading of the electrocardiogram; rheumatic fever seldom left its once unmistakable heart murmurs. Our teachers would then search the child for evidence of erythema marginatum, a rash almost unique to rheumatic fever, and growths along the tendon sheaths. And they would question the parents closely for any evidence of random, involuntary movements, or chorea. These manifestations of rheumatic fever we almost never saw, for they had become rare even when our teachers were in our places as students. Children diagnosed with rheumatic fever were admitted to the hospital in 1970, not so much because of the severity of their current illness but because of the fear of their developing life-threatening heart disease, fortunately by then a rarity. We were instructed to investigate for evidence of prior streptococcal illness, by parental recollection, bacterial culturing, or immunological blood tests, and we were sent off to review T. Duckett Jones's criteria for diagnosis, which had been officially "modified" twice since he published them in 1944 based on his years of experience at the House of the Good Samaritan.[6] To our surprise as students, the older physicians still debated therapy and long-term management, unusual we thought for a disease that appeared "conquered." Even more unusual was that the debaters came from many walks of medicine: pediatrics, internal medicine, cardiology, and surgery. In the highly specialized world of medicine that we were entering, discussion across disciplines at the bedside happened infrequently.

Remnants from rheumatic fever also remained on the medical, surgical, and obstetrical wards. Our older patients often inquired whether they still had telltale evidence of heart damage acquired decades earlier as children. Occasionally, heart valves, scarred during a childhood bout with rheumatic fever, provided friendly sites for life-threatening infectious endocarditis. Frequently, the origin of the infection stemmed from bacteria released into the bloodstream during a routine dental cleaning or extraction. Our job as medical students was to obtain multiple blood samples for culture and to maintain the intravenous catheters for the prescribed six weeks of antibiotics. Some valves, damaged beyond effectiveness, required replacement. By 1970 surgically repairing or replacing heart valves had become routine on the surgical service, more than twenty years after the "revival" of valvular surgery in the late forties.[7] In some of our patients, the heart's muscle or myocardium simply gave out after decades of smoldering rheumatic inflammation. These victims died, their weakened hearts worn out a decade before routine heart transplantation. Surviving rheumatic fever meant that many victims could expect to lead fuller lives. Women of childbearing years were clear beneficiaries. By 1970 many women—with the reluctant blessing of their obstetricians—conceived and survived pregnancy.

My recollections, while vivid, are scanty, for it was simply not possible to immerse myself in rheumatic fever the way that my teachers had done. What struck indelibly, though, was a disease that touched clinical medicine widely: most age groups, most disciplines. It brought laboratory scientists and clinicians together intellectually and physically. In my experience, laboratory researchers only occasionally joined bedside discussions; one ecumenical reason was a child struggling with rheumatic fever. To be fair, laboratory scientists' interest in bedside medicine was fueled by more than nostalgia, for recent discoveries in molecular biology held out the hope of explaining some of rheumatic fever's age-old puzzles. What also seared my imagination was a disease that ignited controversy even after its death.

Rheumatic fever fascinates me as a historian, because it is a disease that abounds with change. Historians anticipate that medical and public health ideas about a particular illness and how to prevent or treat it will change considerably over time, depending on the disease and on the social settings of patients and physicians. In this regard, rheumatic fever does not disappoint. Its striking complexity lends itself to more changes in ideas and theories than most diseases. It is an illness of skin, brain, heart, connective tissue, blood and serum, tonsils, and joints, all bound intimately to a member of the streptococcus family of bacteria that causes several human diseases. Each component of the disease has its own history; together, as rheumatic fever, they share a collective history. In addition, rheumatic fever has been most responsive to the environment, especially living conditions and physical setting.

Equally provocative have been striking epidemiological changes. Rheumatic fever assumed its modern configuration in the early nineteenth century, rose in prevalence and severity throughout that century and reaching its peak in the last decades, and then steadily declined—in both prevalence and severity—throughout the twentieth century.[8] In the nineteenth century, acute rheumatic fever was largely a disease of children and young adults. In the twentieth century, another remarkable epidemiological change occurred: rheumatic fever shifted its character, became milder, and in doing so allowed its victims to live longer, if handicapped, lives. In other words, rheumatic fever evolved into a chronic disease. As it did so, adults also became victims.[9]

Changing ideas and epidemiology are only part of rheumatic fever's history. Orchestrating these alterations was a disease that mutated biologically. Historically, we see biological change first in the increasing severity of symptoms and in the enlarging number of bodily organs that rheumatic fever injured. In the nineteenth century, all the symptoms of rheumatic fever worsened. Arthritis and chorea, while temporary, rendered victims invalids. Inflamed heart tissues, initially the pericardium, the tissue surrounding the heart, and the endocardium, or heart valves—not components of rheumatic fever until the end of the eighteenth century—killed. In the twentieth century, all symptoms moderated. Arthritis yielded to aches and pains; chorea to nervous twitches; diseased pericardium and the endocardium to a more benign myocarditis, an inflammation of the heart's muscle. By 1970 rheumatic fever, a disease of signs and symptoms, became imperceptible both to patients and to their doctors. Antibiotics rightfully deserved credit for preventing rheumatic fever; antibiotics, however, were neither treatment nor cure, and, as we shall see, did not account for the biological alteration of rheumatic fever. Countless children were still infected with the streptococcus—a disease that has remained an everyday experience despite antibiotics—but virtually none developed rheumatic fever, whether or not they received antibiotics.

As a consequence of these changes, rheumatic fever proved something of a "moving target" for physicians, public health workers, and their patients. The link connecting mutating biology, altering epidemiology, and changing ideas, I think, is the shifting sands of the molecular makeup of one member of the streptococcus family and its ecological relationship with humans. The streptococcus is prone to change, and historians recently have noted a marked weakening in the severity of scarlet fever and erysipelas—both caused by the streptococcus—in the 1930s.[10] For rheumatic fever, the fluid molecular biology resulted in changes of an even more fundamental nature: not only did rheumatic fever change its virulence but it also altered how the disease was expressed. Knowledge of the mutable molecular makeup of the streptococcus and its effects on human communities is still unfolding, but enough is known to enlighten this history of rheumatic fever. Understanding rheumatic fever and its history, then, requires the tools both of historians and of physicians.

Wearing both hats, pediatrician and historian, I was drawn to this study of rheumatic fever as a quest to see how these changes in ideas, epidemiology, and biology played out in the clinical setting of patients and doctors. The core of medicine is this interaction: patient and healer, each bringing an array of backgrounds, experiences, and expectations, forced by the circumstance of disease to make choices. Always challenging, this task proved especially demanding in the case of rheumatic fever simply because it was a "moving target." My argument is that this discourse over rheumatic fever also changed with time, reflecting, as we might expect, alterations in ideas, patterns of disease, and biology. I will also argue that this changing relationship between doctor and patient in turn altered ideas, epidemiology, and biology.

Finally, what drew me to rheumatic fever was the array of places its study took me: laboratory and bedside, clinic and hospital, slums and suburbs, tropics and temperate zones, both sides of the Atlantic.

I have elected to begin this history at the end of the eighteenth century, when I believe rheumatic fever first emerged. I have ended my history in 1965, when rheumatic fever had largely disappeared as an everyday concern of physicians. I confess that this latter date is somewhat arbitrary, for exciting insights about streptococcal/human ecology continued to flow from many laboratories. This ending date also precedes the small epidemics of rheumatic fever that struck several American communities in the 1980s. But history requires perspective. For the most part, the setting is the United States and Britain. In so limiting the geographical range, I have elected not to discuss areas in the third world where rheumatic fever still occurs.[11]

Rheumatic fever's researchers have also been its historians. Understandably, the disease which challenged physicians at the bedside, in the laboratory, or in the making of health policy has also stimulated historical reflection. Many of the cardinal studies of rheumatic fever written over the past hundred or more years have contained rich historical sections. Walter Butler Cheadle, Thomas John Maclagan, Alfred Mantle, Frederick J. Poynton, Alexander Paine, Carey Coombs, Homer F. Swift, Gene H. Stollerman, May G. Wilson, Benedict F. Massell, John R. Paul, George E. Murphy, J. Alison Glover, Alvin F. Coburn, Harry Keil, Maclyn McCarty, Edward F. Bland, T. Duckett Jones, Charles H. Rammelkamp, Jr., Lewis W. Wannamaker, Floyd W. Denny, Jr., and Rebecca C. Lancefield have all provided fruitful accounts. In particular, Gene H. Stollerman, who contributed many of the pioneering insights about rheumatic fever beginning in the 1950s, has published helpful studies for the historian. Most recently Benedict F. Massell, a frontline researcher during the middle third of this century, has published the first book-length work on rheumatic fever, detailing many of the exciting scientific studies that spanned his career. Written by physicians and scientists, these histories—directed to physicians and medical students for the most part—depict the many facets of this disease.[12] These medical leaders have discussed some of the early descriptions and changing symptoms of the disease, analyzed the perplexing relation of the streptococcus to rheumatic fever, detailed some of the social dimensions of rheumatic fever, addressed the value of therapies, and provided thoughtful appraisals of rheumatic fever's disappearance. My history has benefited from each account. While insightful, these histories are necessarily rooted in the exciting contemporary questions and challenges that confronted each researcher. I have not been a participant in rheumatic fever's history or an advocate in any of the richly debated controversies that this disease has spawned. As such, I have been able to stand back and gain the perspective that time and separation from events permit. My history has been freer to roam, and I hope that my understanding of rheumatic fever and how it has touched physicians and their patients will prove useful to members of the medical community.

Physicians have also assembled helpful bibliographies for the study of rheumatic fever's history. Beginning in 1935, Philip Hench, who figured prominently in the therapeutic debates of the 1950s, began publishing his annual "The Present Status of the Problem of Rheumatism" in the *Annals of Internal Medicine*.[13] Arthur Bloomfield, a student of streptococcal illness, compiled an insightful annotated bibliography on rheumatic fever included in *A Bibliography of Internal Medicine*.[14] Benedict Massell's *Rheumatic Fever and Streptococcal Infection*[15] contains ninety pages of notes. These bibliographies attest to the mark that rheumatic fever has left on medicine. Hench's annual review tabulated between 400 and 1,100 books and articles for each year. This abundance of information underscores one problem that faces any historian of twentieth-century medicine: identifying and selecting cardinal events and trends. No history, including this one, can mention all participants or their contributions.

In contrast, historians have mostly avoided rheumatic fever.[16] This is another gap that I hope to fill. Rheumatic fever has much to say to historians of disease. What emerges clearly is: biology matters. Historians of medicine often attribute changes in disease to alterations in patient or physician perceptions, colored by theoretical bent, institutional affiliation, characteristics of the observer, or technologies.[17] Certainly changes in perceptions are part of rheumatic fever's history, and my account seeks to set this disease solidly into its unfolding social context. But social history alone does not do justice to rheumatic fever. It is possible to glimpse in the historical record evidence of the actual biological evolution of rheumatic fever—not merely perceptions of change. Rheumatic fever has not been a static disease which patients and physicians have viewed from different vantages over the past two centuries. Biological change abounded which thrust new and taxing problems into the clinical setting of doctors and patients. In other words, the social and biological histories of rheumatic fever are intertwined. Developments in molecular biology over the past forty years have given some clarity to rheumatic fever's dynamic biological history. The challenge for the historian of rheumatic fever is making sense of the consequences of fluid biology in evolving social contexts. The history of rheumatic fever offers historians the opportunity to study the interface of biology and history, disease ecology in historical perspective, the complex relationship of biological science and medical practice, and the patient-physician relationship in the context of one complex disease. In these ways, I hope that my effort will prove helpful to other historians of disease.

The dynamic interaction of mutating biology, shifting epidemiological patterns, developing ideas, and clinical practice dictates a complex historical argument. To introduce some of the broad themes, I offer a brief prologue, emphasizing moments and events when we can see these interactions most clearly. Then in the main text, I will return to evidence in greater detail. Some readers will be unfamiliar with the medical terms. I have defined these terms when first used and have provided a glossary at the end of the book.

Rheumatic Fever in America and Britain

# Prologue

*I*n the late eighteenth century, rheumatic fever was embedded in the diagnostic category of "rheumatism," a broadly defined group of illnesses characterized by fevers, aches and pains of the limbs, and overall debility.[1] "Rheumatism" was a routine complaint in the eighteenth century. The evidence suggests that the biological nature of rheumatism changed in the late eighteenth century so that the heart, especially two tissues of the heart (the pericardium, or membranous sac surrounding the heart, and the endocardium, or heart valves), became inflamed, a striking wound that had not commonly occurred previously. Shortly thereafter, rheumatism's nature altered once again, this time injuring the brain; its victims now suffered from chorea, a bizarre movement disorder that commanded the attention of patient and doctor. Dramatic heart and brain injury made rheumatic fever visible to contemporaries and to historians.

These biological alterations must remain to a degree speculative. What is without question, however, is that clinicians, by the last years of the eighteenth century, appreciated cardiac involvement in ills also characterized by "rheumatism." William Charles Wells, a native of Charleston, South Carolina, who trained in Edinburgh and later remained loyal to Great Britain after the Revolution and practiced medicine in London, provided an early description of the new face of rheumatism. One of his case histories gave details: Miss A. L., a sixteen-year-old girl who had been well until her current affliction. Her fatal illness began in early August 1806:

> Shortly after remaining some time in a cold cellar, she was seized with pains, swelling, and redness of her joints, and fever. These symptoms lasted only ten days. [A week later] she was attacked with pains in her feet [that] remained only a day or two; immediately upon their ceasing, her heart began to beat with considerable violence. Her right [side of her chest] soon after became painful [which is why her family sent for Dr. Wells on September 17].
>
> The palpitation of the heart, which had never ceased from its first appearance, was distinctly felt in every part of the thorax to which my hand

was applied. . . . The strokes of the heart were one hundred and ninety a minute. . . . She frequently complained of a great and indescribable anxiety in her chest, always lessened by taking a few drops of Laudanum. . . . On examining her feet, I found them edematous.

On the evening of the 19th, I visited her again. The day before, she had been thought better; but many things seemed now to indicate her speedy death. The sickness had increased; her face and hands were cold, the skin pale, and the [pulse] scarcely perceptible, and the strokes of the heart against the ribs of much less force than formerly.

My last visit was on the 21st. . . . In the morning she began to be inattentive to what was passing in her room, and to speak sometimes a little incoherently. At two o'clock in the afternoon she died suddenly.

[An autopsy followed.] The whole of the internal surface of the pericardium was attached to the heart, by means of two distinct layers of solid matter, each having the thickness of the shilling . . . sufficiently tenacious to permit its being torn.[2]

This case demonstrates a simple bout of rheumatism that suffered a disastrous turn of events by provoking a mortal case of pericarditis. The aches of rheumatism were commonplace and, as Wells indicated, would have been cared for at home, most likely without his advice. What was different in this instance was that Miss A. L. suffered a violent heartbeat, severe chest pains, and great apprehension in addition to her joint complaints and fever.

Wells and fellow physicians, who were making similar links between rheumatism and heart disease, thought that their observations were new. Could it be that Wells simply "saw" what other physicians had overlooked in the past? This was unlikely. As a rule, in the eighteenth century, patients almost never died during an attack of rheumatism for any reason. As Wells's report indicates, any death was noteworthy. This girl's chest and heart complaints demanded attention in life and investigation after death. His "hands-on" diagnosis was up to the task while the girl lived; the autopsy technique of his colleague sufficient to confirm Wells's impression of heart injury. In other words, Wells responded to changes in disease and patient; no new technology or theoretical insight permitted him to appreciate cardiac damage that had long been "hidden" from view. During his years of practice, Wells came across only a few similar cases.

Hospital-based physicians in London soon corroborated the growing biological link between rheumatism and heart injury. For example, a physician at St. Bartholomew's Hospital tabulated that 13 percent of all patients admitted between 1836 and 1840 with the diagnosis of acute rheumatism also suffered from pericarditis.[3] The proportion of patients with pericarditis as part of their rheumatism grew to 22 percent at Middlesex Hospital between 1853 and 1859[4] and to 24 percent at Guy's Hospital between 1870 and 1872.[5] As we shall see, the increasing prevalence of endocarditis in some hospitals was even more striking.

These initial reports resulted from external inspection of patients followed by confirmatory autopsies. The stethoscope clarified and refined understanding of the nature of the cardiac injury. Following René Laennec's introduction of the stethoscope in 1816, practitioners' acquisition of auscultatory skills that correlated sounds at the bedside with structural changes at the autopsy table took decades. Initially, sounds emanating from the lungs received most attention; only by the 1830s did clinicians begin to sort out which abnormal heart sounds came from a particular chamber or valve of the heart.[6] Jean-Baptiste Bouillaud, a Parisian clinician who had been a student of Laennec, applied this new instrument to rheumatic patients in 1837, greatly enhancing the ability to describe cardiac injury while the patient lived. Significantly, the stethoscope also permitted Bouillaud to discover patients with *asymptomatic* heart disease.[7] What is important to this discussion is that most of Bouillaud's patients were quite symptomatic from cardiac damage; indeed, heart incapacity brought them to hospital attention. The stethoscope did not create physician appreciation of rheumatic heart disease, but it did provide a convenient method to assess heart injury, and it extended the scope of cardiac involvement to include instances that were unapparent to the patient.

There was a similar historical trail leading from rheumatism to chorea. Beginning in the 1830s, doctors began commenting on patients with rheumatism, some of them with heart disease in addition, who also suffered from uncontrollable movements, or chorea. One early example came from Dr. Yonge of Plymouth, England, in his 1840 description of Francis Hill, a nineteen-year-old boy who had suffered from rheumatism for two weeks before developing severe chest pains. What caught Dr. Yonge's attention was:

> irregular twitching of the muscles of the mouth and right side of the face; which is increased by speaking, and occasions some hesitation: seemed unconscious of this till it was noticed, but says, on being asked whether it was habitual that it has come on during the previous week.
>
> [One week later] Has walked from his lodgings; but with great difficulty, from the very uncontrollable state of the voluntary muscles throughout the body: great difficulty in making himself understood; cannot remain for any time in one posture; and although there is no spasm or violent action of the muscles, he is very unmanageable, and gives his friends a great deal of trouble. . . . His gait is unsteady and tottering, and he drags rather than lifts his feet.
>
> [Francis worsened the next day and was hospitalized] The muscular agitation continues to increase; he occasionally strikes himself against objects, from inability to control or regulate movements. [His] articulation is almost unintelligible; the tongue is jerked out. . . . [Of note, one doctor heard a heart "bruit" on auscultation with a stethoscope, but Francis's violent movements prevented accurate description of the heart's injury.]

Over the next week, his chorea deteriorated. He required a "strait waistcoat" for his own safety, and his tongue and facial movements prevented eating or drinking. He died eleven days after entering the hospital. At autopsy, Dr. Yonge concluded that the cause of death was the marked pericarditis (the cause of the chest pain) and endocarditis (which had produced the bruit, an extra sound heard when listening with a stethoscope that indicated disease). His brain appeared entirely normal. Chorea was a most dramatic punctuation of Francis's rheumatism, but it did not kill him.[8] Similar descriptions increased over the next decades until chorea joined heart injury as another new feature of rheumatism.

Could it be that Dr. Yonge and others observed what doctors before them had disregarded? It is unimaginable that an affliction that required a straitjacket, prevented ambulation, eating, and drinking, and distorted facial and bodily features could be easily missed when treating a patient for rheumatism. In its nineteenth-century form, chorea overwhelmed the observer. Rheumatism was on a march to expand into other parts of the body.

## Clinical Thinking

Changes in rheumatic fever's biological character are difficult to prove, but they are nonetheless likely as evidenced by the changing makeup of the disease found in case reports. Less speculative were the distinctive shifts in clinical thinking about the illness, brought about by its evolving complexity. As rheumatic fever changed over the course of the nineteenth century, patients experienced and physicians observed an expanding array of complaints. A variety of joints were swollen, inflamed, and painful. Some patients had rashes, others fever, but in no easily perceived sequence. Some, like Francis Hill, behaved peculiarly. Some were mildly discomforted; others died rapidly in great pain, like Miss A. L. In some families, several would be sick at one time. In other families, many generations suffered. Some patients were sick for days, others for weeks or months. Some endured one bout, others more than ten. Some were noticeably sick from other illnesses before rheumatism struck (scarlet fever, for example), others not. Some responded to therapy, others got better without therapy. Still others died despite all measures.

Repeatedly over the nineteenth century, rheumatic fever's changing biology forced physicians to sort out common and useful patterns in a disease that was becoming increasingly complex in its presentation. This sorting out occurred in distinct phases, clearly reflected in clinical reporting. Early in the century, practitioners, such as Wells and Yonge, wrote about individual cases that stressed elements peculiar to that patient. The focus centered on fever and the joint disease, but other manifestations, such as cardiac damage and chorea, were added to the picture in a supporting role (figure P.1; see also chapter 1). In midcentury, hospital-based physicians in Great Britain, with access to hundreds of patients with the new biologically expanded rheumatism, were able to analyze more carefully rheumatic fever's changing character. Using numbers and statistics, these physicians enumerated precisely how often heart injury and chorea joined fever and arthritis; what age groups were most vulnerable; what time of year rheumatism was most likely to attack; and which therapies were most likely to succeed (chapter 2). Large hospital-based studies also noted that rheumatism was continuing to change: subcutaneous nodules sometimes appeared; erythematous rashes joined in some cases;

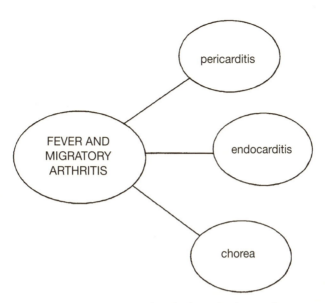

F<small>IGURE</small> P.1. Rheumatic fever in the early nineteenth century

tonsillitis had struck most victims. Significantly, these hospital-based reports recorded that heart disease gravely sickened patients.

The final third of the nineteenth century witnessed another shift in clinical thinking about rheumatic fever. Individual case histories showed the considerable variability of the illness; hospital-based analyses demonstrated in a general way how rheumatic fever affected populations. Neither approach was entirely helpful to the practitioner when confronted with sick patients and a mutating disease. What emerged in the 1880s was the concept of the "typical" case, which allowed for the necessary biological variability yet possessed common elements. Employing an epidemiological approach, which clustered elements from many cases, enabled physicians to make a certain diagnosis in a disease that was most uncertain in its presentation. Another advantage of this strategy was to follow patients over longer periods of time, demonstrating that rheumatic fever was an illness of relapses and remissions, with increasing debility with each episode. Pioneering in this strategy was Walter Butler Cheadle, physician to the Hospital for Sick Children, Great Ormond Street, London.

From the mass of individual cases and hospital studies available, Cheadle identified rheumatic fever's common elements in 1886: fever, arthritis, pericarditis, endocarditis, pleurisy, tonsillitis, erythematous rashes, chorea, and nodules. This expanded list of symptoms alone signaled how far rheumatic fever had traveled in a century. Over the course of this relapsing illness, Cheadle believed that most patients would suffer from most symptoms. Despite this expectation, Cheadle understood that not every patient experienced every possible complaint. He organized

CHART P.1   *Cheadle's Series VIII*

---

1. Chorea probably accom. by endocarditis  (Nov. 1886)

    Interval of 11 months

2. Arthritis (Oct. 1887)

3. Chorea (second attack), subcutaneous nodules, endocarditis, erythema marginatum
   (Nov. 1887)

4. Emotional attacks, chorea (continued), fresh nodules  (Dec. 1887)

5. Erythema marginatum, fresh eruption of nodules, chorea (relapse), arthritis (second
   attack) (Jan. 1888)

6. Fresh eruption of erythema, fresh crop of nodules, tonsillitis   (Feb. 1888)

7. Death, March 1888

SOURCE: W. B. Cheadle, "Harveian Lectures on the Various Manifestations of the Rheumatic State: As
Exemplified in Childhood and Early Life," *Lancet* (1889), 1: 821–827, 871–877, 921–927.

---

these symptoms, or "manifestations," into ten common temporal sequences, or "series." For one example, in chart form he described the case of W. S., aged $4^{1}/_{2}$, that Cheadle thought "typical" of many who suffered from rheumatic fever (chart P.1). Cheadle's clinical organization of thinking about rheumatic fever provided practitioners with a helpful guide to diagnosis. Indeed, no one has improved upon his general approach. Even T. Duckett Jones's diagnostic criteria created in response to rheumatic fever's continuing biological evolution in the twentieth century, which medical students began to memorize after 1944, were solidly based on Cheadle's efforts.

Over the nineteenth century, rheumatic fever's biological changes and the progression of clinical thinking shifted emphasis from fever and joints to the heart. Individual cases showed that cardiac injury was part of rheumatism; hospital studies showed that most debility and death resulted from heart disease; the "typical" case demonstrated that heart involvement was the most vital element in rheumatism from the point of view of prognosis (figure P.2; see also chapter 3).

## Theory

Evolving biology, and the complicated clinical thinking it provoked, challenged physicians to create a unifying explanation. Cheadle thought that tonsillitis differed from other aspects of rheumatic fever in that it often preceded the other manifestations. Sequencing suggested cause, and much of the history of ideas about rheumatic fever over the next half century puzzled over how sore throats led to the array of symptoms that doctors called rheumatic fever. Eventually, investigative epidemiology in the 1930s left little doubt that infection with a specific bacterium, the Group A beta-hemolytic streptococcus (GABS), had to precede rheumatic fever. Sequence alone proved unsatisfying as an answer. Frankly stated,

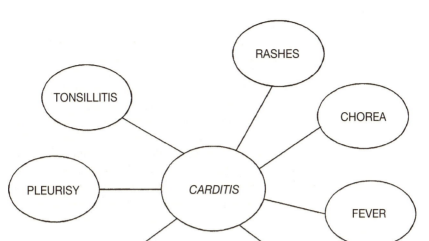

FIGURE P.2. Cheadle's rheumatic state (1889)

what conceivable pathological mechanism connected a simple throat infection to injury of the brain, heart, skin, tendons, and joints? Mutating biology stretched imaginations. The notion of blood-borne infection, or sepsis, carrying germs or poisons from the throat to all parts of the body, was attractive, thoroughly investigated between 1890 and 1920, and found lacking, both at the bedside and in the laboratory (chapter 4). Later, in the 1930s, the fledgling science of immunology provided an attractive alternative. The streptococcus (GABS) served as a "trigger," goading the body to produce antibodies. Initially used as evidence to prove prior infection, these antibodies became potential purveyors of widespread bodily damage (chapter 6). In 1936, Alvin F. Coburn tied together streptococcal epidemiology and immunology to refine Cheadle's scheme in a way that suggested a causal sequence (figure P.3). In Coburn's conception of rheumatic fever, a simple, often clinically asymptomatic, streptococcal sore throat triggered an immunological response leading to symptomatic rheumatic fever. Essentially, Coburn's conception persists to this day.[9]

## Epidemiology

Epidemiologists in the 1930s did more than just provide evidence that streptococcal sore throats preceded rheumatic fever. They recorded how prevalent the disease had become and, as startling, showed that its continuing biological evolution had started its march toward extinction. In an exhaustive study that summarized virtually all relevant epidemiological knowledge in 1930, John R. Paul

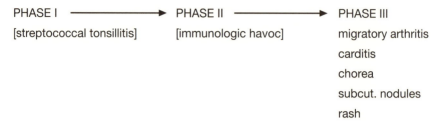

FIGURE P.3. Coburn's phases of rheumatic fever (1936)

determined that approximately 840,000, or just less than 1 percent of Americans, suffered significant and permanent heart damage from rheumatic fever.[10] A decade later, Philip Hench estimated that the number had grown to one million, with an estimated 40,000 deaths each year.[11] Mortality did not tell the whole story. School health doctors in the United States and Britain calculated that between 1 and 2 percent of all school-age children had perceptible cardiac scars with varying degrees of handicap,[12] impediments that mandated special educational programs in most communities.[13]

British epidemiologists first detected rheumatic fever's retreat. Nearly the same year that Cheadle reorganized clinical thinking, Arthur Newsholme, studying data from hospital admissions, discovered that rheumatic fever had reached its peak in the 1870s. In far more detailed studies beginning in the 1930s and based on better sources, J. Alison Glover documented more fully the declining mortality of rheumatic fever for England and Wales (table P.1).

Changing biology moderated mortality rates. Deaths from rheumatic fever in the nineteenth century came from pericarditis and endocarditis. Late in the nineteenth century, physicians detected that the heart's muscle, or myocardium, was a new target of the disease, an injury given pathological energy when Ludwig Aschoff described in 1904 the precise cellular derangement.[14] Pericardial and endocardial injury ceased to be the sole hallmarks of rheumatic heart disease in the twentieth century, joined by myocardial damage that some physicians now thought accompanied virtually all cases of the illness. Of course, pericardial and endocardial disease did not vanish entirely; there were many heart valves in need of repair after surgical techniques became available in the late 1940s. But life-threatening pericarditis and endocarditis shared company with rheumatic fever far less commonly in the twentieth century. The new myocardial insult, often clinically unapparent, was easily documented with the electrocardiogram that detected subtle changes in the electrical impulses of the heart.

Was myocardial injury new at the end of the nineteenth century? I believe that it was. There were certainly a few reports before Aschoff, one or two from early in the century. But virtually all autopsies failed to report myocardial inflammation even though this inflammation would have been clearly visible to microscopic and even visual inspection. This contrasted sharply with autopsy reports at the end of the century which reported that nearly all fatal cases of rheumatic fe-

TABLE P.1   *Mortality from rheumatic fever in England and Wales*

| Year | Deaths/100,000/year |
|------|---------------------|
| 1851–92 | 8.8 |
| 1901 | 7.7 |
| 1928 | 3.8 |
| 1937 | 2.2 |

SOURCE: J. Alison Glover, "Milroy Lectures on the Incidence of Rheumatic Diseases," *Lancet* (1930), 1: 499–505; and Glover, "Rheumatic Fever," *Lancet* (1939), 1: 465–468.

ver had evidence of myocardial injury. Clearly, recognition of rheumatic myocarditis preceded clinical application of the electrocardiogram, which did not become widely available until the 1920s. This is not to dismiss the importance of this new clinical technology. The electrocardiogram became one of the tools which physicians used to monitor myocarditis in patients after 1920; but the electrocardiogram did not "discover" myocarditis.

In contrast to pericardial and endocardial damage, myocardial injury seldom caused death acutely. But rheumatic myocarditis smoldered, producing a chronic debility, reflected in mortality statistics which demonstrated that victims of rheumatic heart disease in the twentieth century died, not as children or young adults, but as older adults in their fifties, sixties, or even seventies (chapter 7). Autopsies revealed that the myocardium was still mildly inflamed, decades after the initial bout with the disease. As the century wore on, even this cardiac injury waned, and rheumatic fever ceased to be a significant cause of death or debility. So complete was the demise of rheumatic fever that pediatrician-epidemiologist Leon Gordis's 1985 T. Duckett Jones Lecture before the American Heart Association was entitled "The Virtual Disappearance of Rheumatic Fever in the United States: Lessons on the Rise and Fall of Disease."[15] That same year Milton Markowitz delivered the Lewis W. Wannamaker Memorial Lecture, speaking on "The Decline of Rheumatic Fever: Role of Medical Intervention,"[16] and the 86th Ross Conference was dedicated to the clinical problem of "Management of Pharyngitis in an Era of Declining Rheumatic Fever."

The moderating severity of rheumatic fever begs explanation. Although some observers credited sulfonamide and later penicillin, these drugs played only a small role in the changing biology of rheumatic fever. Nonetheless, antibiotics, widely used for rheumatic fever after 1945, eliminated the streptococcal trigger from the throats of susceptible people (Coburn's Phase I). At midcentury, antibiotics were crucial to prevention and public health programs. Indeed, the possibility of prevention ushered in a revolution in the way in which physicians and parents evaluated colds and sore throats in children and adolescents. But antibiotics did not influence at all the course of rheumatic fever, once under way (Coburn's Phases II and III). The sweeping use of antibiotics made rheumatic fever less likely to occur, but sulfonamide and penicillin did not treat carditis, arthritis, chorea, rash, or subcutaneous nodules (chapters 8 and 9). What needs emphasis is that rheumatic

fever was diminishing in prevalence and severity before the discoveries of sulfonamide and penicillin.

Moderating biology of rheumatic fever in the twentieth century is easy to
spot. A close look at the central feature of rheumatic fever—carditis—reveals the
outline. Dramatic pericarditis and endocarditis of the late nineteenth century largely
disappeared, replaced by myocarditis that was often clinically subtle and which
might even smolder for decades with minimal perceived morbidity. In the last third
of the twentieth century, few, if any, streptococcal infections—treated or not—injured the heart. We can see the diminishing of other symptoms. By the time that
Jones published his diagnostic scheme in 1944, painful, migratory swollen joints
had yielded to mildly sore joints without much swelling, or arthralgia, melting away
over the next decades to insignificant aches and pains. Chorea, once a major movement disorder with verbal and even psychiatric involvement, also disappeared, witnessed now, if at all, with only an occasional twitch. Subcutaneous nodules and
erythema marginatum have also largely disappeared. In contrast to Cheadle, who
anticipated that most patients would suffer most symptoms at some point in their
illness, for Jones the clinical problem was the difficulty of making a diagnosis in
a disease of increasing rarity and diminishing severity. Most of his patients suffered from only one or two of rheumatic fever's many symptoms. To surmount
these new hurdles, Jones separated the diverse complaints of rheumatic fever into
"major" manifestations and "minor" manifestations. The presence of only two "major" or one "major" and two or more "minor" manifestations was sufficient to make
a diagnosis (chart P.2).

### Patients and Doctors

Mutating biology challenged doctors and patients. Patients in the early nineteenth century came to physicians with specific complaints: fever that persisted
for weeks or even months, painful and swollen joints, chest pain, and movements
that were beyond their ability to control. Treatment addressed these symptoms, success or failure easily visible to both doctor and patient. Bed rest to ease joint pain
and prevent any damage; opium to dull the aches of chest and limbs; sedatives to
calm jerks and promote sleep. Effective relief from fever eluded doctor and patient. The chest pain in these cases stemmed from the accumulation of pericardial
fluid. Endocarditis was imperceptible to the patient until so severe that it produced
congestive heart failure, which the patient experienced as shortness of breath, rapid
heart rate, and limbs swollen with excess fluid.

Realizing that rheumatic fever was beginning to strike pericardium and heart
valves, physicians began to employ the stethoscope for signs of damage to both
cardiac tissues. As experience mounted, doctors came to understand that these cardiac injuries, often unapparent to the patient, were nonetheless paramount to the
patient's survival. We can imagine the tension between doctor and patient: patient
expectations demanded relief from perceived symptoms while physicians worried
appropriately about the potential fatal consequences of invisible dangers. This fracture between patient expectations and physician concern heightened in the early

CHART P.2    *Jones criteria for the diagnosis of rheumatic fever (1944)*

| Major Manifestations | Carditis |
|---|---|
| | Arthralgia |
| | Chorea |
| | Subcutaneous nodules |
| | Prior bout with rheumatic fever |
| Minor Manifestations | Fever |
| | Arthritis |
| | Abdominal pain |
| | Chest pain |
| | Rashes (erythema marginatum, among others) |
| | Nosebleeds |
| | Lung disease |
| | Abnormal laboratory tests, such as elevated erythrocyte sedimentation rate, high white blood count |

SOURCE: T. Duckett Jones, "The Diagnosis of Rheumatic Fever," *Journal of the American Medical Association* (1944), 126: 481–484.

twentieth century with the biological shift to myocardial damage. In this instance, the cardiac damage, still prognostically most significant, was silent even to the doctor's stethoscope. Patients often needed to travel to a hospital or specialist to obtain an electrocardiogram to document heart injury. An unfavorable report often doomed a child to months of bed rest, now to rest the heart, not the joints, and to years of schools for "cardiac cripples," thus reflecting new concerns from epidemiologists that rheumatic fever was a chronic disease.

The chasm widened further in the 1930s with the appreciation of the streptococcal trigger. Frequent colds and sore throats were part of everyday experience for all children, paling, from the point of view of patients and parents, before the far more distressing complaints of chorea, chest pain, and joint woes. In their evaluation of children with rheumatic fever, doctors now pursued laboratory evidence of sore throats that had long since healed in addition to heart damage that caused no immediate distress.

Bridging the gap came three families of drugs that doctors and patients hailed as miraculous, though frequently for different reasons. Just prior to Cheadle's reorganization of clinical thinking, Thomas Maclagan discovered in 1876 that salicin quickly lowered fever, eased joint pain and swelling, and lessened chest pain by decreasing pericardial fluid.[17] It had no effect on chorea. Shortly, many salicylates with slightly varying chemical constituents became available, including aspirin, which formed a mainstay of therapy for rheumatic fever in the early twentieth century. Relief from joint illness, prolonged fever, and chest pain brought excitement to doctors and patients alike; virtually overnight older therapies were cast aside (chapters 2 and 5). So effective was salicylate in alleviating distress that almost no physician critically analyzed its value to the injury that doctors feared most: endocarditis at the end of the nineteenth century and myocarditis in the twentieth century. When these studies were carried out, some nearly a half century after the introduction of salicylate, the drug was found wanting in healing myocarditis, the heart injury then common. Here we see another consequence of the biological mutation of rheumatic fever. We now know that salicylate effectively lowers fever, reduces joint pain and swelling, eliminates some of the pericardial inflammation that leads to the painful accumulation of fluid, and probably (although doubt still exists) cuts some early endocardial inflammation. In other words, salicylate eased both the distresses that brought patients to doctors and the forms of heart disease that doctors most feared at the end of the nineteenth century. Salicylate did not influence myocarditis, which eventually led to the undeserved conclusion that it was ineffective in rheumatic fever.[18] What had happened was that rheumatic fever itself had changed (chapter 8).

Sulfonamide and later penicillin brought similar enthusiasm. Shortly after Coburn singled out infection with the streptococcus as the triggering event in rheumatic fever (Coburn's Phase I), sulfonamide became available for treating bacterial infections, raising expectations that it was just the drug to combat the disease. Here rheumatic fever's unusual nature confounded early therapeutic attempts. Despite Coburn's well-articulated consensus that rheumatic fever was not a widely disseminated infection, early studies treated symptomatic rheumatic fever (Coburn's Phase III) with sulfonamide. The drug had no effect on heart, brain, or joint symptoms, and serious side effects actually worsened the patient's experience.[19] When physicians correctly targeted the triggering sore throat for treatment, sulfonamide also came up short. It could not prevent Phase I from progressing to Phases II and III.[20] The first success with sulfonamide came in preventing relapses with daily doses of the drug administered throughout the year: in other words, not permitting infection to occur in the first place.[21] Newer sulfonamides produced fewer side effects, and prevention was so attractive to the United States military that hundreds of thousands of seamen received daily sulfonamide starting in 1944. Within months of this massive and very successful program, biological disaster struck: the streptococcus became resistant to sulfonamide and diseases caused by resistant streptococci infected sailors. The U.S. Navy had fewer cases of rheumatic fever, but in the process it altered the germ.[22]

After World War II, the military also tested penicillin. It differed from sulfonamide in key ways. Penicillin produced fewer side effects (although initially it required multiple daily injections). Significantly, it could stop rheumatic fever in its tracks at Coburn's Phase I if the streptococcal sore throat was promptly treated (chapter 9). This success led to public health efforts to shift patient concern from the usual symptoms of rheumatic fever (Coburn's Phase III) to the often trivial triggering infection (Coburn's Phase I). All sore throats now needed culturing to check for the presence of the Group A beta-hemolytic streptococcus. Enthusiasm for antibiotics caught up with rheumatic fever by 1950. Fortunately, the hemolytic streptococcus has yet to develop resistance to penicillin. Fear of streptococcal infection and rheumatic fever led to the prompt treatment, perhaps overtreatment, of many simple colds. This fervor coupled with the widespread use of antibiotics to treat other bacterial infections greatly interrupted the ecological relations that existed between the streptococcus and humans. In this way, what went on between doctors and patients almost certainly influenced the evolving biology of rheumatic fever.

Corticosteroid offered the hope of accomplishing what penicillin and aspirin could not: treating myocarditis. This potent anti-inflammatory steroid hormone ran headlong into rheumatic fever's changing biology and epidemiology. Fewer critically ill patients made drug trials more difficult. Fewer deaths and those occurring decades after initial illness made pathological evidence of success or failure nearly impossible. In some instances, steroids appeared to provide quick relief to myocarditis, but new problems swiftly arose. Side effects were prompt and serious, preventing long-term use. Grave "rebound" occurred when the drug was withdrawn.[23] A careful multinational comparison between aspirin and steroids, carried out by the American Heart Association and the British Medical Research Council, demonstrated no superiority for hormones.

By 1970 rheumatic fever had almost disappeared. For most families, the suffering it once produced took its place in the memory of an afflicted parent or grandparent. Its diminished nature properly dictated its lowered status. Physicians and medical students shifted interests elsewhere as well, for rheumatic fever no longer produced serious health consequences. It lingered a while in lectures, textbooks, and clinical lore and then was largely forgotten. Floyd Denny, who participated in the initial trials of penicillin after World War II, remarked in 1986, "I am impressed that we have raised an entire generation of young physicians who have never seen a case of acute rheumatic fever."[24] Only in the continued exaggerated concern over streptococcal sore throats, precautionary antibiotics before trips to dentists for those with suspicious heart murmurs, and repeated, and largely unnecessary, heart examinations looking for newly acquired heart disease during well-child visits did patients and doctors still meet over the remnants of rheumatic fever.

## Molecular Biology

Interest in rheumatic fever waned, but curiosity about the streptococcus and its fascinating biology continued strong. In the late 1950s, pathologists discovered that antibodies were attached to heart tissue removed during surgical repair of rheumatic heart valves. This provided molecular evidence that myocarditis smoldered long after the initial bout with rheumatic fever and suggested that these antibodies mediated cardiac damage. In the early 1960s came proof that these antibodies were identical to streptococcus-induced antibodies. In other words, a constituent of the streptococcus produced antibodies that "cross-reacted" with heart tissue. These antibodies, in theory, were the agents of cardiac injury.[25] Subsequent laboratory research demonstrated similar cross-reactivity between the streptococcus and glycoprotein in heart valves, heart muscle, neurons in the caudate and subthalamic nuclei of the brain, and joint tissues—molecular evidence linking the streptococcus to each part of the body attacked by rheumatic fever. Different components of the streptococcus, usually classified as M proteins, appeared responsible for antibodies targeting distinct tissues, accounting in theory for the variable symptomatic expression of rheumatic fever in diverse people that has characterized so much of its history (chapter 10).[26]

In the mid-1980s, a brief and unexpected resurgence of rheumatic fever occurred in small isolated epidemics. This unpredicted return sparked conjecture concerning what it was about the streptococcus that permitted the historical disappearance and reappearance of rheumatic fever.[27] Focus centered again on streptococcal M proteins, molecules known to vary widely and to change with time. Gene Stollerman, long a leader in streptococcal research, found that the geographically disparate epidemics of the 1980s all shared streptococci with strains of M proteins that had not been present for years.[28]

These molecular discoveries provided insights that helped to explain puzzling aspects of rheumatic fever's history. What I think likely is that the streptococcus in the eighteenth century contained components that cross-reacted only with human joints, thus leading to disease characterized predominantly by arthritis. Over the course of the nineteenth century, new molecular components transformed the streptococcus so that human antibodies cross-reacted with heart tissues, brain, skin, and tendons, resulting in the symptoms that so distressed Miss A. L. and Francis Hill. Over the twentieth century, the streptococcus lost these provocative elements. The coming and going of M proteins dictated the symptomatic variety of the disease in individual patients and the epidemiological movement through populations and time. It is not possible, of course, to analyze streptococci from the throats of Miss A. L. or Francis Hill for evidence of a recent change in M protein. But the abrupt changes in the clinical presentation of the disease that their cases represented indicate that molecular change occurred.

This is not to argue that the history of rheumatic fever can be reduced simply to an alteration of molecules. Rather, these molecular shifts set into motion biological and epidemiological changes that confronted patients and doctors with an ever-changing health problem that demanded attention. To be sure, technologies, such as the autopsy, the stethoscope and electrocardiogram, the progression of medical thinking (individual case histories, large hospital-based studies, Cheadle's "typical" series, Coburn's "phases," and Jones's "major/minor" criteria), the organization of medical care into hospitals, and various research strategies— all helped to define and illuminate rheumatic fever. If molecular biologists are correct in their singling out of M proteins as the ultimate culprit, the very nature of the disease lay beyond truly "curative" therapy until the cusp of the twenty-first century. This observation underscores the dilemma that patients and doctors have often faced in history: combating disease with the knowledge and tools at hand at a given moment, knowing full well that their efforts are not wholly adequate.

The complex bond between molecules, disease, epidemiology, and history continues. Insights about the M proteins suggested to Stollerman an additional means for physicians to attack rheumatic fever: a vaccine against M proteins, signaling an effort for humans to alter the molecular makeup of the streptococcus and thus a chance to alter its history.

# PART I

## The Emergence of Rheumatic Fever in the Nineteenth Century

CHAPTER 1

# The New Face of
# Rheumatism, 1798–1840

✦

*I*n April 1798, Mr. T. M., an eighteen-year-old young man from Scotland, was struck down with rheumatism while traveling in Berkshire, England. He was very familiar with the beginning stages of this illness, for he had been afflicted with rheumatism yearly since the age of nine. It came on in late fall, winter, or early spring. There was a preliminary period of fever and chills, which he and his family attributed to a needless exposure to dampness and cold weather, followed by considerable swelling, redness, and tenderness of his knees, ankles, and wrists. This arthritis had a peculiar twist: it moved from joint to joint, lasting in one spot for a few days or a week before moving to another location. His family put him to bed for several weeks, and he recovered completely after each bout. Despite the considerable debility during the active stage of the disease, he had been left with no permanent handicap. There is no indication that he had ever been attended by a physician.

T. M.'s tenth bout began in the accustomed way: knees and ankles red, swollen, and tender, occurring after an unfortunate submersion into a cold spring pond. What set this episode apart from earlier ones was an "oppression in his chest" and the palpitation of his heart. After three weeks, these chest complaints led to extreme breathlessness and a feeling that he was "about to expire." So different was this addition to his regular rheumatic complaints that he traveled to London to consult a hospital-based physician. There he met Dr. William Charles Wells at St. Thomas's Hospital. Wells listened to the young man's story and quickly confirmed that T. M. had what physicians in the late eighteenth century called "acute rheumatism." What was entirely new in Wells's experience was the history of "oppression in the chest," heart palpitations, and breathlessness. Wells confirmed that the heart was involved by palpating the pulse and feeling the heart bound against T. M.'s chest wall. Wells believed that he was seeing a new aspect of a common disease; he called it "rheumatism of the heart."[1]

### Sydenham and Cullen on Rheumatism

Rheumatism was a quite familiar health concern for patients and physicians at the end of the eighteenth century. Thomas Sydenham, who had turned his revolutionary zeal from Puritan causes to the many epidemic fevers plaguing his practice among London's poor, defined rheumatism in the late seventeenth century in a fashion that continued to serve practitioners a century later:

> This disease happens at any time, but especially in Autumn and chiefly affects such as are in the prime of life. 'Tis generally occasioned by exposing the body to the cold, or immediately after having heated it by violent exercise, or some other way. It begins (1) with chillness and shivering, which are soon succeeded (2) by heat, restlessness, thirst, and the other concomitants of a fever; (3) in a day or two and sometimes sooner, there arises an acute pain in some or other of the limbs, especially in the wrists, shoulders, and knees; which, shifting between whiles, affects these parts alternatively, leaving a redness swelling in the part last affected. (4) In the beginning of the illness, the fever and the aforementioned symptoms do sometimes come together, but the fever goes off gradually whilst the pain continues, and sometimes increase[s], occasioned by the derivation of the febrile matter to the limbs, which the frequent return of the fever, from the repulsion of the morbific matter by external remedies sufficiently shews.[2]

Sydenham's description well fit Mr. T. M.'s complaints for his first nine attacks.

Wells had more precisely diagnosed his young patient with "acute rheumatism," a refinement that William Cullen (1710–1790), a Scottish physician working at the Royal Infirmary in Edinburgh, had incorporated after years of experience treating both rich and poor. Rheumatism was among the most common complaints Cullen was called upon to treat.[3] Cullen had appreciated that joint complaints separated into two distinct clusters: "acute rheumatism" in teenagers and young adults with short-lived arthritis that left no permanent disability, and "chronic rheumatism" in older adults, in their fifties and sixties, with persistent joint complaints that often resulted in crippling arthritis. Ideas about rheumatic fever evolved from what Cullen called "acute rheumatism," a term that others enlarged to "acute articular rheumatism," to place emphasis on the painful joints. In *First Lines of the Practice of Physic,* Cullen stated that rheumatism "seldom appears either in the very young or elderly persons, and most commonly occurs from the age of puberty to that of thirty-five years."[4] He concurred with Sydenham that "the pains affect several joints, often at the very same time, but for the most part shifting this place, and, having abated one joint, become more violent in another."[5] Figure 1.1 represents rheumatism for Sydenham and Cullen.

### A New Outcome for Acute Rheumatism: Death

Mr. T. M., like most sufferers from acute rheumatism, survived even repeated attacks of this disease. Beginning in the middle of the eighteenth century, physi-

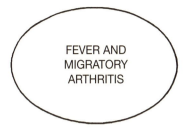

FIGURE 1.1. Rheumatism in the eighteenth century

cians began to record a few who died from their bouts with rheumatism. These deaths contrasted sharply with the complete recovery that both patients and physicians anticipated with acute rheumatism. As with any new phenomenon, these deaths begged explanation. The precise reason for the deaths perplexed physicians because it was not at all clear why a temporary joint complaint should suddenly turn fatal. When this unusual event occurred, physicians would explain that the rheumatism had moved somehow from the joints to a vital organ. For example, Gerhard van Swieten, the great Viennese physician of the mid-eighteenth century, noted in his *Commentaries upon Boerhaave's Aphorisms*, "while the rheumatism attacks only the joints, it is rarely fatal; but when it seizes the brains or lungs, it is highly dangerous, and sometimes occasions sudden death."[6] Van Swieten gave only a cursory explanation of how rheumatism could move around the body. Early in his discussion, he claimed that "rheumatism derives its name from [the Greek word] to flow."[7] He had a vague notion that a misdirected rheumatic "poison" could flow from the joints to produce havoc elsewhere.

Sydenham and Cullen had spoken of diseased joints in a general way. Other observers sought to locate the site of disease more precisely within the joint itself. For example, William Balfour, a physician writing on the pathology of rheumatism early in the nineteenth century, claimed that the location of rheumatism was in the "cellular membrane" of the joints, by which he meant the connective tissue surrounding the joints. Balfour based his notion on his examination of living patients and not on dissection.[8]

Cullen, who was known for his meticulous classification of diseases, had struggled over where exactly to locate "acute rheumatism." It shared many characteristics with inflammation. Acute rheumatism produced swollen, painful joints that appeared to the examiner just like joints in other illnesses that were filled with pus, or suppuration. In these latter conditions, the joints frequently were destroyed, leaving the patient crippled. In contrast, Cullen noted that the affected joints in rheumatism never contained pus and never were permanently damaged: "The acute rheumatism, though it has much of the nature of the other phlegmasiae [inflammation], differs from all these hitherto mentioned in that it is not liable to terminate in suppuration."[9] Acute rheumatism also differed from other forms of inflammation in that it moved from one joint to another without affecting the tissue in between.

William Shearman, senior physician to the Royal West London Infirmary, took issue with Cullen over whether rheumatism should be grouped with inflammatory illnesses at all. Noting Cullen's observation that swelling and pain migrated from joint to joint in rheumatism without leading to crippling, Shearman argued:

> Inflammation, when it has attacked a part, remains confined to that part, or is extending only by progressive continuity; rheumatism attacks and recedes from various parts successively; and we not uncommonly have one joint swelled, hot, and red—whilst another, just previously affected in the same manner, shall become cold, pale, and contracted, exhibiting no signs of inflammation—yet the same joint shall again become hot, red, and swelled; and this alteration we find to take place with several distant parts, whilst no such occurrence is observed in pure local inflammation.[10]

While Sydenham and Cullen remained the guideposts for most discussions of rheumatism, its uncommon features made it difficult for practitioners of the early nineteenth century to define clearly. For example, L. A. Dugas's attempt to provide a contemporary definition of rheumatism for his audience of physicians at a meeting of the Medical Society of Georgia illuminated some of the problems that rheumatism presented physicians. After citing Sydenham, Boerhaave, and Cullen, Dugas strove to provide a contemporary description that would be helpful:

> A disease classed amongst the Phlegmasiae (inflammations), located in the muscular and fibrous tissues of animal life, and attended with the following symptoms: pain, more or less intense, either continued or intermitting, fixed or wandering, and with or without heat, tumefaction, redness, and pyrexia. It usually terminates with resolution, sometimes suddenly followed or not by metastasis, rarely by suppuration, and still more seldom by gangrene.[11]

In addition, practitioners began to realize that the umbrella of "rheumatism" often covered many conditions that Sydenham and Cullen had never intended. Edward J. Seymour, a physician at St. George's Hospital in London, noted that practitioners loosely used the term to cover many ills, both trivial and serious: growing pains in children, the limb pains that accompanied many febrile illnesses, the pains of nerves damaged by hemorrhage, debilitated constitutions, abuse of mercury, any pain stemming from muscles, bones, or joints, as well as the joint pain in rheumatism.[12]

So commonplace and so likely to remit spontaneously was acute rheumatism that patients and physicians often thought that the disease was trivial. Samuel Fish, explaining why a family delayed in sending for him to care for a twenty-five-year-old man with fever and arthritis, stated: "Thinking it 'nothing but rheumatism,' as they expressed themselves, they did not send for a physician as soon as they otherwise would have done."[13]

## William Charles Wells and "Rheumatism of the Heart"

Despite difficulty in defining acute rheumatism precisely, Wells had no trouble diagnosing acute rheumatism in Mr. T. M.[14] What stymied Wells were the heart complaints. Wells recalled that two colleagues, David Pitcairn and Matthew Baillie, had mentioned similar cardiac difficulties in patients with acute rheumatism. After scouring the available medical literature, he could find only one or two additional references. Nevertheless, it is clear from accounts of patients suffering from acute rheumatism that practitioners were becoming aware of the cardiac connection before Wells. For example, van Swieten had reported that "sometimes, when the pain in the limbs ceases, there arise an anxiety in the breast, a palpitation of the heart, an intermitting pulse."[15] Despite this observation, van Swieten did not connect the rare involvement of the heart with the few patients he treated who died from rheumatism. Cullen, too, had called attention to the "full and hard pulse" that accompanied rheumatism on occasion.[16] In the first extensive statistical analysis of rheumatism, John Haygarth noted in 1805 that fifty-five of ninety-three patients with acute rheumatism who had their pulse recorded had a heart rate greater than ninety-six beats per minute. Haygarth did not make the connection between heart damage and rheumatism, and an elevated pulse does not always mean heart disease (fever alone can raise the pulse). But Haygarth's observation indicated that physicians were beginning to look at the heart when confronted with patients with rheumatism. Twelve of Haygarth's patients died. His detailed case histories indicate that three died with either severe chest pain or shortness of breath. While it is not possible to be certain of the exact anatomical cause of the deaths, it is likely that diseased hearts were responsible.[17]

When Wells published Mr. T. M.'s history with thirteen additional cases in 1812, he did not claim priority for his observation linking heart disease with rheumatism. Rather, he credited David Pitcairn, a prominent British physician, with the initial association in 1788. Pitcairn failed to publish his remarks on the subject, so Wells considered his paper to be serving the purpose of recording Pitcairn's idea, to which he added his own cases. Wells also remarked that Matthew Baillie, a Scottish pathologist, had made the initial autopsy investigation of a patient with rheumatism dying from heart disease.[18] In a footnote, Baillie recorded that "Dr. Pitcairn has observed this in several cases."

Wells also called attention to the experience of David Dundas, sergeant-surgeon to the king, who reported in 1809 nine patients with heart disease and rheumatism. Most had suffered chest pains, anxiety, and increased pulse, ascites (fluid in the abdomen), pleural fluid, or peripheral edema following one or more attacks of acute rheumatism. Seven of the nine were under twenty-two years of age; and seven died, usually after a period of several months. He autopsied six and found the heart enlarged in most; excess pericardial fluid surrounded one heart; and in several others the pericardium adhered to the surface of the heart.[19]

Wells presented the experiences of nine of his patients, plus five from colleagues. Miss A. L., the young woman who died from cardiac complications that we met in the prologue, was Wells's fifth case. Eleven of these patients were teen-agers, two were in their twenties, and the oldest was thirty-six. With fever and mi-grating arthritis, each clearly suffered from acute rheumatism. Like the cases of Mr. T. M. and Miss A. L., each had complaints explicitly related to the heart: chest pain, breathlessness, palpitations, irregular heartbeat, forcible or violent heartbeat, or an enlarged heart. In each case, Wells or his colleagues confirmed cardiac in-volvement with examination of the pulse and inspection and palpation of the chest wall. Six patients died, a highly unusual outcome for acute rheumatism. The au-topsies revealed that pericarditis, a collection of fluid resulting from an inflamed pericardium, was the cause of each of the deaths. One of the older patients had the additional finding of "excrescences" attached to the mitral heart valve, indi-cating injury to another of the heart's tissues, the endocardium. Of passing inter-est was Wells's finding that one patient, Martha Clifton, also had "many of the tendons of the superficial muscles . . . studded with numerous hard tumors," the first clear description of subcutaneous nodules, another ailment later associated commonly with acute rheumatism.

Following Wells's lead some practitioners began looking for heart disease in cases of rheumatism. James Russell, a surgeon from Birmingham, provided an example from 1814. Seth Bassett, a twenty-two-year-old wagoner, came to Russell with painful joints. Russell, aware of the writings of Baillie, Dundas, and Wells, took a special interest when Bassett developed chest pain, shortness of breath, and a rapid pulse several weeks later. Russell confidently believed that Bassett had an inflamed heart.[20] In 1821, René Laennec listed "gouty or rheumatic affections" as an occasional cause of pericarditis.[21] William Potts Dewees, a physician from Philadelphia, described the case of A. B., an eight-year-old girl: in mid-Novem-ber, the young girl developed swelling and redness of her wrists and ankles shortly after a sore throat, chill, and cough; suddenly she was overwhelmed by a "great oppression" in her chest and shortness of breath so severe that she could not lie down; a week later she was dead.[22] Similar case reports increased over the next decade so that a Parisian medical student, Joseph-Irénée Itard, was able to sustain a twenty-four-page thesis for graduation from medical school, entitled "Considéra-tions sur le Rhumatisme de Coeur" in 1824.[23]

As observations linking acute rheumatism and heart disease mounted, post-mortem examinations showed that the pericardium was the main site of cardiac injury. An early exception was Dewees's findings at the autopsy of A. B. He dis-covered that both pericardium and myocardium were involved: "Heart twice as large as usual, and adhering by a thick coat of lymph to the pericardium, . . . Two ounces of straw-colored serum in pericardium. The texture of the heart was sensibly al-tered . . . in the crispy semi-cartilaginous manner peculiar to inflamed muscles. I did not detect any inflammation of its lining membrane."[24] Wells's earlier single description of endocardial injury indicated that acute rheumatism was capable of attacking all three tissues of the heart.

### Was Rheumatic Heart Disease New?

Wells believed that his and others' recent observations coupling heart injury to acute rheumatism were new at the end of the eighteenth century. Is it possible that Pitcairn, Wells, Dundas, Dewees, and others simply observed what others had overlooked in the past? This is unlikely. Acute rheumatism was rarely a fatal disease until the end of the eighteenth century. Patients' new chest complaints were striking and demanded attention; physicians confirmed with their usual examinations that the heart was behaving improperly; and autopsies demonstrated definite cardiac injury. Careful physicians could not fail to miss either patient demands for alleviation of symptoms or the result of examination or autopsy. Even Haygarth, van Swieten, and Cullen—who did not associate rheumatism with heart disease—nevertheless did remark on these "unusual" symptoms. In the eighteenth century, patients with acute rheumatism were not discomforted except from their joint pains and fever, and they did not die. A close look at the individual case reports from Wells and Dundas shows that these early patients were dramatically symptomatic:

> Wells (case II): Her pulse was small, but the heart struck the ribs with such force that its beats could be reckoned by applying the hand to the right side of the chest.

> Wells (case III): His pulse was quick, and his heart beat forcibly against the ribs.[25]

> [Dundas]: The patient complains of great anxiety and oppression at the praecordia; has generally a short cough, and a difficulty of breathing, which is so much increased by motion or by an exertion, as to occasion an apprehension that a very little additional motion would extinguish life. There is also frequently an acute pain in the region of the heart, but not always.[26]

What was likely was that acute rheumatism had changed its biological nature to include injury to the heart.

Wells treated only nine patients with the new rheumatic heart complication in the span of twelve years; Dundas encountered a like number of patients over the course of thirty-six years. The observation that took Wells and Dundas years to repeat became commonplace later in the nineteenth century. For example, a physician at St. Bartholomew's Hospital, P. M. Latham, tabulated that 13 percent of all patients admitted between 1836 and 1840 with the diagnosis of acute rheumatism suffered from pericarditis.[27] The proportion of patients with pericarditis as part of their rheumatism grew to 22 percent at Middlesex Hospital between 1853 and 1859[28] and 24 percent at Guy's Hospital between 1870 and 1872.[29] The prevalence of endocarditis in some hospitals was even higher.

### Bouillaud and the Stethoscope

Most initial reports resulted from specific and striking complaints of patients, external inspection of chest and pulse, followed by confirmatory autopsies. The stethoscope changed this. While René Laennec's introduction of the stethoscope in 1816 has been well studied by historians, a great deal less is known about the reception by practitioners of this technological breakthrough. The acquisition of skills among practitioners that correlated sounds at the bedside with structural changes at the autopsy table took time. The best historical accounts demonstrate that the stethoscope received a slow but steady welcome from clinicians, especially among those physicians who had been trained in Paris. Initially, sounds emanating from the lungs received attention, and only by the 1830s did clinicians begin to sort out which abnormal heart sounds came from a particular chamber or valve of the heart.[30]

Using a stethoscope, Jean-Baptiste Bouillaud (1796–1881), who had been a student of Laennec,[31] argued convincingly in 1836 that there was a "constant coincidence either of endocarditis or of pericarditis with acute articular rheumatism."[32] In September 1835, he had been called to consult in the case of a nineteen-year-old boy who had been admitted to La Charité Hospital two weeks earlier. The boy's admitting physician asked Bouillaud's advice when the young man developed chest pains in addition to his joint complaints. On this initial visit, Bouillaud placed his hand on the chest and felt a "very distinct vibration which immediately led me to announce the existence of the bellows, file, or saw sound," which he confirmed when he applied his ear to the boy's chest. He interpreted his findings to mean that the boy had the valvular damage of endocarditis. He visited weekly, each time recording his cardiac findings. A month after his initial visit, he found the boy improved. This time he examined his patient with a stethoscope and discovered that the abnormal heart sounds had largely disappeared.[33] This and other experiences led Bouillaud to observe that "in auscultating the sounds of the heart in some individuals still laboring under, or convalescing from acute articular rheumatism, I was not a little surprised to hear a strong, full, saw or bellows sound . . . such as I had often met in chronic or organic induration of the valves, with contractions of the orifices of the heart."[34] In a short monograph devoted entirely to the subject, Bouillaud gave a systematic approach to examining the heart in patients with rheumatism. Like other members of the Paris School, the term often used by historians of medicine to describe the extraordinarily creative hospital-based medicine which grew out of educational and clinical innovations of the French Revolution, Bouillaud made extensive use of percussion and auscultation, and he followed unsuccessful cases to the autopsy room.[35] Hospital-based, Bouillaud saw enough cases to estimate that nearly one-half of people with acute rheumatism suffered from either pericarditis or endocarditis or both. Bouillaud's observation of the frequency of cardiac injury was another piece of evidence of the malignant transformation and increasing severity of acute rheumatism.

What the stethoscope permitted Bouillaud to discover was the location of cardiac injury while the patient still lived. For example, chest pains resulted from pericarditis; shortness of breath from a damaged mitral heart valve. Even more significant, the stethoscope allowed Bouillaud to identify patients with heart disease that was unapparent to the patient. Bouillaud's volume and its translations convinced practitioners of the value of examining the heart in all patients with

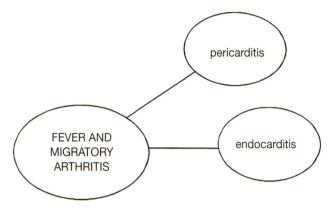

Figure 1.2. Acute rheumatism in the 1830s

acute rheumatism. When Alfred Stillé discussed the death of a twenty-three-year-old man from rheumatism, he stated to his listeners at the Pathological Society of Philadelphia in 1839 that examination of the heart in rheumatism had become routine.[36] In the same year that Bouillaud published, Henry Shuckburgh Roots (1785–1861) described a man he admitted to St. Thomas's Hospital in London who suffered from acute rheumatism and pericarditis, a diagnosis he made with the use of a stethoscope.[37]

Technology thus confirmed rheumatism's change in biological character. Bouillaud's use of the stethoscope followed Wells's observation by more than a quarter of a century and initial reports of cardiac involvement by nearly fifty years. This is not to argue that technology played no role. The stethoscope cemented cardiac damage to acute rheumatism in the minds of many practitioners by contributing fresh bedside evidence. And it extended the link between heart injury and rheumatism to include the many *asymptomatic* cases in which the injury was so mild that it went unnoticed by the patient. By midcentury, then, experience and technology were available to diagnose whether the pericardium or endocardium was involved in acute rheumatism; the stethoscope was not, of course, as helpful in determining myocardial damage, which was often silent.

Despite the growing association of heart disease with acute rheumatism, clinicians still gave central importance to fever and joint pains. These were the complaints that brought the patient to the practitioner; these were the criteria needed to make a diagnosis; these were the objects of therapy. But heart damage had joined fever and joint pains as an associated manifestation (figure 1.2).

## Acute Rheumatism Mutates Again: Chorea

There was a comparable path leading from acute rheumatism to chorea, a dramatic movement disorder. In the middle third of the nineteenth century, chorea began to afflict some patients of acute rheumatism, another indication that rheumatism was changing its biological character. Again, it was Thomas Sydenham who gave chorea its classic description in 1686:

This is a kind of convulsion, which attacks boys and girls from the tenth year to the time of puberty. It first shows itself by limping or unsteadiness in one of the legs, which the patient drags. The hand cannot be steady for a moment. It passes from one position to another by a convulsive movement, however much the patient may strive to the contrary. Before he can raise a cup to his lips he makes as many gesticulations as a mountebank; since he does not move it in a straight line, but has his hand drawn aside by spasms, until by some good fortune he brings it at last to his mouth. He then gulps off at once, so suddenly and so greedily as to look as if he were trying to amuse the lookers-on.[38]

In Sydenham's practice, chorea and rheumatism did not occur together in the same patient.

In 1838 Richard Bright (1789–1858), a prominent London physician who had studied at the same Royal Infirmary where Cullen had encountered so many patients with rheumatism, called attention in his Lumleian Lectures at the College of Physicians to the occasional association of chorea with diseases of the pericardium.[39] Each patient also suffered from acute rheumatism. The following year he reported in detail three case histories. The initial case was a seventeen-year-old boy who twelve days earlier "had begun to complain of general rheumatic symptoms; pains in the limbs, with puffiness and swelling of the wrists, and some other joints." Six days later, he developed chorea: "his head was constantly thrown from one side of the bed to the other; his lips were closed, and opened with a smacking sound, and when desired to put out his tongue it was protruded with all the forced grimace and difficulty observed in chorea." A rapid and irregular heartbeat "led to suspicions" that the heart was also affected. Sixteen days later, the boy died. At autopsy, Bright discovered that both the pericardium and the endocardium were involved. Careful dissection of the brain failed to yield any perceptible abnormalities.[40]

Bright's evaluation of these cases prompted him to scour the literature looking for prior references. As in most "discoveries," Bright found a few earlier allusions.[41] What Bright accomplished was to suggest a linkage between acute rheumatism, heart disease, and chorea. This observation confronted him with a conundrum similar to the one that had faced Cullen and Wells: how to explain the connection between a minor, self-limited form of arthritis and a serious brain injury. Bright believed, although his post-mortem dissections failed to demonstrate it, that rheumatic inflammation spread from the pericardium to the spinal cord then on to the brain, leading to chorea.

Prompted by Bright's observation, Dr. Yonge of Plymouth consulted Bright in 1840 about the case of Francis Hill, a nineteen-year-old gardener whom we met in the prologue, who struggled with his bout of rheumatism, endocarditis, and chorea.[42] Francis was so afflicted with his chorea that he could not walk, eat, or drink and required a straitjacket to prevent him from harming himself. After Francis's death, Yonge and Bright discovered that his mitral valve was seriously damaged; the spinal cord and brain, while carefully dissected, yielded no visible abnormalities.

Three years later Dr. Hughes, at Guy's Hospital in London, encountered S. M. and S. F., teenage girls:

> On admission [S. M.] was suffering from acute rheumatic swelling of the right knee. Her hands and arms were constantly in motion from chorea, the irregular movements being considerably increased when she was spoken to, or particularly noticed . . . she had considerable pain on pressure in the praecordial region.

> [S. F.] The chorea had now so much increased that it was necessary to place boards by her side to prevent her falling out of bed; and it was utterly impracticable to examine her heart and lungs.[43]

Richard Bright thought his linkage of chorea with the now-cardiac-expanded acute rheumatism was a new observation. Could it be that Drs. Bright, Yonge, Hughes, and others "saw" what other practitioners had overlooked previously? It is unimaginable that an infirmity which called such attention to itself as to require confinement and restraint could be easily missed when treating a patient for acute rheumatism. In its nineteenth-century form, chorea overwhelmed the observer. Rheumatism had altered its biology again.

## Patients and Doctors

At midcentury, changing biology dictated a significant shift in the way practitioners approached patients with acute rheumatism. When confronted with patients with fever and joint pains, physicians routinely examined the heart—often with a stethoscope—whether or not the person complained of chest pains. In addition, practitioners anticipated the possible onset of chorea. James Richard Smyth, confronted by a case that showed rheumatism in its full glory, confidently proclaimed: "The diagnosis, not withstanding that it was formed necessarily from complicated symptoms of a plurality of diseases, was not a matter of much difficulty; we did not hesitate on first, and but a cursory examination, in pronouncing the case to be one of rheumatic fever with rheumatic pericarditis."[44]

At St. Bartholomew's Hospital, Dr. Burrow matter-of-factly reported on the heart examination of a nineteen-year-old boy suffering from repeated attacks of rheumatism and chorea.[45] Before the Boston Society of Medical Improvement, Dr. Hodges claimed that his patient, a seventeen-year-old boy, displayed "no physical signs about the heart" at initial examination, but sixty hours later he developed a great "oppression" in his chest that subsequent autopsy revealed to be the result of pericarditis.[46]

What was important was that physicians began to assign greater significance to heart damage. The rising prominence of the heart in rheumatism came from the growing clinical appreciation, backed up by autopsy reports, that deaths from acute rheumatism resulted not from arthritis or fever but from injury done to the heart. Chorea, although seldom a cause of death and never accompanied with an autopsy finding, added complexity, misery, and certainly drama to acute

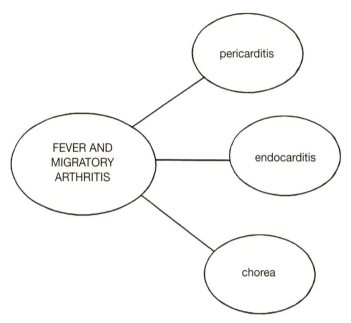

FIGURE 1.3.  Acute rheumatism in 1850

rheumatism. While neither heart disease nor chorea occurred in every case of rheumatism, their presence was anticipated in the minds of practitioners (figure 1.3).

## The Social Setting of Acute Rheumatism

Changing biology challenged physician explanations. Practitioners in the eighteenth century, before the advent of heart disease and chorea, observed that people who succumbed to rheumatism often belonged to families who seemed to have a constitutional weakness that predisposed them to this disease. Several children in one house would have rheumatism at the same time; parents had suffered similarly when children themselves. In people so prone, rheumatism was thought to follow a chill brought on by exposure to cold and wet, reflecting the usual onset of the disease in fall, winter, or early spring. In many instances, an unwise, often youthful, usually inadequately dressed laborer immoderately worked up a sweat in cold weather. Physicians thus noted a social dimension to rheumatism. Not too infrequently, the victim, often poor and living in crowded circumstances, was described as intemperate in drinking, eating, or sleeping. For example, Lionel Beale, physician to King's College Hospital, claimed that victims of acute rheumatism were "weak, ill-nourished, overworked and often underfed and insufficiently clad, unhealthy . . . children, students, and young people."[47] As such, physicians thought that rheumatism had seasonal, familial, and social dimensions.

The new injuries, especially those to the heart, fit nicely into emerging theories of disease in the early nineteenth century and engrafted onto older concerns for the hereditary, social, and climatic dimension of acute rheumatism. Following the lead of the Paris School with its focus on anatomical alterations in disease, physicians described structural changes in the bodies of patients dying from rheumatism. In particular, the major pathological concern centered on changes in the tissues of the heart. Minor changes in joints and elusive alterations in the brain occupied less attention, because they failed to leave identifying marks for the pathologist. Through anatomical analysis of those who died from rheumatism, "acute rheumatism" became an inflammatory illness in most classification schemes. Yet it never comfortably fit into any nosological niche, largely because the joints and brains of victims, clearly diseased in life, appeared normal at autopsy.

Acute rheumatism, often with some of the severest cases of heart disease, occurred occasionally in small epidemics. These sporadic outbreaks normally occurred in fall, winter, or early spring, and physicians were struck by coincidental outbreaks of other diseases that were present in the community at about the same time. Of note, Dr. Knight of New York, reflecting on nearly three decades of practice, recalled that he did not see many cases of acute rheumatism in the 1820s. After that, he saw more cases each year, which he linked to outbreaks of scarlet fever and erysipelas (illnesses, like rheumatic fever, now known to be associated with the streptococcus). "It is true also," Knight claimed, "that during the time in which we enjoyed an almost immunity from rheumatism, scarlet fever was not seen at all. . . . The same remarks will apply to erysipelas."[48]

## Therapy for Acute Rheumatism in the Early Nineteenth Century

Changing biology challenged therapeutics with its new injuries, but initially led to only a few fundamental changes. Until the end of the eighteenth century, doctors and patients addressed the complaints that brought patients to physicians: joint distress and fever. In addition, doctors worried about an underlying, but poorly defined, phlegmasiae, or inflammation. Bed rest, always a pillar in the care of any debilitating illness, formed the mainstay of treatment for acute rheumatism. Enforced rest, it was thought, prevented permanent damage to hurting joints. Physicians also directed attention to local, external care. Painful joints were frequently wrapped. Some doctors preferred linen; others flannel; still others a variety of plasters.[49] Opium became the prime drug for alleviating joint pain and, after the march of acute rheumatism to the heart, for chest pain as well.[50] Reports from the first years of the nineteenth century indicated that opium was administered in doses large enough and frequent enough [often hourly] to relieve pain. Whether opium speeded the course of acute rheumatism or merely lessened troublesome symptoms was a debated point.[51]

Physicians at the end of the eighteenth century also treated acute rheumatism with depletive therapies commonly employed to lessen any form of inflammation: bleeding, purging, sweating, and local irritation. These measures continued during the first decades of the nineteenth century. Although he had altered how physicians thought about rheumatism, Bouillaud advocated these traditional treatments. Significantly, Bouillaud directed some of these customary remedies at heart injury, for example, cupping the chest wall over the heart in an effort to draw off inflammation around the heart. Pericarditis and endocarditis thus were treated both systemically with bleeding and locally with application of leeches or other locally applied medicines to the chest wall.[52] Physicians treated chorea with bed rest, restraint, and occasionally sedatives.

Doctors normally administered opium in conjunction with various depletive measures. Although Bouillaud supported substantial bloodletting, other physicians worried that such measures actually weakened their patients. Dr. D. J. Corrigan found support for his concerns in the writings of Thomas Sydenham:

> As to the cure of rheumatism I have often been troubled that it could not be performed without the loss of a great deal of blood, by which the patient is not only much weakened for a time, but if of a weakly constitution he is most generally rendered more obnoxious to other diseases for some years.[53]

In opium Corrigan found a drug that worked well. In 1840 he treated a colleague, Dr. J. Aldridge, who wrote him a grateful letter detailing his experience with a relapse of acute rheumatism. His letter was a testimonial to the relief from the pain of arthritis:

> I confess that I was somewhat afraid of what appeared to me very large doses of this powerful drug, especially as my head always had a tendency to be affected whenever I had fever of any kind. It was therefore with some misgiving I obeyed you, but soon I had reason to congratulate myself on the effects of your advice, for during the remainder of my illness, i.e., from the second day after being forced to succumb, the pains, although they visited me occasionally were by no means intolerable; I slept much, my intellect remained clear, except when occasionally I took an overdose of the opium (for as soon as I began to experience its good effects, I became quite enamored of it) and, in fine, I was enabled to walk down the stairs the fourteenth day after taking to bed.[54]

Some physicians turned to cinchona bark to treat the fever of acute rheumatism. This use was prompted by the perceived similarities between rheumatism and malaria: high fever and a tendency to recur. After John Haygarth published his favorable experience using cinchona bark with 170 patients with rheumatism in 1805, the drug enjoyed several decades of popularity.[55]

Many physicians combined standard therapies for inflammation with drugs for pain and fever. For example, Bouillaud treated a woman suffering from rheumatism complicated by endocarditis with bed rest, compresses applied to the joints, opium, general bleeding, and scarified cups over the chest.[56] Another illustration was Dr. Taylor's treatment of Thomas Vardy in 1841. Vardy, a thirty-one-year-old blacksmith, developed his third bout of acute rheumatism, which Taylor attributed to exposure to cold after overworking and considerable drink. In his successful course of treatment of Vardy, Taylor used bleeding, purgatives, leeches, calomel, and narcotics. Of course, he also prescribed bed rest.[57]

Reflecting the new cardiac emphasis of acute rheumatism, physicians altered their reasons for advising bed rest, transferring their advocacy of this treatment from arthritis to heart involvement. Bed rest, in this view, would avoid strain on the heart, leading to less permanent cardiac damage.

Perceptions of physicians and patients that a variety of therapies worked quite well in acute rheumatism were enhanced by the nature of the disease to remit frequently on its own. In general, physicians stuck by traditionally favorite remedies, and normally the patient recovered. When confronted with a patient who developed a serious case of chorea or heart disease, most physicians "threw the book" at the patient, hoping that one or all remedies would prevent death. A case in point was Dr. O'Connor of the Royal Free Hospital. In 1861 he was faced with an eleven-year-old-girl who did not respond as expected. Dr. O'Connor eventually treated the girl with depletives (castor oil and calomel), several chemical remedies (bicarbonate of potash, nitrate of potash, and acetate of ammonia), and opium for pain. He wrapped her joints, applied leeches to her chest, and eventually gave her a mixture containing additional depletives. One can sense O'Connor's relief when the month-long ordeal ended with the girl's leaving the hospital.[58]

The treatment of acute rheumatism was very much an open question in midcentury. Some physicians were beginning to question whether traditional therapeutic approaches squared with rheumatism's new nature. Dr. James Alexander, an English physician, voiced his concern: "I was never able to prescribe for a case of rheumatism without feeling that I was committing legalized quackery."[59] Therapy was an issue that practitioners treating individual patients addressed on a case-by-case basis. Acute rheumatism was evolving into a disease that was too complicated for effective therapy to be sorted out in the setting of a patient's home or within a single physician's practice. It required pooling experiences in hospitals.

In 1864, John Roberton, in his review of the state of therapy for rheumatism presented to the Manchester Medical Society, shifted emphasis from a focus based on individuals to one centered on larger groups. Using actuarial data from John Gibson Fleming's *Medical Statistics of Life Insurance*, he discovered that fifty-seven members, covered by the Scottish Amicable Life Assurance Company, had died of heart disease over the preceding thirty-five years, many the result of acute rheumatism. On analyzing the published literature, Roberton learned that nearly one-half of all patients with rheumatism now suffered from the recent biological complication of heart injury and that it was cardiac disease that killed them. After looking at the broad array of available therapy, Roberton asked, "What we may now inquire is the treatment best fitted to arrest the disease and so prevent heart affection."[60] With his statistical analysis of a large number of patients, Roberton previewed a new approach to studying acute rheumatism that was to occupy much of the next decades.

CHAPTER 2

# *Acute Rheumatism and Hospitals, 1840–1880*

+⹀

$\mathcal{V}$ictims of acute rheumatism, complicated by either heart disease or chorea, found their way to hospitals. Often considerably more debilitated than those who suffered only from migratory arthritis, patients with pericarditis, heart failure, or poorly controlled movements outstripped the care that family or friends were able to provide at home.[1] Treatments, recommended by physicians and sought by patients, called for therapeutic interventions, such as restraint, opium or other drugs, depletives, local irritation applied to the chest, and bandages to hurting joints, as often as every two or three hours.[2] As the nineteenth century wore on, the daily regimen for acute rheumatism, especially with its new biological face, became even more intrusive. Hospital-based physicians, of course, saw acute rheumatism in its severest forms, the patients most critically ill and most likely to die. Patients who suffered only from fever and joint ailments seldom ended up in hospitals. New technologies, such as the stethoscope, enhanced appreciation of the most serious cases of acute rheumatism. Advocates of auscultation were often found in the wards of hospitals, where patients with the most dramatic murmurs were victims of the newly mutated acute rheumatism. For example, Henry Marshall Hughes (Guy's Hospital), Henry Gawen Sutton (London Hospital), Edmund Lyon (Manchester Royal Infirmary), and Samuel West (St. Bartholomew's Hospital) were all pioneers in auscultation and students of acute rheumatism.

Hospitals provided an imperfect lens to view acute rheumatism. Not all sufferers, even those with chorea or heart disease, ended up in hospitals. In London's hospitals, for example, only the "deserving poor" were admitted, those with steady employment who nevertheless failed to earn enough to provide for around-the-clock care at home. The more affluent patients and the very poor were excluded from hospital care.[3] Hospital patients, then, came from crowded environments later found to be most hospitable to the streptococcus. Without knowing of the bacterial worry, hospital physicians nonetheless became critically aware of the importance of patients' physical surroundings. Also excluded from hospital care were fever cases, because of the fear of contagion. Here a certain irony existed. Until the end of the nineteenth century, acute rheumatism was not considered a contagious disease. Even then, the question of its infectious nature sparked heated debate. By the time a patient developed heart disease or chorea—reasons for admission to a hospital—the fever had been gone for weeks, lessening any suspicion of contagion. Unknown to patients and physicians, the streptococcus lingered in the throats of victims, ready to spread from patient to patient in close hospital quarters. Thus sufferers of acute rheumatism left their contagious home environment for the equally contagious and dangerous company of fellow patients. A further insalubrious factor was that many hospitals in mid-nineteenth-century Britain played host to lethal epidemics of erysipelas, an often-fatal skin and soft tissue infection, found later to be caused by the streptococcus.[4] Additionally excluded from hospitals were patients with incurable diseases. Acute rheumatism, even complicated by chorea or heart disease, abruptly killed its victims only in a minority of cases: patients were seriously incapacitated but usually not at death's door.[5]

Despite shortcomings, British hospitals, especially those in London, provided a rich, if imperfect, source of information about acute rheumatism in the nineteenth century. In 1800 Britain had thirty-five hospitals supplying nearly four thousand beds; London's hospitals accounted for almost one-half of the total.[6] Eighteenth-century London had undergone a marked upsurge in population, from roughly 700,000 in 1700 to one million in 1800; the population would double by 1840. Such growth taxed public health measures such as water supply, waste disposal, and care for the sick.[7] In the eighteenth century, five general hospitals joined St. Thomas's Hospital and St. Bartholomew's Hospital to help in providing respite for the sick: Westminster Hospital (1720),[8] Guy's Hospital (1724),[9] St. George's Hospital (1733), London Hospital (1740), and Middlesex Hospital (1745).[10] Other cities followed suit, including Liverpool,[11] Manchester (1752),[12] and Edinburgh, where William Cullen had so frequently encountered rheumatism at the Royal Infirmary (1729). For physicians, one solid step on the path of professional success was appointment to a hospital staff.

Patients with complicated courses of acute rheumatism entered in great numbers to hospitals, often accounting for one of the leading reasons for entry. For example, at St. Bartholomew's Hospital, acute rheumatism was the admitting diagnosis of 7 percent of all patients; at St. Thomas's Hospital, acute rheumatism was frequently the most common recorded reason for admission.[13] In marked contrast to the practices of physicians such as William Charles Wells or David Dundas, when it took many years—even decades—to accumulate several cases of acute rheumatism with its new biological manifestations, hospital physicians easily managed to amass many cases, often within the space of a year or two. Hundreds of patients provided an abundance of information about acute rheumatism but necessarily dictated an entirely different format for reporting on medical experience: large charts that reduced individual cases to tabular outline (table 2.1), reflecting a numerical trend introduced by Pierre-Charles-Alexandre Louis in France.[14] Gone were the long and intimate individual case histories that had characterized Wells's reporting. The new charts, frequently massive in size, often extended to more than ten pages in length, tabulating symptoms, gender, class, age, autopsy findings, seasons, climatic variables, therapies, length of hospital stays, and outcomes.

TABLE 2.1    *British hospital studies of acute rheumatism, 1840–1888*

| Hospital | Cases | Year | Source |
|---|---|---|---|
| Manchester Royal Infirmary | 291 | 1840 | Lyon, *Trans. Prov. Med. Surg. Assoc.* 9: 338–344. |
| Guy's Hospital | 100 | 1846 | Hughes, *Guy's Hosp. Rep.* 4: 360–395. |
| University College Hospital | 51 | 1855 | Garrod, *Med-Chir. Trans.* 38: 111–156. |
| St. Mary's Hospital | 31 | 1857 | Sibson, *BMJ* 2: 1000–1004. |
| Middlesex Hospital | 476 | 1861 | Bury, *Brit. & For. Med-Chir. Rev.* 28: 194–198. |
| Hospital for Sick Children/St. George's Hospital | 164 | 1861 | Dickinson, *Med-Chir. Trans.* 45: 343–354. |
| St. Mary's Hospital | 243 | 1862 | Chambers, *Lancet* 2: 199–201. |
| St. George's Hospital | 663 | 1868 | Fuller, *St. George's Hosp. Rep.* 3: 1–13. |
| Guy's Hospital/ London Hospital | 25 | 1869 | Sutton, *Guy's Hosp. Rep.* 11: 392–428. |
| Guy's Hospital | 400 | 1874 | Pye-Smith, *Guy's Hosp. Rep.* 19: 311–356. |
| St. Thomas's Hospital | 161 | 1875 | Peacock, *St. Thomas's Hosp. Rep.* 10: 1–20. |
| Liverpool Royal Southern Hospital | 431 | 1881 | Carter, *Liverp. Med.-Chir. J.* 1: 88–101. |
| St. Bartholomew's Hospital | 693 | 1887 | Church, *St.Barts.Hosp. Rep.* 23: 269–287. |
| Westminster Hospital | 500 | 1888 | Syers, *Lancet* 1: 1292. |
| St. Bartholomew's Hospital | 1137 | 1888 | West, *Practitioner* 41: 104–113. |

## Hospitalized Patients with Acute Rheumatism

Sheer numbers permitted hospital doctors to reach conclusions that had eluded physicians practicing alone. Hospital studies demonstrated who were the victims of acute rheumatism. Edmund Lyon (1790–1862), a physician who brought auscultation to the Manchester Royal Infirmary during his nearly twenty-five-year tenure (1817–1841),[15] tabulated his experience: women and men were equally vulnerable to attacks of acute rheumatism; and, underscoring Cullen's observation, virtually all were under thirty-five years of age. Those old enough to work were employed as outdoor laborers, weavers, and smiths.[16] At Guy's Hospital, half the patients were under twenty years of age,[17] an observation supported by experience at Middlesex Hospital.[18] Nearly one-fourth of the patients at Guy's Hospital came from families who numbered at least one additional victim from acute rheumatism. Lyon's analysis in Manchester confirmed Sydenham and Cullen's impressions that most cases occurred in winter and early spring, although sporadic cases might happen at other times of the year.

Hospital studies helped to sort out how frequently heart disease and chorea occurred together, calling attention to the tendency of rheumatism's recent injuries to afflict at quite varying rates. For example, Henry Marshall Hughes (1805–1859), a physician at Guy's Hospital known as an "ardent cultivator of auscultation" and author of *Clinical Introduction to the Practice of Auscultation and Other Modes of Physical Diagnosis*,[19] found that only 9 percent of patients suffered with both chorea and heart disease in 1846.[20] The proportion grew more than three times when Philip Henry Pye-Smith (1840–1914), a physician who taught physiology and dermatology and was the author of the authoritative *Principles and Practice of Medicine*,[21] analyzed patients at Guy's Hospital thirty years later.[22]

Heart injury, as the cause of death in acute rheumatism, received considerable attention. Half of all patients at Middlesex Hospital,[23] Guy's Hospital,[24] and St. Bartholomew's Hospital[25] suffered from heart disease. At all three hospitals, the younger the patient the more likely the chance of serious heart illness. Eighty percent of children with acute rheumatism at St. Bartholomew's Hospital suffered from cardiac disease. All three hospitals recorded that, among patients with heart disease, endocarditis had become the most common site of cardiac injury (Middlesex Hospital–78 percent, Guy's Hospital–58 percent, St. Bartholomew's Hospital–89 percent); pericardial injury, the more common cardiac injury earlier in the nineteenth century, afflicted fewer patients (Middlesex Hospital–42 percent, Guy's Hospital–42 percent, St. Bartholomew's Hospital–11 percent). At Middlesex Hospital, nearly one-third of patients had both endocarditis and pericarditis.

Acute rheumatism tended to relapse. For example, Mr. T. M., William Charles Wells's patient we met earlier, suffered nine bouts before the one that injured his heart. Thomas Bevill Peacock (1812–1882), a physician who trained at the Royal Infirmary in Edinburgh and became one of Britain's leading authorities on valvular heart disease,[26] found that 60 percent of patients at St. Thomas's Hospital had suffered at least one prior attack. Ten percent had two relapses; one patient endured eight.[27] Risk for serious heart complications increased with each relapse.

For example, at St. Bartholomew's Hospital, 65 percent of patients with acute rheumatism suffered heart injury on relapse compared with 50 percent during the initial bout.[28]

Deaths were few but always the result of heart disease. Pye-Smith found that just under 5 percent of patients with acute rheumatism died at Guy's Hospital. William Carter, a socially active physician at Liverpool Royal Southern Hospital who championed temperance, sanitation, and the registration of midwives,[29] recorded just over a 2 percent mortality rate.[30] At Westminster Hospital, Henry Walter Syers, a medical registrar who later died from a wound received while performing an autopsy,[31] tallied a 3 percent mortality rate.[32] Only 1 percent of patients died at St. George's Hospital.[33] These figures need a note of clarification. One reason for the low mortality rate was that the numbers reflected deaths that occurred during the hospital stay. The statistics did not take into account patients who survived an initial bout with acute rheumatism but later succumbed to a weakened heart.

Analysis of large groups of hospitalized patients, then, provided physicians with considerable information about acute rheumatism. Sheer numbers did not always illuminate the changing character of the disease. Tabular appraisals were considerably less successful in answering some questions. For example, averaging the temperatures of hundreds of patients with acute rheumatism yielded an unhelpful mean because a mathematical average obscured the daily fluctuations of temperature that each patient experienced. Similarly, looking for common abnormalities in the urine of large numbers of patients failed to find common properties.[34] An added concern was that the individual patient simply got "lost" amid the press of so many victims.

## Changes in Therapy in Hospitalized Patients

Therapy, the reason patients sought physicians' advice, was one area where the experience with large groups of hospitalized patients offered promise. Opium, the mainstay for the alleviation of joint and chest discomfort, was among the first targets for scrutiny. Here shifting biology altered how physicians appraised the value of the painkiller. It was heart injury that killed; so physicians switched their measure of any drug's efficacy to cardiac injury. The question which Ernest Hart, dean of St. Mary's medical school at only twenty-nine years of age before becoming the socially minded editor of the *British Medical Journal*,[35] and his colleague Francis Sibson, an authority on pericarditis and endocarditis (as well as on the blowhole of the porpoise),[36] addressed was whether opium lessened rheumatism's damage to the heart. They conceded that opium diminished joint and chest pain and enhanced a general sense of well-being—the prior gauge of therapeutic success for both patient and physician—but they concluded that opium was entirely unhelpful in diminishing cardiac complications.[37]

For hospital physicians, a disease that caused fever, arthritis, chorea, and heart disease implied a pathological connection among symptoms. Earlier students of the disease, such as van Swieten and Cullen, had suggested that an imprecisely defined rheumatic poison or inflammation flowed from hurting joints to vital organs. Nineteenth-century doctors hoped that the emerging field of medical chemistry would provide a chemical link. Specifically, many singled out a derangement in the body's acids, a notion that offered a ready therapeutic solution: basic or alkalinic medicines which would neutralize excess acids.

Contemporary participants credited the "acid" theory of acute rheumatism to a chance comment "thrown out by [William] Prout in a lecture at the College of Physicians."[38] Prout (1785–1850), who is known to chemists for his eponymous hypothesis that elements possess atomic weights which are integral multiples of the atomic weight of hydrogen, had trained as a physician at the Royal Infirmary in Edinburgh before setting up a practice in London that included treating patients at St. Thomas's Hospital and Guy's Hospital.[39] Although Prout never published specifically on acute rheumatism, it is safe to assume that he encountered the disease often in his training and practice. Prout was intrigued with the chemical reflection of diseases in the urine and was among the first to isolate urea from urine in 1814. In his text published seven years later, he commented that many diseases, especially those with fever, caused the body to produce excess lithic, or uric, acid. To compensate, the body secreted the surplus acid in the sweat and urine. This suggested to him a benefit from alkaline medicines.[40] In his view, alkaline drugs would neutralize or counteract excess acid. Prout's notion also served as a backdrop for another observation, again not specifically pertaining to rheumatism. In 1848 Alfred Baring Garrod, a physician at University College Hospital, found that patients with gout had excess uric acid both in their blood, and, more to the point, crystallized in their joints, causing arthritis. By analogy, Garrod proposed that patients with acute rheumatism also had an acidic derangement.[41] To some, the acrid smell of the profuse sweat from patients with acute rheumatism leant support to the notion that some acid, perhaps lactic acid, was in oversupply. Lessons that Garrod learned from the study of gout played an additional role in the treatment of acute rheumatism: in the laboratory, alkaline solutions kept uric acid from crystallizing, suggesting that a similar approach might work in the suffering rheumatic patient. When the dust settled decades later, surrounding the introduction of salicylate, patients with acute rheumatism were found not to produce excess acid in the blood, urine, or sweat.[42] Before this understanding became commonplace were years of therapeutic enthusiasm, dosing patients with sufficient alkaline drugs to render urine, which is normally slightly acidic, alkalinic. As one physician explained in 1858: "[There is] every reason to hope that we may be enabled by a very simple chemical operation to reason backwards from the urine to definite conclusions as to the quality and composition of the blood, and by the aid of which the physician may ascertain the changes in the composition of the blood in disease."[43]

Virtually all theoretical and therapeutic discussions about acute rheumatism in midcentury centered on the oversupply of acids. William F. Channing, an American physician, stated in 1855: the "marked characteristic of rheumatism [is] an acid condition of the fluids and secretions."[44] Specifically, most doctors speculated that elevated lactic acid was the culprit. For example, J. H. Salisbury, a professor of histology and physiology at Charity Hospital Medical College in

Cleveland, Ohio, argued that rheumatism followed an accumulation of lactic acid in the blood and connective tissues following "exposure" to cold and damp surroundings or an indiscretion in lifestyle.[45] Peter Wallwork Latham, a physician at Westminster Hospital in London, disagreed about the lactic acid.[46] In an elaborate argument, Latham named excess uric acid as the offender. Applying contemporary ideas about the chemistry of uric acid to neurophysiology, he claimed that muscles and connective tissue produced large amounts of uric acid in acute rheumatism and that this surplus poisoned the vasomotor center in the brain stem. In an intricate if imprecise manner, Latham claimed that the vasomotor center, so altered, produced the various symptoms of acute rheumatism by sending harmful impulses along nerves.[47] In supporting various views about proposed acid derangements in acute rheumatism, physicians reported that patients had acidic sweat, urine, and saliva. What was missing from these chemical analyses were data comparing the acidity of bodily fluids in other diseases or from people during the healthy periods in their lives. As it turns out, urine, saliva, and sweat are almost always acidic; acid is the norm and not a sign of disease.[48]

Not all physicians adhered to the prevailing acidic theory. For example, J. M. DaCosta, a doctor at Pennsylvania Hospital, objected:

> I believe that this entire question of excessive acidity, acid sweats, etc. has been overstated. I feel convinced that there are a large number of cases in which the skin does not yield these excessive acid perspirations, and in which the acid in the urine is not what one might suppose from reading books. . . . In other words, the so-called acid theory of rheumatism which assumes that there is an extreme condition in the system and that such acid must be eliminated fails to convince me that it is the real and only solution of the so-called rheumatic diathesis or production of the phenomenon of acute articular rheumatism.[49]

### Alkaline Therapy Replaces Older Treatments for Acute Rheumatism

Notions about acids in acute rheumatism directly influenced therapy. Physicians had at hand several drugs that could neutralize bodily acids, and these received careful testing in hospitals. The aim of all alkalinic regimens was to give sufficient oral drug to alter the normally acidic urine to become alkalinic, often requiring the administration of medicine every one or two hours. One of the first tests came not from a London hospital but from the United States. A resident physician at New York Hospital, John B. Chapin, conducted a trial in 1854 giving drugs which would "alkalinize" patients with acute rheumatism. When he did so for a period of three weeks, Chapin's twenty-five patients recovered from joint complaints. What particularly excited him was that only three developed heart disease, or less than one-fourth the number he anticipated.[50] The following year, Alfred Baring Garrod achieved similar beneficial results when he added alkaline drugs to his former regimen of opium and depletives in treating patients at University College Hospital in London.[51]

TABLE 2.2   *Therapy for patients with acute rheumatism*
*at St. Mary's Hospital in 1866*

| Therapy | Number of patients | Hospital stay (in days) | Heart disease number (%) |
|---|---|---|---|
| Nitrate of potash | 26 | 40 days | 5 [19.2%], 4 deaths |
| High dose bicarbonate of potash | 141 | 34.3 days | 9 [5.3%], 0 deaths |
| Low dose bicarbonate of potash | 33 | 40 days | combined with higher dose |
| No treatment | 11 | 30 days | 0 |

SOURCE: Thomas K. Chambers, "Statistics of the Treatment of Rheumatic Fever," *British Medical Journal* (1863), 2: 237.

William Howship Dickinson (1832–1913), a physician who began his career at St. George's Hosptial before joining the medical staff at the Hospital for Sick Children, Great Ormond Street, London,[52] used his experience with patients at St. George's to compare the outcomes of treatment with alkaline drugs with traditional therapy. Dickinson divided his 164 patients into fourteen separate groups, distinguished by minor differences in regimen. For example, four of his groups received some form of alkaline therapy. Adding a further complexity, his groups varied in size from twenty-eight patients to only three. His study, while illustrating a commendable investigative spirit, nevertheless created too many categories for detailed analysis. Despite these shortcomings, only 10 percent of Dickinson's patients receiving alkaline drugs developed heart disease, less than one-third the tally of those undergoing the traditional regimen. No treatment shortened the patient's stay; patients in all groups spent about forty days in the hospital.[53]

Physicians had several alkalinic drugs from which to choose, usually selecting either nitrate of potash or bicarbonate of potash; and either could be given at several doses. Thomas K. Chambers at St. Mary's Hospital attempted to sort out drug and dosage in 1866. His measure was development of heart disease and length of hospital stay (table 2.2). A number of issues immediately emerged. The sizes of Chambers's groups were not comparable. He made no comment on his selection of patients for each group: were all similarly afflicted at the start of therapy? Length of hospital stay was a difficult criterion because patients often sought medical help at different points during their illness. Nevertheless, Chambers concluded that any regimen that incorporated bicarbonate reduced the proportion of patients who developed heart disease. Of note, the group that fared best received no specific therapy other than bed rest, a result Chambers elected not to comment upon.[54]

Austin Flint, the distinguished physician who was largely responsible for

TABLE 2.3    *Dr. Henry Fuller's comparison of "older" therapy and alkaline therapy for acute rheumatism at St. George's Hospital*

| Therapy | Number of patients | Patients with heart disease | Deaths |
|---|---|---|---|
| "Older" | 246 | 119 | 17 |
| Alkaline | 417 | 9 | 0 |

SOURCE: Henry William Fuller, "On the Treatment of Rheumatic Fever," *St. George's Hospital Reports* (1868), 3: 1–13.

popularizing percussion and auscultation in the United States, reflected in 1863 on the state of therapy for acute rheumatism there.[55] Alkaline drugs had largely replaced older treatments, Flint claimed, because of the English hospital successes.[56] Specifically, Flint singled out the experience of Henry Fuller at St. George's Hospital. Fuller, the author of *On Rheumatism, Rheumatic Gout, and Sciatica*, which a reviewer of the second edition (1856) called the "standard work on rheumatism for the use of the British practitioner,"[57] became a stirring champion of alkaline therapy as the result of his remarkable successes with it (table 2.3). As Austin Flint had commented, Fuller's results seemed hard to beat.

Not all hospital physicians were quick to replace objectional older remedies that consisted, in part, of debilitating depletives with newer alkalinic therapy. A few physicians in the 1850s simply stopped the depletives and elected to allow acute rheumatism to run its course without any provocative therapy. Dr. G. Owen Rees, a physician at Guy's Hospital with an interest in urinary chemistry, advocated treating acute rheumatism with bed rest and large volumes of lemon juice.[58] With citrus and rest, Rees achieved results that equaled both older and alkaline therapies.[59] These encouraging results prompted an attack on the dominant alkaline therapy more than a decade later. William Withey Gull (1816–1890), a Guy's Hospital physician known to contemporaries more for his work with acute rheumatism than for his early description of anorexia nervosa that has gained him fame among historians a century later,[60] and Henry Gawen Sutton, a meticulous, if somewhat withdrawn, collaborator at London Hospital,[61] demonstrated that bed rest and a "light" diet alone worked about as well, perhaps better, than loading up patients with alkaline drugs. To this expectant regimen, Gull and Sutton added only mint water. By every clinical criteria (length of hospital stay, development of heart disease, and mortality), Gull and Sutton argued that "our cases appear to teach us that the rheumatic process runs its course under the expectant plan as favorably as under the treatment of drugs."[62] Understandably unpersuaded, Henry Fuller, who was present in the audience when Gull and Sutton delivered their views, adamantly criticized the expectant approach. Also present was Francis Sibson, who had helped to show that opium failed to prevent heart damage in acute rheumatism. Sibson reasonably surmised that both alkaline and expectant regimens, with emphasis on "rest, care, and nurture in the hospital," shared advantages over more intrusive depletive measures.[63]

The editors of the *British Medical Journal* believed that the arguments Gull and Sutton put forth had dealt a "severe blow" to the alkaline therapy. To assess what they expected to be an erosion of support, the editors conducted a survey in 1869 of thirteen hospitals. To their surprise, only at Guy's Hospital, where Gull worked, was the expectant approach followed.[64] The editors of the *Medical Record* in New York conducted a similar but less extensive survey in 1873 to see how doctors in American hospitals treated rheumatism. As in the British investigation, alkaline therapy predominated.[65] Speaking for many practitioners, R. Clement Lucas commented in 1874: "There are few diseases that have [been] so variously and at the same time successfully treated as acute articular rheumatism; and not a few reputations have been built upon the number of undoubted recoveries which have followed the many and diversified methods of treatment that have been recommended."[66] Two years later, Thomas Maclagan announced his discovery of salicin, which fundamentally altered the course of therapy for acute rheumatism.

## Salicylate and the Treatment of Acute Rheumatism

In 1876 Thomas Maclagan, a Scottish physician who practiced in Dundee, employed salicin to treat eight patients suffering from rheumatic fever. Salicin, a component of willow bark, was known in the ancient world as a treatment for gout and fever.[67] Earlier in the nineteenth century, salicin had been extracted from willow bark and salicylic acid, a more active form, synthesized.[68] Salicin enjoyed a degree of popularity in the nineteenth century in treating a variety of ailments: taken internally for fever, worms, or as a general tonic; or applied on the skin as an astringent. By 1876, Maclagan reported that salicin had largely fallen from common usage among practitioners.[69]

Maclagan's reasoning for trying salicin in rheumatic fever was curious. He pointed to the similarities that he perceived between malaria and rheumatism, for example, recurring fevers. He noted that the cinchona bark, which contained quinine and was the major therapy for malaria, was found in areas where malaria was prevalent. By analogy, he argued that some naturally occurring plant should be found in areas where rheumatic fever was commonplace. The willow tree fit the bill.

Maclagan gave salicin to his initial patient, a forty-eight-year-old man, on 26 November 1874. By the following day, his fever had fallen to 99.6 degrees Fahrenheit from 103 degrees Fahrenheit; his pulse declined to 100 beats per minute from 120 beats per minute; and his aching, swollen joints were nearly free from pain, swelling, and redness.[70]

At virtually the same moment, German physicians prescribed salicylic acid and sodium salicylate in the treatment of rheumatism, with equally dramatic results.[71] As is typical in the history of medicine after any discovery, a heated battle for priority followed with physicians from both countries claiming credit for their countrymen. An immediate infatuation with the therapy ensued, with dosage, frequency and duration of treatment, and clinical measures of assessing outcome hotly debated.[72] When the smoke lifted a decade later, salicylate had replaced both salicin and alkaline drugs, although doubts had emerged on the effectiveness of salicylate in preventing or treating rheumatic heart disease.

A comment by W. H. Broadbent, a physician at St. Mary's Hospital and authority on rheumatic heart disease,[73] gives a sense of the enthusiasm from an early supporter of salicylate:

> Few diseases have had brought against them a heavier armament of drugs than has acute rheumatism. It has been stormed by alkalies and saline, attacked by acids, assaulted by perchloride of iron and by quinine, surprised by propylamine . . . , drained by venesection and purgatives, flooded alternatively with hot and cold water, alarmed with blisters, blasted with hot air, lulled by opium, and appeased by chloral hydrate. In addition to these, it has been constantly harassed by the raids of lesser foes, such as lemon juice, citric acid, belladonna, and iodide of potassium. Now another powerful enemy has appeared, salicylic acid. . . . The beneficial action of the drug was constant and unequivocal.[74]

From the first, physicians directed their therapy with salicylates at the reduction of fever and cessation of joint pain. Even though doctors had understood for decades that what mattered in terms of patient survival was damage to the heart, painful joints and fever—symptoms that brought patients to doctors—dictated treatment. Even Maclagan stated, "Regarding the action of salicin on the cardiac complications of rheumatic fever I have no experience." It was hard for practitioners to ignore the joints. A case in point was Willie T. C., a seventeen-year-old boy from Boston whose joints were so painful during his third bout with acute rheumatism in 1875 that he required ether to get to sleep. His doctor, S. L. Abbott, gave him salicylic acid to relieve his joint pain, with dramatic results.[75]

Salicylate became very quickly what one French clinician called "la grande vogue du jour."[76] Almost immediately physicians reported small trials on a few patients, usually with moderate success. In the view of some, salicylate proved revolutionary. To others, salicylate showed no advantages. Others found that salicylate produced annoying side effects, such as tinnitus or deafness, later shown to be signs of overdose.[77]

Dosage varied greatly. Albert Wood of Worcester employed six grains every two hours (72 grains in a day); Henry Clark used ten grains every hour for twelve hours then spaced to every two hours (180 grains in a day); D. W. Hodgkins gave five grains every two hours that he increased to every hour (80 grains a day); Ralph Huse asked his patients to take only two grains every two hours (24 grains in a day). In these early reports, no physician compared the benefits of differing doses. With hindsight, we know that an adult requires approximately fifteen grains every six hours (60 grains each day). It is clear that early dosage schedules both under- and overshot the mark. In addition, James Russell at the Birmingham General Hospital complained that it was very hard to know whether salicylate worked at all because of the nature of rheumatic fever to remit and relapse.[78]

Hospital-based physicians were among the first to compare salicylate with alkaline therapy. Very quickly surveys of hospital practices appeared. How were cases of rheumatic fever treated? Was salicylate being used, if so how, and at what dose? How effective was the new drug? As might be expected, these early surveys revealed that physicians usually began treating a patient with the "standard" alkaline therapy but that they shifted to salicylate in difficult cases.[79] William Howship Dickinson never forgot that alkaline drugs lessened cardiac complications for his patients; when salicylate came along, he simply added it to alkaline.[80] Distinguished workers in the field also rendered an early judgment on the salicylates. For example, Germain Sée of Paris, who had studied chorea years earlier, tested salicylate promptly after its introduction and found it superior to other therapies.[81]

Hospital studies comparing the effectiveness of salicylate with that of other therapies soon showed both advantages and shortcomings. These studies were difficult to compare because they varied in the amount, frequency, and duration of dosage as well as over which parameter to measure success or failure. In the initial comparative studies, physicians often chose duration of fever, joint pain, and length of stay in the hospital as the litmus.

At St. George's Hospital, doctors found that adding salicylate at high, moderate, or even low doses lessened the period of fever and the total length of illness but did not cut the length of hospitalization. Length of stay within the hospital was a tricky measure in that many factors went into making a decision to discharge a patient, such as compliance in taking salicylate, general debility, and presence of supportive home life.[82]

Patients receiving salicylate at St. Bartholomew's Hospital suffered less joint pain than did those receiving alkaline therapy but remained in the hospital a similar length of time and were as likely to develop cardiac complications.[83] Middlesex Hospital reported similar benefits of shorter periods of fever and joint pain for patients on salicylate but no difference in heart complications.[84] At East London Hospital for Children, patients getting salicylate had shorter periods of fever, less joint pain, and slightly less time in bed;[85] Westminster Hospital reported similar results.[86] When physicians at Guy's Hospital compared the results of 1,200 patients given various treatments for rheumatic fever, they found that those receiving salicylate had shorter periods of fever and joint pain.[87] Just how short the period of fever could be was demonstrated at Birmingham General Hospital. Patients receiving alkaline therapy suffered 248 hours of fever on average; those getting salicylate only 38 hours.[88]

Early observers of salicylate also noted serious complications. William Osler reported a women who developed delirium. Of seventeen patients who received salicylate at Massachusetts General Hospital in 1879, five developed nausea and gastric distress, eight deafness, and five delirium, symptoms attributed to the new drug.[89]

Most physicians agreed with Thomas Maclagan that salicylate was beneficial in alleviating fever and arthritis and that it had clear advantages over either expectant therapy or alkaline.[90] A few physicians cautioned that salicylate was not clearly superior, especially in treating cardiac injury, and that inflated claims had muddied the therapeutic debate. Robert Sinclair, physician to the Dundee Royal Infirmary, blasted Maclagan:

Dogma like this [salicylate cure] cannot be sufficiently deplored. It hinders the progress of therapeutics, imperils human life, and in the long run injures the cause it is intended to help. Unfortunately, the student of the history of medicine is no stranger to confident assertions; some with good foundations, some with marvelously little, and some with none.[91]

Sinclair called attention to the peculiar nature of rheumatic fever to remit spontaneously: "It is probable . . . that there are cases which yield to every kind of treatment, or to no treatment, and some which pursue their destructive career in spite of all artillery in the pharmacopoeia and out of it."[92] Alfred Stillé of Philadelphia went so far as to say that "no treatment was ever invented which stopped a case of acute articular rheumatism."[93]

Other physicians, understanding that avoiding damage to the heart was key to survival, cautioned physicians to assess the value of salicylate therapy in preventing or treating heart disease. A physician from Auburn, New York, W. S. Cheesman, claimed that doctors were misdirecting their therapy by focusing on fever and joint pain.[94] In 1882 members of the London Medical Society debated the question of the value of salicylate in treating rheumatic heart disease: "The importance of this question is apparent, seeing that the chief element of danger, present and future, in this disease is imparted to it by the great liability that exists to inflammatory processes in and around the heart."[95] One member of the society, T. Gilbart-Smith, found no protective value to the heart with salicylate therapy. Present at the discussion was Thomas Maclagan, who had capitalized on his discovery by setting up a successful London practice. Maclagan explained that he now believed that salicylate would indeed protect the heart, but only if started early enough: "Every hour is of importance, for it needs no argument to show that the danger to the heart is less in a case in which the course of the disease is arrested within twenty-four hours than it is in one in which three or four days are expended in the process."[96] Charles H. May, a physician at Roosevelt Hospital in New York, published the most detailed early comparison of therapies in 1884. May agreed with many British physicians that salicylate shortened the duration of fever and joint pain. Unfortunately, salicylate did not appear to influence heart damage.[97]

Ten years after Maclagan first announced his trial of salicin on rheumatic fever, William Osler responded to a survey from the editors of *Medical News* of Philadelphia about his approach to the treatment of rheumatic fever. Osler claimed that he treated less serious cases of acute rheumatism with alkaline and opium. But for grave cases, those with fever higher than 103 degrees Fahrenheit and with many painful joints, he used salicylate. Osler confirmed that he did not believe that salicylate shortened the illness or modified in any way damage done to the heart. Nevertheless, salicylate therapy did make patients feel better.[98]

Therapy for acute rheumatism thus followed a circuitous path in the hands of hospital-based physicians. Changing biology altered the nature of the disease, and doctors responded appropriately by assessing the treatment of heart disease as one measure of clinical outcome. Initially physicians, such as Bouillaud, responded to cardiac injury by directing established therapy, for example cupping, to the chest, where they hoped it would draw off pericardial fluid. They added opium, an effective painkiller, to alleviate both chest and joint distress. Alkaline therapy, also combined with opium, replaced the older therapeutic measures, in part based on theory and in part based on superior results attained by hospital-based physicians. Hospital doctors compared alkaline drugs with depletive measures and, despite serious flaws in their studies, interpreted the results as showing clear advantages in diminishing damage to the heart. No study that has come to light advocated depletives after 1860. Other hospital-based doctors attained similarly improved cardiac outcomes with simple bed rest and improved diet without either depletive regimens or alkaline drugs. As surveys of physician practices in London and New York City demonstrated, most doctors elected to ignore these studies and continued to prescribe alkaline drugs.

There was no question that these physicians believed, and their tabulated experiences supported, that alkaline drugs benefited patients. In hindsight, we know that around-the-clock oral dosing of patients with alkaline drugs, even in large amounts, did not alter the acid–alkaline balance of the body. In particular, these drugs would not change the acidic content of joint or pericardial fluids. The kidney, detecting an increase of alkaline substances in the body, would immediately excrete excess alkaline in the urine in order to maintain a steady state. The urine did change to alkaline—the alteration that physicians employed as their measure of efficacy—but this change did not mean that the rest of body had undergone fundamental modifications. Alkaline drugs, then, did not work as physicians hoped they would, and twentieth-century pharmacology has not shed light on any reason why they might have been helpful in acute rheumatism. Perhaps hospital physicians unwittingly divided patients into groupings that prejudiced outcomes. Francis Sibson's rationale for perceived alkaline efficacy makes a good deal of sense: alkaline therapy—which has no harmful side effects—was an improvement over depletives from the patient's point of view. An insight from the twentieth century does help in understanding therapeutic claims: once the ravages of rheumatic fever start, no drug yet discovered has halted its cardiac or neurological onslaught. Physicians who did less for their patients with acute rheumatism almost certainly helped them more.

Salicylate was a striking improvement from the point of view of patient comfort. It dramatically lessened fever and quickly alleviated joint pain, two reasons why patients sought medical attention. So effective was salicylate that it replaced opium. Salicylate was far less dazzling with heart disease. Discerning physicians thought they could see a pattern: salicylate helped more with pericarditis than with endocarditis. Twentieth-century evidence has confirmed that salicylate lessens pericardial fluid, and subsequently chest pain. Quickly changing biology tended to obscure this observation. By 1885, endocarditis had surpassed pericarditis as the primary cardiac injury. Salicylate was less helpful with endocarditis, which may have led to the undeserved conclusion that salicylate was not efficacious in the treatment of any form of rheumatic heart disease.

One therapeutic accomplishment of these hospital physicians that cannot be denied was their establishment of the method of any claim. Any therapy needed to be tested on a large number of patients in order to show its value in reducing or preventing heart injury (a measure of mortality) and decreasing of hospital stay (a measure of morbidity).

## Mortality from Rheumatic Fever Declines

Nineteenth-century hospital physicians' tabulations made one additional contribution to the epidemiological understanding of rheumatic fever. Arthur Newsholme, a leader in British public health who in 1895 was medical officer of health for Brighton, carefully pieced together the experiences of many of the nation's hospitals.[99] Newsholme found that mortality from acute rheumatism had peaked in Britain in 1875 and had begun a discernible decline. Hospitals in Paris and Berlin documented a similar peak and recession. Decline in mortality signaled a decline in life-threatening heart injury and indicated that rheumatic fever's biological march continued. But now the retreat had begun. In contrast, cases of acute rheumatism remained essentially constant but continued to ebb and flow according to a pattern, which suggested to Newsholme an epidemic contagion.[100] It is very difficult for the historian to determine whether alkaline or salicylate contributed significantly to the overall decline in mortality, despite the encouraging conclusions from hospital studies. Meticulous research in the twentieth century has revealed that aspirin—the commonly used form of salicylate after 1925—even when carefully used, saved few, if any, lives. What is more likely is that the streptococcus altered in ways that damaged fewer hearts critically.

What needs stressing is that variability in acute rheumatism was the major clinical issue that faced hospital physicians in the middle third of the nineteenth century. Studying large numbers of patients in hospitals was the initial manner by which doctors dealt with the wide range of experiences of both patients and their physicians. In this fashion, doctors grasped more precisely the number of patients who were expected to suffer from heart disease or chorea. The method alerted them to the shift in the prime cardiac target from pericardium to endocardium. And it helped to shelve a few of the older therapies. Simple numerical analysis, however, proved to be of only limited help to clinicians when struggling with the individual diagnostic and treatment needs of their patients.

## CHAPTER 3

# Walter Butler Cheadle and the "Typical Case," 1880–1890

━━

$\mathcal{T}$he second half of the nineteenth century witnessed more changes to acute rheumatism. In contrast to chorea and heart injury which were brought about by biological alterations in the disease, the newer aspects of acute rheumatism—tonsillitis, subcutaneous nodules, and erythematous rashes—joined acute rheumatism after traversing more complicated paths which included both biology and physician perception. The result was a complex disease with eight components (fever, migratory arthritis, pericarditis, endocarditis, chorea, subcutaneous nodules, erythematous rashes, and tonsillitis) that challenged physician thinking in ways that only a few diseases—such as syphilis—did. At issue was the beguiling nature of the elements to appear in several different combinations. "Individual" case histories of the sort William Charles Wells employed to describe the illnesses of Miss A. L. and Mr. T. M. showed the variability of acute rheumatism as the disease was beginning to alter its nature. Large hospital studies demonstrated how the new injuries of acute rheumatism touched populations. Neither approach was entirely helpful to physicians when confronted with the added complexity of the disease. Bluntly stated, the issue was whether a patient who suffered from fever, migratory arthritis, and pericarditis had the same illness as one who complained of subcutaneous nodules, sore throat, and chorea. What emerged at the end of the century was the diagnostic concept of the "typical" case that allowed for considerable variability yet possessed common elements. The typical case benefited from both individual case histories and hospital-based amalgams. In addition, the new approach injected new dimensions: natural history and epidemiology. The new strategy followed rheumatic fever from onset to conclusion—through relapses and remissions and possible death—and it pursued rheumatic fever across generations and geography. The typical case permitted physicians to make a certain diagnosis in a disease that could be most uncertain in a clinical setting. Pioneering in this strategy was Walter Butler Cheadle, physician to the Hospital for Sick Children, Great Ormond Street.[1]

Acute rheumatism changed in other ways. Victims became younger and more likely to suffer heart disease. Another metamorphosis, which virtually escaped comment, was the gradual shift to the term "rheumatic fever," away from both "acute rheumatism" and "acute articular rheumatism." In shifting the term, clinicians continued their switch in emphasis away from the dramatic, yet fundamentally less serious, fever and migratory arthritis to a broader conception of the disease that also included insults to heart, brain, tendons, and skin in addition to joints. The elimination of "acute" heralded an understanding that damage done, especially to the heart, persisted in many cases long after the initial phase of the disease had receded. Of note, "acute" returned in the twentieth century to distinguish aspects of rheumatic fever that occurred during the initial phases of the disease from permanent injuries that left "chronic" disabilities.

## Tonsillitis

In the 1870s tonsillitis joined fever, migratory arthritis, carditis, and chorea as a commonly associated manifestation of rheumatic fever. Insights from the twentieth century make certain that a streptococcal sore throat necessarily had always been present, long before physicians noted its appearance. Tonsillitis had been "obscured" from physicians' sight most likely because its ubiquity, especially in children, did not set the complaint clearly apart and because the more attention-grabbing symptoms of arthritis, chorea, and carditis occurred weeks after a sore throat had receded from memory. What made tonsillitis different from the other symptoms was the observation that a sore throat normally preceded problems of the joints and heart and could, therefore, be viewed as an inciting event. It is important at this point not to get ahead of the story. The subsequent understanding that the streptococcus causes tonsillitis and in the process triggers a complex immunological reaction that results in what we now call rheumatic fever was decades in the making. To physicians in the 1870s, tonsillitis was one of the various elements of rheumatic fever that occurred often enough for physicians to single it out as a helpful guide to diagnosis.

The association of tonsillitis with rheumatic fever was not entirely new in 1870. As case histories have demonstrated, many physicians commented that individual patients suffered from a sore throat, a catarrh, or upper respiratory infection before coming down with rheumatism. Upon examination, doctors on occasion noted a "furred tongue," a colorful term used to describe the white lingual coating that now and then appears in streptococcal infection.

In particular, physicians singled out the sore throat that accompanied scarlet fever, a dramatic illness with its characteristic red rash that was far more lethal in the nineteenth century than it has since become, as a successful inciting event for rheumatic fever. Again, it is crucial not to let the benefits of hindsight provide more clarity to the picture than nineteenth-century events permitted, for scarlet fever, even as late as the 1890s, was not clearly understood to be a streptococcal disease. But sequence was critical. Scarlet fever, when it occurred, always preceded rather than followed rheumatic fever. Linking rheumatic fever with scarlet fever was Dr. Knight's observation in 1847, which we encountered earlier, that New York was free from rheumatism when it was also free from scarlet fever.[2] Still earlier was a report from the West Indies in 1830 of an epidemic of scarlet fever that provoked acute rheumatism in some of its victims.[3] Nathaniel J. Haydon, a physician in England, investigated an epidemic of scarlet fever during the summer of 1850. Several people later developed rheumatic fever, leading Haydon to conclude that the two illnesses were loosely linked. In addition, he called on a personal experience: "A friend of my own, a young medical man, while a pupil in London, had scarlatina [scarlet fever] very slightly, but it was followed by a most acute attack of rheumatic fever. . . . Within a few months he had a second attack of rheumatic fever, with pericarditis, and there was at the same time a great functional disturbance of the brain [perhaps chorea]."[4] Providing an example from 1854, Hughes Willshire reported that he "coincided with the views generally held with respect to the connexion of rheumatism with abnormal states of the joints and heart and with scarlatina."[5] While examination of the literature does not quite reflect such widespread dissemination of the notion, Willshire's comment does indicate that some physicians were beginning to think that scarlet fever often preceded rheumatic fever. A doctor at the Royal Free Hospital, Dr. O'Connor, conceded the association between scarlet fever and rheumatic fever in 1861, but he claimed that it was the unusual case. Further, O'Connor provided a theoretical understanding for the association: "It is well known that in scarlatina the serous membranes lining the great cavities of the body are not infrequently attacked with inflammation, and we see no reason why others, such as the pericardium, should escape."[6] A particularly distressing case was reported by Dr. Bolles to the Roxbury, Massachusetts Medical Society. A seven-year-old girl developed a distinct case of scarlet fever with its characteristic sore throat, rash, "strawberry tongue," and subsequent peeling of the palms and soles. Eleven days later, rheumatic fever struck, attacking wrists and ankles, producing fever and tachycardia. Two days later, Dr. Bolles discovered the auscultatory findings of pericarditis in the girl, who was now complaining of severe chest pain. On the twenty-fourth day of her illness she developed a new heart murmur, and three days later the valves of her heart were so damaged that she suffered from severe congestive heart failure. After seven weeks she died. At autopsy, Dr. Bolles found typical evidence of rheumatic heart disease: pericarditis and endocarditis with destruction of the mitral valve.[7]

Clusters of rheumatic fever occasionally followed scarlet fever. Typical of these small epidemics was a household of cases that T. F. Raven investigated. Following a romantic affair with a lover who was recovering from a sore throat, a domestic servant developed scarlet fever. Three children in the house then developed scarlet fever, and three adults later suffered from scarlet fever and rheumatic fever.[8]

In most cases of rheumatic fever, the preceding sore throat stood alone, unaccompanied by scarlet fever. For example, in 1874 Dr. J. Kingston Fowler,[9] who was serving as house physician at King's College Hospital, contracted a case of rheumatic fever. Archibald Garrod, the ardent advocate of alkaline, attended him. During Garrod's initial evaluation, he asked Dr. Fowler if he had suffered previously from tonsillitis. Fowler remembered a bout a month earlier. The association stuck. Taking his cue from Garrod after he recovered, Fowler began to inquire of his own patients with rheumatic fever whether tonsillitis had also preceded their illnesses. Fully 80 percent reported that a sore throat, with or without scarlet fever, had occurred from a few days to a month before.[10]

Drawing on several decades of experience, in 1887 Alfred Mantle put forth a hypothesis that a throat infection always predated rheumatic fever;[11] by 1890, B. Mayston Bond claimed that "everyone knows that rheumatism is an occasional complication of scarlet fever."[12] To be sure, there were some doubters. Henry Ashby, a physician in Manchester, believed that the aches and pains following scarlet fever were different from true rheumatic fever, urging physicians to maintain rigorous diagnostic standards before linking the two diseases.[13] William Osler, in his widely read textbook, criticized the cement binding tonsillitis to rheumatic fever from a different vantage. Osler observed that sore throats were so commonplace that their association with rheumatic fever might be due to chance alone.[14] Despite such reservations, tonsillitis joined carditis, arthritis, and chorea as a definite, if not constant, part of rheumatic fever.

### Subcutaneous Nodules

Small nodules, located on the subcutaneous tendons, were also linked to rheumatic fever. William Charles Wells commented on the appearance of nodules in Martha Clifton, one of his patients with rheumatism of the heart, in 1812.[15] It is more difficult for the historian to determine whether these nodules were new to rheumatic fever about the time Wells described them. Physicians believed that they were. Rheumatic nodules varied in size from a pea to a walnut. Being painless, certainly the smaller ones could escape the notice of both patient and physician. The disappearance of nodules from rheumatic fever in the twentieth century attests to the possibility of marked change occurring over a brief historical span. In the years after Wells's initial portrait, there were many descriptions of such nodules, but not until the 1880s were they included as a common, if not invariable, component of rheumatic fever. Oval in shape, rheumatic nodules were well circumscribed and did not promote an inflammatory response from the surrounding tissues. Nodules were always subcutaneous, arising from the tendon sheaths. They occurred most frequently about the elbows, knees, ankles, and wrists, but even the tendons about the skull could be involved, giving the victim a distorted appearance. The presence of nodules was never common, occurring in fewer than 10 percent of patients. Afflicted patients would normally have three or four nodules, but physicians, on occasion, reported unfortunate children with hundreds. Physicians could not fail to notice nodules when they occurred in such large numbers or when they deformed the appearance of patients (illustration 1). In the usual case nodules appeared about two weeks after arthritis struck.

While some physicians understood that these painless bumps often went unnoticed, other practitioners, such as Thomas Barlow, a physician at the Hospital for Sick Children, credited subcutaneous nodules with both diagnosis and prognosis.[16] Since the nodules did not occur in other diseases, their presence was a

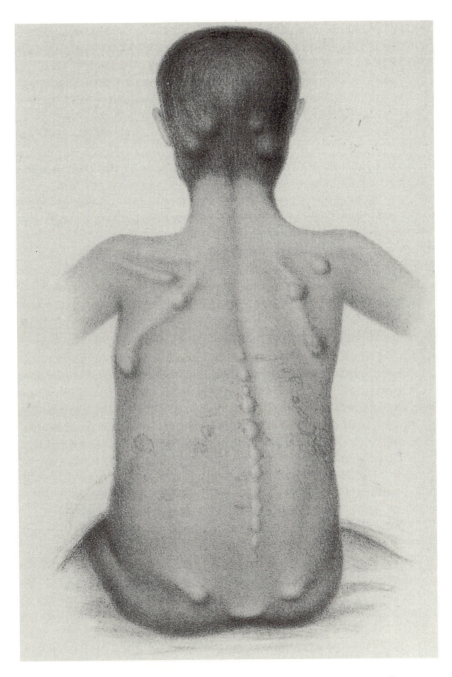

ILLUSTRATION 1. Numerous large subcutaneous nodules. Reprinted from W. B. Cheadle, *Various Manifestations of the Rheumatic State as Exemplified in Childhood and Early Life* (London: Smith, Edler, 1889).

boon to the diagnosis of rheumatic fever. Nodules carried an ominous prognosis. Barlow noted that nodules nearly always accompanied severe carditis: one-third of his patients with nodules died.

## Rashes

Various rashes, too, became associated as a clinically less important manifestation of rheumatic fever in the 1880s. Specifically, physicians reported erythema marginatum, erythema nodosum, and erythema multiforme, among several others, with isolated cases of rheumatic fever. Each of these rashes later became associated with streptococcal infections. Whether these rashes were entirely new to rheumatic fever in the nineteenth century is another difficult question for the historian. Erythema marginatum, the rash later found to be virtually unique to rheumatic fever, was often quite faint in appearance and, in failing to provoke either pain or itch, did not call attention to itself. Both patient and physician could easily miss this rash amid the other, more striking complaints. Erythema nodosum and erythema multiforme were different. Both were highly visible and painful and unlikely to be missed. Unlike nodules, rashes carried no prognostic significance. Even when present, rashes seldom played a key role in disease from either the patient's or the physician's point of view.[17]

## Epidemiological Alliances

Adding further complexity to rheumatic fever were three epidemiological issues that arose in the 1870s and 1880s. The first was the question of rheumatic fever's communicability. To many practitioners, rheumatic fever "ran in families." This observation sparked a series of inquiries over the next century that attempted to unravel what "running in families" meant in the context of rheumatic fever. The problems were several. Rheumatic fever often struck several, but not all, children in a family. It could afflict members in different generations. And rheumatic fever could attack families, either of one or more generations, at a single episode, or repeatedly over months, years, or decades. Clouding the issue, rheumatic fever could strike in families that lived together in the same dwelling or who lived apart. In other words, rheumatic fever raised theoretical issues of heredity, proximity, and possible infectious agents or pollutants—working alone or together. These epidemiological questions proved hard to tackle.

The initial issue raised was whether rheumatic fever was hereditary. At Guy's Hospital, Philip Henry Pye-Smith asked three hundred patients with rheumatic fever whether a parent or sibling also had suffered from rheumatic fever. Sixty-eight, or 23 percent, replied affirmatively. Forty-five reported one or both parents; twenty-eight claimed rheumatic siblings. Forty-five claimed a single additional relative with rheumatic fever; sixteen identified two additional relatives; seven related three or more.[18] Pye-Smith interpreted his findings to show a genetic tendency.

James F. Goodhart believed that "liabilities incurred by children of rheumatic parentage" were even higher. Nearly 30 percent of his patients at Guy's Hospital had a close family relative with rheumatism.[19] Critics of such surveys were quick to point out that rheumatic fever was so common in the general population that causal connections between generations were difficult to determine. To assess the increased risk borne by family members of rheumatic sufferers, Archibald E. Garrod and E. Hunt Cooke asked five hundred patients at St. Bartholomew's Hospital, who were admitted for reasons other than rheumatic fever, whether any family member had ever had rheumatic fever. One hundred five, or 21 percent, replied affirmatively. Garrod and Cooke then asked one hundred patients admitted with rheumatic fever the identical question. Thirty-five percent, or nearly double, answered yes.[20] On the basis of these studies and commonplace observation in many doctors' practices, most physicians concluded that rheumatic fever had a familial link. These early investigations, of course, did not clearly separate issues of inheritance, proximity, and environmental pollutant, whether infectious or chemical.

A second epidemiological issue was whether rheumatic fever preferred certain climates or geographical locations. August Hirsch, in his *Handbook of Geographical and Historical Pathology* (1886), addressed questions of the spatial distribution of rheumatic fever. Hirsch claimed that rheumatic fever was "universally diffused and one of the commonest of complaints." Nevertheless, most cases occurred in colder northern areas in winter or spring.[21] A decade later, Arthur Newsholme reached similar conclusions about the climatic and geographical distribution of the rheumatic fever.[22]

A third epidemiological issue addressed in the 1880s was whether rheumatic fever was evolving into a childhood disease and, in a closely related question, whether rheumatic fever was a different disease when it struck children. Earlier in the century, individual case histories had included many children and adolescents, and later statistical reports from hospitals broke down elements, such as heart disease, by age. In stressing that rheumatic fever "ran in families," initial genetic studies necessarily also focused on children. These varied sources all pointed to rheumatic fever—especially its first attack—as a disease primarily afflicting those between the ages of five and twenty-five years. Although the span was large, most first attacks in the second half of the nineteenth century occurred before adolescence. Hospital-based reports included more and more children as the nineteenth century progressed. Whether this increase indicated that rheumatic fever was preferentially afflicting more children is yet another difficult question. Children are particularly susceptible to streptococcal infection, and detailed family studies in the twentieth century documented a steadily lower age of first attack. Certainly, the advent of children's hospitals in the middle of the nineteenth century provided a focal point of children's diseases. At the Hospital for Sick Children, Great Ormond Street, Thomas Barlow, a physician who studied the unique aspects of rheumatic fever and scurvy in children, argued from his experience that certain features of rheumatic fever were different in childhood.[23] He stressed that arthritis was less severe but that heart disease, chorea, nodules, and rashes were more prominent in children than in adults. Reflecting doubts that some physicians held about the inclusion of sore throat as an element of rheumatic fever, Barlow denied that any causal connection existed between a preceding "catarrh" and rheumatic fever because "catarrh" was so common in children, a sentiment that was shared by other prominent physicians, such as Luther Emmett Holt.[24] Holt's fellow New Yorker, Abraham Jacobi, echoed the increasing importance of rheumatic heart disease for children, pointing out that it was the leading cause of heart injury in young people.[25]

### Walter Butler Cheadle

When Walter Butler Cheadle confronted rheumatic fever in the 1880s, he found a disease that was more complicated and challenging than earlier in the century. Rashes, sore throats, nodules, younger victims, and the clear possibility of contagion and inheritability made rheumatic fever a more complex illness. Effective therapy with salicylate may have placed a measure of urgency on clearly defining the clinical entity. While salicylate did not satisfactorily treat all aspects of rheumatic fever, for example, heart disease or chorea, without question in the minds of all observers salicylate greatly reduced the period of fever and joint distress. Salicylate was useful in fevers caused by any disease, but this was not the case for all forms of arthritis. Joint disease caused by the tubercle bacillus or bacteria did not respond to salicylate, and chronic crippling arthritis in older people responded only poorly. Salicylate was highly and uniquely effective in treating the migratory arthritis of rheumatic fever, and as such almost certainly helped to define the disease.

The diagnostic problem for Cheadle was that each patient with rheumatic fever experienced the disease differently. A variety of joints might be swollen, inflamed, and painful, but rarely in any perceived pattern. Some patients had rashes, most—but not all—suffered fever, but in no common sequence. Some, stricken with chorea, behaved peculiarly. Some were mildly discomforted; a few died rapidly in great pain. In some families, several members would be sick for days, others for weeks or even months. Some patients suffered one bout, others as many as ten. Some were noticeably sick from other illnesses before rheumatism struck (scarlet fever, for example), others not. Some responded to therapy; others got better without therapy; still others died despite all measures. Rheumatic fever required physicians to sort out common and useful patterns in a disease that was intricate in its presentation. What Cheadle accomplished was a new way of organizing clinical thinking about rheumatic fever that preserved a degree of individual variation that was missing in the hospital statistical accounts and at the same time sifted out elements common to most cases that individual histories—limited to consideration of a single patient—lacked.

Cheadle (1836–1910) attended Cambridge, where he received his bachelor of medicine in 1861. Following graduation, he explored western Canada with Viscount Milton. Their popular account, *The Northwest Passage by Land,* went through many editions.[26] Upon his return to England, he completed his degree for doctor of medicine. From 1866 until his death, Cheadle was an attending physician at St. Mary's Hospital. After 1869, he also treated young patients at the Hospital for Sick

Children, Great Ormond Street, where his interests included scurvy and infant feeding.[27]

When asked to deliver the prestigious Harveian Lectures in 1889, Cheadle chose to tackle the complexity of rheumatic fever. The question he asked was how could a practitioner recognize what he called the "various manifestations of the rheumatic state." His solution was to describe "typical" cases, which Cheadle grounded on his experiences with individual patients and on the large hospital-based series.

The idea of the typical case did not spring forth entirely new from Cheadle. Thomas Barlow, who also treated patients at the Hospital for Sick Children, suggested in 1883 that one way to escape the semantic entanglements of "acute rheumatism" was for physicians to agree on a typical case.[28] He suggested an illness of fourteen days, with fever, painful migratory arthritis in large joints, sweating, pericarditis, endocarditis, and pleurisy. While Barlow's attempt was pioneering, his single typical case did not encompass the wide spectrum of rheumatic fever. One physician remarked: "It would rather seem that rheumatism might be regarded less as a disease than as an expression of a series of disturbed conditions—morbid states, however manifest in decided relationship one to the other, and presenting phenomena which, although sometimes existing in an isolated manner, are oftentimes grouped together."[29] Not all of the "morbid states" needed to be present to make a diagnosis, and the temporal order need not be rigidly fixed. As Henry Dwight Chapin explained to the New York Academy of Medicine in 1886, "the diagnosis of rheumatism generally depend[s] on the considerable number of corroborative symptoms, rather than the marked severity of one or two."[30] That same year Angel Money, who also worked at the Hospital for Sick Children, suggested a typical time course for rheumatic fever in children, which included an erythematous rash, arthritis, nodules, chorea, and endocarditis.[31] Cheadle built upon the examples of Barlow and Money. First—reflecting the increased biological complexity of rheumatic fever—he identified the common elements:

> the claims of endocarditis, of pericarditis, of pleurisy, of tonsillitis, of exudative erythema, of chorea, of subcutaneous nodules, will hardly, I think, be seriously disputed.[32]

Cheadle's inclusion of pleurisy needs a note of explanation. Pleurisy, or lung congestion, occurred as a late complication of mitral valve injury. As such, most physicians considered pleurisy as an end phase of endocarditis.

What Cheadle did next was revolutionary. He claimed that each element was separate and could appear in nearly every combination or in almost any order during a bout with rheumatic fever. In children the variation was more extreme than in adults. In Cheadle's experience, most patients suffered from most manifestations of rheumatic fever at some point in their illness. Cheadle's natural history approach—which followed children through many bouts and relapses—taught him that rheumatic fever did not always return with precisely the same manifestations. For example, H.B.K., a nine-year-old boy (see table 3.1) suffered from migratory

TABLE 3.1 *Walter Butler Cheadle's Series, I, II, and X (1889)*

| Series I, H.B.K., boy age 9 | Series II, C.H.B., boy age 5 | Series X, John T., age 7 |
|---|---|---|
| Arthritis, endocarditis, 1882 | Endocarditis, date unrecorded | Chorea, Nov. 1886 |
| Arthritis, endocarditis, 1884 | Arthritis, nodules March 1888 | Chorea, Aug. 1887 |
| Arthritis, endocarditis, 1885 | Nodules, pleurisy, pericarditis, June 1888 | Arthritis, nodules, endocarditis, Nov.-Dec. 1887 |
| Arthritis, endocarditis, 1886 | Nodules, fresh endocarditis, fresh pericarditis, July 1888 | Chorea, nodules, endocarditis, pericarditis, pleurisy, June 1888 |
| Arthritis, endocarditis, 1887 | Pleurisy, pericarditis, August 1888 | Endocarditis, pericarditis, July 1888 |
| Arthritis, chorea, 1888 | | Death, Aug. 1888 |

SOURCE: Walter Butler Cheadle, "Harveian Lectures on the Various Manifestations of the Rheumatic State: As Exemplified in Childhood and Early Life," *Lancet* (1889), 1: 821–827, 871–877, 921–927.

arthritis and endocarditis for all bouts except his last, when he suffered from chorea and arthritis. In contrast, C.H.B., a five-year-old boy, exhibited far greater complexity. He suffered from endocarditis on his first bout; arthritis and nodules during his initial relapse; nodules, pericarditis, and pleurisy on his second relapse; nodules, endocarditis, and pericarditis on his third relapse; and pleurisy and pericarditis on his final relapse. Cheadle called this variation "phases in the rheumatic process or series." Each manifestation, such as chorea or carditis, had causes other than rheumatic fever, but rheumatic fever was one of the most common, if not the most common, predisposing cause.[33] Lest this variation become too unmanageable and unhelpful clinically, Cheadle offered the ten most common "series" or patterns from his practice, three of which are given in table 3.1.

Cheadle reinforced Barlow's contention that rheumatic fever was different in children. In Cheadle's practice, youngsters had more carditis and less arthritis. Each element of the disease behaved more independently than in adults. Drawing from family studies, he also strongly believed in a heredity component of rheumatic fever, "with a family history of acute rheumatism in an immediate blood relative the chance of an individual with such hereditary tendencies contracting acute articular rheumatism is nearly five times as great as that of an individual who has no such hereditary trait."[34] Cheadle then discussed at length each element in the rheumatic series. Arthritis was nearly always present but less prominent in children. Fever almost always accompanied rheumatic fever, but in children it seldom exceeded 101 degrees Fahrenheit. Although Cheadle argued that any el-

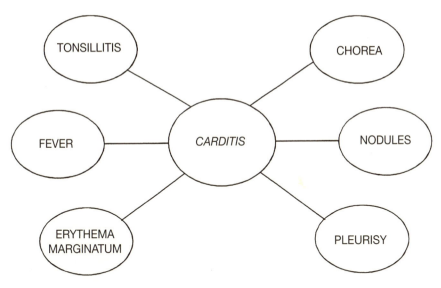

FIGURE 3.1. Cheadle's view of rheumatic fever, 1889

ement of the series could occupy any temporal space during the disease, he claimed that tonsillitis, if present, "always precedes the articular affection." Cheadle sorted out the rashes of rheumatic fever, stating that erythema marginatum was the most common. Though not trying to set a firm rule, Cheadle argued that chorea, if present, followed the arthritis. Subcutaneous nodules had special meaning for Cheadle. Contrasting nodules with all other elements, Cheadle believed that nodules occurred only in rheumatic fever. When they were present, a clinician could be absolutely certain of a diagnosis. He thought that nodules were more common in children with rheumatic fever (he had five children with nodules in his care at that very moment). For Cheadle, heart disease always accompanied nodules, and death always followed the growth of large nodules. Pericarditis normally occurred early and rapidly in the illness; endocarditis later and more insidiously. Cheadle enthroned heart injury as the key element of rheumatic fever. Carditis became the element that mattered most for physicians (figure 3.1).

Cheadle hardly discussed theory except to offer a general notion that the inflammation which provoked nodules in all likelihood was capable of yielding similar inflammatory changes in heart valves. His discussion on therapy was also brief. He focused on the prevention of heart injury as the only measure of effective therapy. Cheadle accepted the generally held view that salicylate, while useful in reducing fever and joint pains, did not influence the course of heart disease.

Cheadle's accomplishment was clinical: case recognition for the practitioner. More precise than those before him, Cheadle did not simplify at all. It might appear that Cheadle solved the problem of diagnosis by offering a smorgasbord instead of a prix-fixe meal. There was no alternative to rheumatic fever's evolving complexity. Cheadle's conception helped physicians get a handle on a disease that was changing before their eyes. Doctors needed guidance, and Cheadle's method illuminated the path.

Walter Butler Cheadle's clinical organization of thinking about rheumatic fever largely settled the difficult task of diagnosis. Leading physicians quickly adopted Cheadle's scheme, and nearly every discussion at meetings and lectures, in textbooks, and in scholarly papers showed clear evidence that his method swiftly reached both practitioners and prominent workers in the field. No one has improved upon Cheadle's general approach. Even T. Duckett Jones's criteria, which medical students began to memorize after 1944, must be understood as responding to a disease that continued to change during the fifty years after Cheadle.

## Rheumatic Fever at the End of the Nineteenth Century

One point bears repeating. Of all the changes that rheumatic fever underwent, it was heart injury that altered rheumatic fever fundamentally—both biologically and in the way clinicians thought about the disease. Carditis pushed aside joint pain as the cardinal manifestation of the illness. It became key to diagnosis, therapy, and prognosis. Mutated biology of rheumatic fever, however, was not the whole story. Shifting patterns of clinical thinking and institutional changes collaborated as well. For the most part, individual practitioners described individual case histories from experiences at the patient's bedside—normally at home. This type of practice dictated the smaller number of cases and the longer period between cases, as the practices of Wells and Dundas demonstrated.

Hospital-based practice, which often included hundreds of patients, reinforced the conclusion that damage done to the heart was the clinical event of most concern. Almost certainly, there was a selective bias. Contemporary reports make clear that only the sickest patients were admitted to hospitals; "sickest" usually meant patients suffering from pericarditis or endocarditis. Less-common reasons for admission were extreme joint pain or poorly controlled chorea. In other words, nineteenth-century hospital practice tended to concentrate those patients suffering from heart disease in the hands of hospital physicians who were frequently leaders, authors, and educators. Those dying of rheumatism invariably died from heart complications, findings detected with the autopsy techniques available to nineteenth-century pathologists. During an autopsy, evidence of pericarditis and endocarditis could be seen easily with the naked eye; they did not require either special stains or even a microscope.

Climate and geography may also have played a role in the emergence of rheumatic fever. As is obvious from this account, much of the writing on rheumatic fever came from Britain and northern France—northern latitudes with a generally cold and damp climate. Was this just coincidence? In 1886, August Hirsch found evidence of rheumatic fever at all latitudes and climates, but he confirmed the generally held view that rheumatism was more prevalent in northern, cold, and damp locations. That rheumatic fever occurred most frequently in a region of the world that both introduced the stethoscope and organized the practice of medicine in hospitals could only have reinforced the clinical and pathological recognition of heart damage.

The shift in clinical spotlight to the heart was not without its ironies. Even after physicians recognized the prognostic significance of heart disease, fever and joint pain were often the symptoms that brought patients to doctors. Yet it was just these obvious complaints that physicians were asked to ignore, focusing instead on potential dangers, often unperceived by the patient, that had to be detected through a new technological device—the stethoscope. This disparity between what was clinically apparent and what was pathologically relevant did not die easily. An example came from therapeutics. In the early nineteenth century, physicians treated fever and joint pain. Both patient and physician were satisfied if these both-ersome symptoms were ameliorated. This pattern of gauging successful treatment did not cease with the introduction of salicylate after 1876. Fifty years later physicians still debated whether salicylate, then in the form of aspirin, benefited carditis, in addition to lowering fever and easing joint pain, in part because there were few carefully crafted clinical studies measuring the value of salicylate in reducing cardiac damage. Nearly all investigations had gauged dosing and its effects on the benefits to the joints and fever.

What I argue is that acute rheumatism evolved into rheumatic fever over the course of the nineteenth century as the result of distinct biological changes that provoked injury to several parts of the body, the most important of which was the heart. Clinicians appreciated this alteration through the assimilation of technological changes (stethoscope and autopsy), refinements of clinical thinking ("typical" case), and the concentration of these invalids in hospitals. Quite possibly, there was also the serendipitous influence of geography and climate.

The historical record indicates the progression of injuries to heart, brain, skin, and connective tissue. Insights from the molecular biology of the streptococcus, gained in the last thirty-five years, lend support to the hypothesis that historical alterations in the signs and symptoms of rheumatic fever had at their root a molecular explanation. A question that this notion begs is whether similar injuries may have occurred from time to time before the nineteenth century.[35] This is a distinct possibility, just as reasonable as the prospect of such injuries returning in the future.

In the decades after Cheadle, the predominant focus of medical attention shifted from the bedside to the laboratory. In particular, Cheadle's observation that tonsillitis preceded rheumatic fever challenged physicians to find a bacterial cause.

# PART II

# *The Clinical and Scientific Challenges of an Evolving Disease*

*F*ollowing Walter Butler Cheadle's clinical formulation of rheumatic fever at the end of the nineteenth century, the historian easily senses a shift in the "gaze" of physicians from the bedside to the laboratory in order to gain clarity regarding the disease's root cause. Of course, rheumatic fever did not sit still while physicians redirected their efforts. In particular, all rashes which had once been associated with rheumatic fever—except erythema marginatum—faded. The heart's muscle, the myocardium, became the primary cardiac target, supplanting the pericardium and endocardium. These biological alterations challenged physicians. In response, clinicians refined diagnosis with blood tests and the electrocardiogram, modified treatment, and with tonsillectomy sought to prevent the disease from striking children in the first place. Despite these biological changes and clinical responses, the great weight of medical effort shifted to the laboratory.

Any disease with fever suggested contagion. In striking so many parts of the body, rheumatic fever was far more complex than most infections. While pneumonia sickens only the lungs and a boil distresses merely the flesh, rheumatic fever injured heart, brain, skin, joints, and tendons. This complexity challenged existing views of the nature of simple infection. With the concept of sepsis—where bacteria course though the body in the bloodstream—physicians initially believed they had a ready explanation for rheumatic fever's protean nature. Blood-borne infection made good sense, and physicians on both sides of the Atlantic spent two decades and enormous energy before concluding that the sensible solution was not the correct one.

Frustrated, researchers struck out in different directions. Some looked more closely at victims: children and young adults were often members of families where parents or siblings had also suffered from rheumatic fever. Vulnerability to rheumatic fever ran in families. What constituted "vulnerability" was an extraordinarily challenging question in the first third of the twentieth century. Early answers came from the new science of immunology. Using skin tests and laboratory means of detecting antibodies, immunologists described a crucial characteristic: victims of rheumatic fever greatly overreacted to simple streptococcal throat infections.

Other physicians looked to environmental and social settings that promoted rheumatic fever. Cold damp climates, northern latitudes (or more southerly ones in the southern hemisphere), and crowding were clearly most conducive to the spread of rheumatic fever. Crowding gave clarity not only to rheumatic fever's attraction to poverty and poor housing but also its appeal for boarding schools and military barracks.

To most physicians, rheumatic fever still "smelled contagious." Epidemiology eventually pointed to a simple streptococcal throat infection not as a portal for sepsis but as the instigator of immunological overreaction in susceptible people. Environmental and social settings that enhanced the spread of streptococcal infections—cold, damp, northern, crowding—in turn proved to be seedbeds of rheumatic fever. What emerged was a complex ecological entanglement: streptococcal instigator, genetically vulnerable population, conducive environmental and social settings. Rheumatic fever became the prime example of an immunological and ecological disease.

## CHAPTER 4

# Rheumatic Fever as Sepsis, 1890–1920

✦

*W*alter Cheadle had singled out tonsillitis as the necessary trigger for rheumatic fever. Over the next thirty years, this observation fueled the notion that rheumatic fever was an infectious disease. Just prior to Cheadle's masterly work, Arthur Mantle, an English physician, was the first to state clearly the belief that rheumatic fever likely followed bacterial tonsillitis.[1] Epidemiologists soon joined clinicians in supporting the notion that rheumatic fever should be added to the ever-growing list of illnesses of bacterial origin. In 1895, Arthur Newsholme, in the pioneering study on the epidemiology of rheumatic fever that heralded its milder course, had argued in favor of the "infective character" of rheumatic fever.[2] Newsholme's case was largely circumstantial. Rheumatic fever was associated with a sore throat, a condition that many physicians thought infective. Its fever, a characteristic found in many infectious diseases, also argued in favor of contagion. To these slender threads, he added several negative arguments. That rheumatic fever often relapsed (survival of a single bout not conveying life-long immunity), Newsholme believed, should not automatically remove it from the infectious group of diseases. Tuberculosis could recur, as could syphilis. That rheumatic fever ran in families also should not negate an infectious etiology in favor of a genetic or an environmental one, because it was a commonplace observation that infections could be passed easily among family members.[3]

Additional associations pointed to the infective nature of rheumatic fever. In 1891, G. B. Longstaff noted that the incidence of rheumatic fever paralleled that of scarlet fever—an observation made earlier in the century—erysipelas (a serious skin and soft tissue infection that occasionally followed injury or surgery), and childbed fever, illnesses commonly believed—but not yet proved—to be bacterial in origin.[4] Cheadle, responding to Mantle, Newsholme, and Longstaff, accepted these arguments in 1896, but he was quick to point out that no specific germ had been identified.[5]

Because tonsillitis preceded the other rheumatic manifestations, it seemed logical that the bacterial infection must start in the throat.[6] Just how frequently tonsillitis and rheumatic fever overlapped was debated. In his Wesley M. Carpenter Lecture in 1899, Frederick A. Packard claimed that there was a 70 percent association.[7] Major Charles F. Kieffer, a surgeon in the U.S. Army stationed at Fort D. A. Russell in Wyoming, claimed that about one-fifth of recruits with sore throats developed rheumatic fever within a month.[8] In other words, all sore throats did not lead to rheumatic fever, and clinicians could not always identify a preceding bout with tonsillitis even when looking for one.

## The Bacteriological Setting

Cheadle had settled on his clinical organization of rheumatic fever amid the first years of the search for specific bacterial causes of disease. In the preceding five years, tuberculosis, diphtheria, and lobar pneumonia, among other diseases, had each been found to have a unique bacterium as a causative agent. In the next decades, many more diseases would follow. Robert Koch, the acclaimed bacterial pioneer, and his students had set forth a method for establishing certainty of germ causation. Koch's "postulates," studied by medical students to this day, appeared deceptively straightforward: a germ must be found in all cases of the disease, the germ must be a living organism distinguishable from other germs, the distribution of the germ must match the distribution of the disease, the germ must be grown independently outside the diseased person or animal, and the germ when reintroduced into an animal must re-create the same disease.[9] What this scheme camouflaged was the mountains of painstaking work in developing culture media, establishing which bacteria required which nutrients, determining how to stain bacteria so that they could be seen with microscopes, and the often difficult task of finding susceptible animals. To many, rheumatic fever seemed a likely candidate to meet Koch's postulates.

That a bacterium might be responsible for triggering the sequence of events leading to rheumatic fever proved to be a most attractive hypothesis. A "sepsis model" proposed that bacteria entered the bloodstream after an inciting bout of tonsillitis and then circulated around the body, causing damage to the heart, skin, central nervous system, joints, and tendon sheaths. An alternative proposal, actually a corollary to the sepsis hypothesis, was consideration of a bacterial poison or toxin model. This proposal, similar to the proven mechanism of disease in diphtheria and tetanus, proposed that a bacterial poison, released after a throat infection, would circulate in the blood, provoking havoc in distant bodily locations. These were not idle speculations in the years between 1890 and 1920. In many respects, the medical spirit of the times was decidedly bacterial, with one disease after another found to be incited by a specific microorganism.[10] The hope of finding a germ ignited optimism that a specific treatment might be found. Reason for such optimism abounded. Nearly all physicians were beginning to use antitoxins to treat diphtheria and tetanus;[11] other antisera would soon follow as treatment for additional bacterial illnesses. The turn of the century also witnessed the advent of bacterial vaccines, in particular one to prevent pneumococcal pneumonia.[12] Quite simply, rheumatic fever appeared to be part of this general sweep of medical history.[13] Clinical and laboratory research in rheumatic fever initially pursued a "sepsis" model but, when frustrated after 1920, followed alternative paths, searching for destructive elements circulating in the blood, investigating hereditary vulnerability of victims, and exploring the nature of hospitable social and physical environments.

Attempts to isolate bacteria from the blood, pericardial fluid, or joint fluid in patients suffering from rheumatic fever came at a turbulent time in the history of microbiology. For example, physicians were struggling over whether and under which conditions germs were normally present in the living human. They understood that certain parts of the body were swimming with bacteria, such as the mouth, the skin, and the intestines. Bacteria in these places did not signal disease. Other sites of the body were normally sterile. The blood, joint fluid, and pericardial fluid did not contain bacteria in healthy people. When germs were discovered in these fluids, they were invariably responsible for infection. Also, most internal tissues of the body, such as the valves of the heart, were sterile during health. Finding bacteria lodged on a heart valve signaled infection. When a person died, however, these sterile bodily fluids and structures were quickly overrun with microorganisms. Cultures obtained after death, then, did not reflect health or disease while the patient lived. These understandings, coupled with technical difficulties in obtaining cultures, were to plague attempts to isolate bacteria in rheumatic fever.

Research on rheumatic fever was also thrust into an ever more sophisticated classification of bacteria. In the early years of bacterial study, physicians normally described the shape of a bacterium, whether it was a coccus (ball-shaped) or bacillus (rod-shaped), large or small, with or without a flagellum. Problems arose when researchers tried to compare results. How did a physician in London know for certain whether the germ under his microscope was the same as the one under a similar microscope in Paris? For example, too many bacteria formed chains of cocci for this simple designation to be helpful. To aid in distinguishing bacteria, scientists developed stains to differentiate among bacteria. Physicians also made distinctions between bacteria that required oxygen to grow (aerobic) and those that did not need oxygen (anaerobic). Some bacteria emitted chemicals during their life cycle; others required specific nutrients, such as sugars. Others triggered the breakup of red blood cells, or hemolysis. The importance of these considerations for the history of rheumatic fever was that researchers sought bacteria when the science of microbiology was still immature. Classification was still evolving, and the perils of contamination faced even the most fastidious worker.[14]

The initial bacterial experiments were quite simple in design. Blood, joint fluid, or pericardial fluid was obtained from a patient hospitalized with rheumatic fever. In selecting only the sickest patients for study, physicians introduced a bias to their results that would take a decade to become clear. Obtaining these samples was fraught with peril. Imperfect sterile technique marred the collection of many specimens by inadvertently contaminating samples with bacteria from the patient's skin or from germs on the researcher's fingers. It is often difficult for the historian to be certain exactly how a physician obtained a sample. Descriptions of technique were frequently absent except for a phrase that a culture was obtained "in the usual way" or that the researcher was "careful to avoid contamination." Unaware of any bias introduced by selection of patients for study or method of securing specimens, these early researchers placed their samples of bodily fluids onto various culture media. When bacteria grew, they would be identified by staining, shape, and biochemical properties.

### "Malignant" Endocarditis and Rheumatic Fever: Overlapping Diseases

That any bacteria grew from the blood, joints, or pericardial fluid of patients with rheumatic fever highlighted the intersection of the disease with another illness which ultimately was called "infectious" or "bacterial" endocarditis. Four years before Cheadle's seminal work on rheumatic fever, William Osler, reflecting upon his experience with over two hundred patients at Montreal General Hospital, summarized the state of knowledge of what he called "malignant endocarditis." Malignant endocarditis was a rare disease, uniformly fatal, that was characterized by fever, signs of endocarditis (such as a heart murmur), and embolization. When pathologists dissected the hearts of these patients, they discovered the reason for the emboli. The heart valves were covered with friable growths that broke off into the bloodstream, lodging in the brain, kidney, or other organs where they would prevent cell metabolism. Victims, then, might show signs of a stroke or have blood in their urine after months of suffering from a nagging but undiagnosed fever.

Pathologists also noted that the heart valves in malignant endocarditis had been damaged *before* they became hosts to the peregrinous vegetations. Here was the overlap with rheumatic fever. Many of Osler's patients had suffered from acute rheumatism years or decades earlier which had left them with scarred heart valves. A few of Osler's patients had gone on to suffer from malignant endocarditis during a bout with rheumatic fever, in other words without a significant delay between the two diseases. In these cases, rheumatic fever and malignant endocarditis blended. Still other cases of malignant endocarditis occurred in the context of overwhelming postoperative surgical infection or pneumonia, seemingly without a prior experience with rheumatic fever. In the early years of bacteriology, physicians gave greater precision to the vegetations lodged on scarred heart valves: they were filled with bacteria.

To Osler's eye in 1885, rheumatic fever and malignant endocarditis were very different illnesses. Rheumatic fever was common, rapid-fire, highly dramatic with its varied symptoms, and seldom fatal; malignant endocarditis was rare, subtle (even in his practice only one-half of patients were diagnosed while living), lingering, and always fatal. The diseases were linked by the scars that rheumatic fever left on heart valves. Even more significant to this discussion, most of the patients selected by various researchers for bacterial study actually had rheumatic fever complicated by malignant endocarditis.[15] Conclusions drawn were often more valid for malignant endocarditis than for rheumatic fever.

## Clinical Research

In the same year Cheadle delivered his lectures, Alfred Mantle, consultant physician at the Royal Halifax Infirmary, was struck with the similarity between rheumatic fever and other diseases, such as scarlet fever, tonsillitis, and erythema nodosum, which physicians had suspected, but not proved, to be bacterial in origin. Wanting to culture the blood and joint fluid from his patients with rheumatic fever but having no skills in bacteriological technique, he studied briefly with Watson Cheyne, a pupil of Joseph Lister, who was then exploring surgical infections. So trained, Mantle isolated from joint fluid "small bacilli and a few micrococci" and from blood a "bacillus" in most cases and a "micrococcus" in a few instances. We know nothing of the clinical details of his patients except that they were "marked" cases and nothing at all of Mantle's technique.[16]

### Early Bacterial Isolates from Paris

The first sustained bacteriological investigation into rheumatic fever began in Paris in the 1890s. In July 1891, a twenty-nine-year-old patient died, a victim of a second attack of rheumatic fever that was complicated by chorea. At autopsy, the pericardial fluid possessed "l'odeur de putréfaction." The heart valves were severely damaged. Pierre Achalme cultured pericardial fluid, blood, and cerebral spinal fluid on both aerobic and anaerobic media. On the anaerobic medium, he grew a pure culture of a bacillus that had a similar "odeur âcre," a sour odor. Achalme initially raised the issue—prophetically as it turned out—whether this bacillus could be a post-mortem contaminant. He dismissed the possibility because he believed that he had conducted the autopsy a reasonably short interval after the patient's death.[17]

It took nearly six years for Achalme to report another case: a thirty-six-year-old man who died of rheumatic endocarditis. Once again his aerobic cultures of joint fluid and blood were sterile, while those cultures planted on anaerobic media grew out a bacillus that looked similar to the "bacille de charbon," or anthrax. Achalme thought that this bacillus was the identical to the one he had isolated in 1891.[18]

Prompted by Achalme's work, J. Thiroloix initiated a research program beginning in 1895. He cultured the blood from a patient who died from rheumatic fever with chorea and obtained a similar bacillus that he termed an "anthrax-like bacterium."[19] Beset by doubts that this bacillus was merely a post-mortem contaminant, Thiroloix set out to culture patients who were still living. In November 1895 and January 1896, Thiroloix cultured the blood of two patients with endocarditis. In both he grew on anaerobic media a large, poorly mobile bacillus, which possessed an "odeur butyrique," a buttery odor. He argued that this bacillus could not be a post-mortem contaminant because the patients had both been alive when he obtained the samples. In Achalme's honor, Thiroloix named the germ "bacille d'Achalme."[20] Thiroloix reported three more isolates of the "bacille d'Achalme" from living patients in 1897. He did not include detailed case histories or descriptions of his technique in obtaining cultures.[21]

From the start, other workers had difficulty reproducing the work of Achalme and Thiroloix. Henri Triboulet, known more for his temperance work than for the study of rheumatic fever, and Amand Coyon cultured the blood of five living patients with rheumatic fever.[22] In marked contrast to Thiroloix, they found diplococci (two ball-shaped bacteria stuck together) which grew on aerobic cultures. These discrepancies troubled Triboulet and Coyon. They wondered whether the "bacille d'Achalme," recovered from dead patients, might be responsible for the most severe cases of rheumatic fever. Perhaps their diplococcus caused milder cases. They also raised the question whether the "bacille d'Achalme" was a post-mortem contaminant,[23] a contention that Achalme rejected.[24]

In 1898 Triboulet and Coyon reported five additional cases. In each instance they failed to find the "bacille d'Achalme," but in every case they isolated their diplococcus from the blood of patients with rheumatic fever. Buoyed now by ten isolations, they proclaimed that rheumatic fever resulted from bacterial sepsis.[25]

From Vienna another approach emerged: culturing the urine in patients with rheumatic fever. Results conflicted. Gustav Singer found that many patients had bacteria in their urine, often *staphylococcus albus*,[26] a result that others disputed.[27] Even though an editorial writer at the *Boston Medical and Surgical Journal* praised Singer's work as a step forward in understanding germs in rheumatic fever, it puzzled some workers in the field who argued that urinary abnormalities normally played no role in the disease.[28] Reviewing the entire subject at century's end, A. S. Wohlman, a physician from Bath, concluded that Achalme's work was the most persuasive to date.[29]

In an effort to explain the conflicting isolates, R. Oppenheim and A. Lippmann obtained blood cultures from ten patients with rheumatic fever. In four whom they considered less ill, they grew no bacteria. In the six sicker patients, they grew a diplococcus that they believed was the same as that cultured by Triboulet and Coyon. These results confirmed the presence of the diplococcus. But what about the "bacille d'Achalme"? Oppenheim and Lippmann suggested a laboratory error. They claimed that Achalme and Thiroloix's anaerobic cultures might have used a milk-based medium and that spores from the "bacille lactique de Pasteur" survived the sterilization process. In this view, these spores were the source of the "bacille d'Achalme" and not bodily fluids cultured from patients. It would also explain why it took so long to grow the "bacille d'Achalme." Indeed, this was an attractive argument to settle two widely divergent claims. Unfortunately, a careful reading of Achalme and Thiroloix's several reports shows that they obtained their bacillus in anaerobic cultures on both milk-based and bouillon media.[30]

### Frederick Poynton and Alexander Paine in London

In another attempt to settle the rival claims between the "bacille d'Achalme" and the diplococcus, Frederick J. Poynton, a physician at the Hospital for Sick Children in London and St. Mary's Hospital who had studied with Cheadle, and Alexander Paine, a bacteriologist at St. Mary's, initiated a series of experiments that would last a quarter century. In their first effort, Poynton and Paine cultured the blood, heart valves, and pericardium of eight patients who had died from rheumatic fever. In every case, they found a diplococcus that could exist alone or form short chains, characteristics that they attributed to the streptococcus family of bacteria. They believed that their diplococcus was the same one Triboulet and Coyon had isolated. Significantly, Poynton and Paine extended the Parisian studies in efforts to produce rheumatic fever in animals by inoculating them with the diplococcus.[31]

Almost from the start, Poynton and Paine's work came under fire. Critics claimed that their bacterial isolate was a post-mortem artifact and that Poynton and Paine lacked sophistication in the methods of identifying bacteria. Poynton and Paine acknowledged that only one of eighteen isolates came from a living patient and that their experimentally induced arthritis failed to mimic the peculiar arthritis of humans in rheumatic fever.[32] Buoyed by their repeatedly successful attempts at isolation and with their initial animal experiments, Poynton and Paine, despite criticism, confidently proclaimed in 1901 that they had found the bacterial cause of rheumatic fever: "diplococcus rheumaticus."[33]

Independent confirmation was soon at hand. Newton Pitt, at Guy's Hospital, grew streptococci from the blood of a woman who died of endocarditis later that year.[34] Colleagues at Guy's Hospital, E. W. Ainley Walker and J. Henry Ryffel, also isolated a coccus. They believed it closely related to *streptococcus pyogenes,* the bacterium responsible for a number of human illnesses, including erysipelas. Despite similarities, they thought it sufficiently different to give the germ a separate name, "micrococcus rheumaticus."[35] By 1903 Walker had isolated his streptococcal "micrococcus" in fifteen additional patients, eight near death from endocarditis and seven at autopsy.[36]

Confusion ensued. Poynton and Paine argued that their "diplococcus rheumaticus" was different from Walker's "micrococcus rheumaticus." Adding to the fray came the announcement of the discovery of another streptococcus from Germany, isolated from a patient dying with chorea, appropriately called "streptococcus aus chorea." In an attempt to make sense of the rival claims, W. V. Shaw, working at the Wellcome Physiological Research Laboratories, requested each claimant to submit a bacterial specimen. After testing each bacterium, Shaw concluded that all were almost certainly identical members of the streptococcus family.[37] A question arose: was the microbe isolated from patients with rheumatic fever unique or was it shared with other illnesses caused by the streptococcus? James M. Beattie, a pathologist at the University of Edinburgh, argued that the "micrococcus rheumaticus" was specific to rheumatic fever, basing his claim on the shorter length of its chain and its slightly different culturing characteristics.[38]

Not all workers found microbes in rheumatic fever. Thomas McCrae reported on forty patients admitted to Johns Hopkins Hospital between 1901 and 1903. These patients, sick enough to require admission but not nearing death, had cultures taken of blood, joint fluid, and urine. McCrae reported that all cultures were "practically negative," which he acknowledged was frustratingly "disappointing, and we regret that thus far we have been unable to confirm the observation of foreign observers."[39]

Poynton and Paine responded to criticism that their findings were not always reproducible. They claimed that in some cases the body's defenses simply over-whelmed the bacteria, thus rendering the culture sterile. Only in more serious cases, the victim overpowered by sepsis, did the culture yield bacteria. In this way they explained why so many cases at autopsy had positive cultures while many living patients had sterile cultures.[40] Relapses, they argued, occurred when "the diplo-coccus, only partially defeated, lies quiescent in the rheumatic lesion, as does the bacillus in the tubercular gland, and is ready to become virulent again under these mysterious influences which confer virulence."[41] Poynton and Paine staunchly be-lieved that their "diplococcus rheumaticus" was distinct and causative in rheumatic fever, but they conceded in 1904 that they had some difficulty characterizing it, largely because of the "futility of bacteriological methods."

### *Rufus Cole: Critic*

Evidence mounted that contradicted Poynton and Paine. Rufus Cole, then a medical resident at Johns Hopkins Hospital before he left to become the distin-guished director and researcher at the Rockefeller Institute, reported that he had cultured the blood and joint fluid of all patients with rheumatic fever at Johns Hopkins—both outpatients and those admitted to the hospital—over a three-year period. Like McCrae before him, Cole discovered that all cultures were sterile.[42] From Edinburgh, James Beattie, though convinced that rheumatic fever resulted from sepsis caused by the "diplococcus rheumaticus," confessed that only once had he actually cultured the organism himself from a patient. For his laboratory studies, he had relied on Poynton and Paine's providing him with samples of the bacteria.[43]

Rufus Cole continued to pick away at Poynton and Paine's work. Working at Johns Hopkins, Cole had the benefit of William Osler's continuing study of what Osler now called "chronic infectious endocarditis." Most of these patients had suf-fered from rheumatic fever years, perhaps decades, earlier, leaving them with scarred heart valves that served as friendly hosts to bacteria. Culturing the blood of a patient with infectious endocarditis virtually always yielded bacteria.[44] In 1906 Cole reaffirmed that all patients diagnosed at Johns Hopkins with rheumatic fe-ver continued to have sterile cultures. Thoughtfully, he observed that Poynton and Paine had obtained all of their cultures from dead or nearly dead patients. In con-trast, cultures from Johns Hopkins Hospital were obtained from much healthier victims of rheumatic fever. Cole reasoned that Poynton and Paine's autopsy cul-tures were contaminants, and he questioned whether their focus on patients who died from rheumatic fever, an outcome that was becoming rarer in the first de-cade of the twentieth century, should now be considered "typical." Perhaps these unfortunate patients had become *secondarily infected* as a result of damage done to heart valves. In other words, rheumatic fever caused the original injury to the heart valves, but the ultimate reason for death was infectious endocarditis.[45]

At this point, there was something of a stalemate. Walker,[46] Beattie,[47] and Poynton and Paine[48] repeated their work and stuck to their guns. Observers ana-lyzing the work of the participants reached different conclusions. Lewis A. Conner, professor of clinical medicine at Cornell Medical College, believed that Poynton and Paine's work made the most sense.[49] Charles Hunter Dunn of Harvard Medical School, Ludwig M. Loeb at Rush Medical College, and J. Ross Snyder concluded that the inability of workers in the United States to culture any organism undermined Poynton and Paine's theory.[50] In 1910 Poynton and Paine once again answered their critics directly. To those who claimed that their cultures came from agonal or post-mortem contaminants, Poynton and Paine countered that at least some of their cultures derived from patients who lived for months. To those who stated that the "diplococcus rheumaticus" was unrelated to the pathogenesis of rheumatic fever, they explained that their bacteria had some success in producing arthritis in laboratory animals. To those who expressed doubt because others could not find bacteria, Poynton and Paine confidently proclaimed that they were just more fortunate in selecting cases.[51] Despite their vigorous defense, the tide was beginning to turn against the notion that rheumatic fever was a form of bacterial sepsis.

### French Studies

In spite of doubts in some quarters, French bacteriologists pressed on. Thiroloix, now working with Georges Rosenthal, continued to find the "bacille d'Achalme." For example, they recovered the bacillus from the blood of an apprentice *charcutier* in 1907. The man, who eventually recovered, had arthritis, but neither chorea nor endocarditis. They described the bacillus as taking Gram's stain, which bacteriologists would now term "Gram positive." Thiroloix and Rosenthal believed it to be the "bacille d'Achalme," but they also claimed that it was virtually identical to the "bacille perfringes," a non-disease-producing saprophyte that resided in the gut and skin. They acknowledged how difficult it was for others to find their bacillus. Although Thiroloix and Rosenthal believed that this young man suffered from rheumatic fever, the absence of heart disease and his occupation, apprentice butcher, suggests that his illness might have been either anthrax or brucellosis.[52]

Later that July, Henri Triboulet, physician at Hôpital St. Antoine, again suggested a compromise between his micrococci and the "bacille d'Achalme." Triboulet now believed that Thiroloix's bacillus was a gut saprophyte, in other words, a normal, non-disease-producing intestinal bacterium. He suggested that their bacillus migrated from the gut and lessened the body's resistance, setting it up for infection with micrococci, a process that led eventually to rheumatic fever. No doubt bacterial diplomacy at its height, Triboulet's hypothesis, nevertheless, stood on very thin ice.[53]

Thiroloix and Rosenthal persevered. In the fall of 1907, they presented a remarkable biological property of their microbe. Under anaerobic conditions, their cultures yielded a bacillus. When they forced the microbe to grow on aerobic media, they claimed they found cocci, occasionally diplococci. This phenomena seemed to explain for them how different researchers had achieved such disparate results. It is certainly difficult for the historian to understand how they converted a bacillus into a coccus, unless we postulate that the "bacille d'Achalme" was a spore-producing bacterium. Under an adverse environmental stress, such as a profound change in culture medium, the microbe produced spores that Thiroloix and Rosenthal interpreted as cocci.[54] Nevertheless, Triboulet readily accepted Thiroloix's argument.[55]

The similarity of the "bacille d'Achalme" to the commonly recognized saprophyte "bacille perfringens" worried Georges Rosenthal. Indeed he pointed out their congruence when he proved that antiserum to "bacille d'Achalme" neutralized both bacilli.[56] Despite this observation, he insisted that one was a true pathogen while the other was "banal."[57] Still the rarity of finding the "bacille d'Achalme" perplexed Thiroloix. He reported that various workers had isolated it only 11 times in 240 cases since 1897. Even so, he insisted that the bacillus was not a post-mortem contaminant.[58]

### Flaws in Obtaining Cultures

At this point came an attack that completely undermined the work of Thiroloix, Rosenthal, and Triboulet. In 1913 F. G. Bosc claimed that all previous cultures had not been obtained "after a 'surgical' cleansing of the patient's skin, the instruments, and the physicians' hands." Proper technique yielded sterile cultures. The "bacille d'Achalme" was a "faute de technique."[59] Bosc cultured the skin of healthy humans and found that the bacillus was a normal resident, identical to the "bacille perfringens," a nonpathogen.[60] Achalme, who had not entered the debate in a decade, conceded that position.[61]

Both major bacteriological contenders, one French and one British, were untenable by 1913. The "bacille d'Achalme" was most probably just what Bosc claimed it was, a skin contaminant. Very few workers had been able to culture it, and, as we shall see, when injected into animals, it failed to produce a rheumatic fever-like illness. The claims for the diplococcus were stronger. Yet it seems likely that virtually all of these bacterial cultures came from gravely ill patients or corpses. People who died from rheumatic fever invariably died from the complications of infectious endocarditis. In their selection of patients to culture, Poynton and Paine chose people whose heart valves had been damaged, predisposing them to infectious endocarditis. The isolated diplococcus was a vital part of infectious endocarditis but of no consequence to rheumatic fever.

Rufus Cole's work undermined the argument that rheumatic fever was a bacterial form of sepsis. His uniformly sterile cultures at Johns Hopkins Hospital also beg explanation. It is difficult to imagine that none of his patients had both rheumatic and infective endocarditis. One explanation is that cardiac complications from rheumatic fever were far less common in the United States than they were in Britain.[62] A more likely explanation was that patients with endocarditis at Johns Hopkins were segregated from patients with uncomplicated rheumatic fever. Osler's clinical interest in infectious endocarditis may offer a clue. Osler and Cole must have split patients, which London physicians grouped together, into two separate categories.

Simple culturing of patients' bodily fluids did not yield a bacterial etiology. What was astonishing was that this failure did not lessen the conviction that rheumatic fever had a bacterial origin. Perhaps the sheer weight of so many reports of positive cultures—all inaccurate—nevertheless strengthened the claim for a bacterial source. Undaunted, researchers now shifted the focus from culturing patients to experimental efforts to produce rheumatic fever in animals.

## Laboratory Research

Culturing fluids and tissues from patients with rheumatic fever failed to yield a creditable bacterium. Nevertheless, conviction remained strong that rheumatic fever was bacterial in origin, buoyed primarily by its epidemiological associations with other illnesses thought infectious and by its clinical similarities with illnesses of known bacteriological causes. Rheumatic fever proved just as elusive in the experimental laboratory. The historian must step back once again to appreciate the problems facing these first laboratory researchers. The complexity of the disease stymied them. Cheadle had described a disease that injured the skin, joints, heart (pericardium and endocardium), tendon sheaths, and brain. Was there an animal disease which was roughly equivalent to this human illness? How many of these organs and tissues should a researcher attempt to target? As a practical matter, all initial researchers greatly simplified rheumatic fever, normally satisfied when they could produce any form of arthritis or carditis.

All of the initial experiments were quite simple in design. Bacteria, isolated from patients with rheumatic fever, were injected intravenously into animals, typically rabbits. At first workers did not set the high standard of producing the peculiar migrating, nonsuppurating arthritis or the carditis that damaged the several tissues of the heart. In the early years, there were no attempts at all to induce chorea, rashes, or nodules, and none that came close to re-creating the entire spectrum of the disease. Despite some early perceived successes, laboratory re-creation of rheumatic fever eluded researchers. With hindsight, we know that the whole enterprise was doomed. The bacteria employed to produce rheumatic fever were either contaminants or isolates from infectious, not rheumatic, endocarditis. The technique of inoculating animals—intravenous injection—while convenient for the researcher, had no counterpart in tonsillitis, the suspected point of bacterial entry into the human body. And no laboratory animal was found to suffer from a disease remotely similar to rheumatic fever.

In the initial experimental forays, researchers inoculated animals with the two rival bacteria, the "bacille d'Achalme" and the diplococcus. In October 1897, Thiroloix injected the "bacille d'Achalme" into a laboratory animal. He produced endocarditis, convincing him that he was on the right track. He was disappointed in his failure to induce arthritis.[63] Months later Triboulet and Coyon injected their diplococci into rabbits. They, too, damaged heart valves, which was evidence enough to persuade them that rheumatic fever was a form of bacterial sepsis.[64]

### *Poynton and Paine's Laboratory Experiments*

Experimental rheumatic fever produced by diplococci received a tremendous boost from Poynton and Paine. In 1899 they injected their "diplococcus rheumaticus" into rabbits, producing arthritis, endocarditis, and ultimately death. This was the closest approach yet to laboratory re-creation of a multisystem disease.[65] By 1901 they could regularly and reproducibly create arthritis and complex carditis (both pericarditis and endocarditis).[66] A closer look at their results demonstrates clear reasons for excitement. Much, but not all, of the arthritis they produced was transient, nonsuppurative, affecting several of the large joints: all characteristics of arthritis in human rheumatic fever. In each instance, Poynton and Paine were able to culture their diplococcus successfully from the joint fluid of the animal, a finding that neatly supported their hypothesis that rheumatic fever was a form of bacterial sepsis.[67]

### *Rufus Cole: Once Again the Critic*

Rufus Cole, critic of Poynton and Paine's clinical research, took aim at their animal studies as well. At Johns Hopkins, Cole had failed to isolate a single bacterium from the blood or joint fluid in patients with rheumatic fever. He believed that Poynton and Paine had obtained their isolates from atypical cases, those either close to death or already dead, in any event suffering from a secondary infection with "diplococcus rheumaticus." Cole, believing that he had identified the error underpinning their research, sought to identify the "proper" inciting germ of rheumatic fever. He also looked to the streptococcal family of bacteria, choosing the *streptococcus pyogenes* because this germ was thought to cause human diseases such as erysipelas. His intravenous injection of this strain of streptococcus also produced arthritis, pericarditis, and endocarditis in animals. *Streptococcus pyogenes*, when compared with the "diplococcus rheumaticus," proved to be considerably more virulent, provoking a suppurative form of arthritis and a suppurative endocarditis, very different from rheumatic endocarditis.[68] It was curious that Cole, the opponent of Poynton and Paine's sepsis hypothesis, nevertheless investigated sepsis, merely selecting a different bacteria.[69]

James Beattie, the pathologist from Edinburgh, was quick to criticize Cole. Beattie correctly noted that Cole had injected into animals bacteria that he had collected from patients who had diseases other than rheumatic fever. This violated Koch's postulates, the standard method of proving disease causation. Beattie also pointed out that the arthritis that Cole produced was suppurative. By 1906 the experimental arthritis provoked by Poynton and Paine (as well as other workers) with the "diplococcus rheumaticus" or "micrococcus rheumaticus" was nearly always nonsuppurative in nature.[70] Poynton and Paine, dissecting their laboratory animals, discovered their "diplococcus rheumaticus" in joint fluids and heart, a finding that reinforced their belief that rheumatic fever was a form of sepsis. For the historian is left the puzzle of how the "diplococcus rheumaticus" got into the joint fluid and cardiac tissues of experimental animals. The most obvious explanation is that Poynton and Paine, by injecting the bloodstream with the "diplococcus rheumaticus," created sepsis, thus sending bacteria everywhere in the body, including to the joints and heart. In essence, what Poynton and Paine had accomplished was an experimental model of infectious endocarditis, not rheumatic fever.

Oscar M. Schloss, a pediatrician at Bellevue Hospital and Babies' Hospital in New York, took a different tack in trying the prove the infectivity of rheumatic fever. In 1912 he injected whole blood from patients with rheumatic fever into rhesus monkeys. What Schloss's experiment hoped to show was whether there was anything infective in the blood of patients with rheumatic fever—not just bacteria—and whether an animal closer to humans in an evolutionary sense might prove a better experimental target. The monkeys did not become ill, which Schloss interpreted as support of Cole's contention that rheumatic fever was not a form of bacterial sepsis.[71]

## Streptococcus and Experimental Rheumatic Fever

Despite claim and counterclaim, nearly all researchers agreed that some form of streptococcus was likely involved, remarkable indeed given that able critics disputed the notion from many sides. Perhaps one reason for the lure of the streptococcus stemmed from the growing epidemiological association between tonsillitis—one of Cheadle's rheumatic manifestations—and the understanding that infection with *streptococcus pyogenes* produced human tonsillitis. Cole's work added evidence that *streptococcus pyogenes* could incite arthritis and carditis, even though it was not precisely the same type found in rheumatic fever. Along similar lines, Leila Jackson isolated in 1911 *streptococcus pyogenes* from a milk-borne epidemic of tonsillitis and arthritis in Chicago. She then injected *streptococcus pyogenes* into rabbits, producing, like Cole before her, suppurative arthritis.[72]

At this point something of a paradox existed. *Streptococcus pyogenes*, which caused tonsillitis in humans and was linked epidemiologically to rheumatic fever, failed to produce the right kind of arthritis when injected into the bloodstream of experimental animals. "Diplococcus rheumaticus," never found as a cause of human tonsillitis, nevertheless produced an experimental arthritis that was far closer to the nonsuppurative arthritis in rheumatic fever. In 1915 Harold Kniest Faber carefully reviewed the puzzle. Faber argued that the rapid death with suppurative endocarditis and arthritis that occurred after intravenous injection with *streptococcus pyogenes* was very different from rheumatic fever in humans. In contrast, Faber concluded that the experimental arthritis and carditis which less virulent strains of the streptococcus family, such as the "diplococcus rheumaticus," produced in animals was the closest laboratory approximation to date to human disease. In particular what struck him was that it often took researchers several intravenous injections with the "diplococcus rheumaticus" before the animal developed the nonsuppurating arthritis. This suggested to Faber that a process of "sensitization" was occurring. In his hands, the *streptococcus viridans,* an organism similar to "diplococcus rheumaticus," produced a convincing experimental arthritis. Faber believed this period of sensitization best explained the clinical delay between acquiring tonsillitis and the development of the other symptoms in rheumatic fever, as well as the span between relapses.[73]

## Homer F. Swift

In 1917 Homer F. Swift and Ralph A. Kinsella, both at Rockefeller University, took stock of the experimentally produced arthritis. Swift, a 1906 graduate of Bellevue Medical College whose distinguished career also included appointments to Cornell University Medical College and Columbia University, was a leader in American research on rheumatic fever until 1950.[74] In this first effort, Swift and Kinsella pointed out that many of the earlier claims were not interpretable because the streptococcus involved had not been typed in a way that made sense to researchers in 1917. Swift and Kinsella explained that contemporary bacteriologists divided members of the streptococcal family according to the ability to break down, or hemolyze, red blood cells. The nonhemolytic group could be further subclassified on whether it metabolized hemoglobin into methemoglobin. Swift and Kinsella believed that Poynton and Paine's "diplococcus rheumaticus" was almost certainly the same as the *streptococcus viridans* or *mitis,* a nonhemolytic, methemoglobin-positive streptococcus. *Streptococcus pyogenes* was a member of the hemolytic branch.

Using this more precise classification, Swift and Kinsella cultured the blood in fifty-eight hospitalized patients with rheumatic fever. Specimens from seven patients grew bacteria. They also cultured joint fluid in twenty-five patients, all of which was sterile. Swift and Kinsella characterized the isolates from the blood as members of the *streptococcus viridans* group.[75] Swift, now working with Ralph H. Boots, took up Faber's suggestion to employ hypersensitization to the non-hemolytic streptococcus as a means of producing experimental arthritis. This idea proposed that the arthritis in rheumatic fever was actually a form of allergy, produced by repeated exposure to bacteria. Swift and Boots injected nonhemolytic streptococci into the joints of laboratory animals, then followed these injections with intravenous inoculations with the same bacteria. The anticipated allergic arthritis failed to occur.[76] For Swift, hypersensitization remained an attractive hypothesis for decades, but one that was far from proved in 1917.

## Myocarditis: A New Component of Rheumatic Fever

The ever-changing biology of rheumatic fever served as an additional challenge to researchers. Myocarditis, an occasional aspect of rheumatic fever in the nineteenth century, became increasingly common. This new cardiac injury thus provided an additional—but frustratingly elusive—experimental target. In the last decades of the nineteenth century, clinicians began to describe cases in which patients suffered from myocarditis that occurred either alone or in conjunction with either pericarditis or endocarditis. For the clinician, myocarditis was a difficult diagnosis, usually entertained when a patient had signs of an enlarged heart without the auscultatory findings of endocarditis or pericarditis. This rare finding became much more common in the twentieth century, eventually becoming the primary cardiac injury in rheumatic fever. Pathologists confirmed the clinical finding of myocardial injury. In 1878 Samuel West at St. Bartholomew's Hospital reported microscopic changes in the heart muscle in patients who showed no evidence of either pericardial or endocardial illness.[77] Five years later Angel Money,[78] a young physician at the Hospital for Sick Children in London, reported the autopsy of a ten-year-old girl who died after bouts with both scarlet fever and rheumatic fever that had produced multiple relapses of chorea and myocarditis. At autopsy, he found "some nodules about the size of a millet seed . . . in the wall of the right ventricle."[79]

In the 1890s, several pathologists argued that hearts "failed" in rheumatic fever more from muscular damage than from valvular injury.[80] In 1904 Ludwig Aschoff described a peculiar microscopic inflammatory response in the myocardium of patients dying from rheumatic fever. He interpreted these degenerative collections of cells, Money's millet-sized nodules, as being responsible both for the myocardial damage and for the disruption of cardiac rhythm that patients were beginning to suffer and physicians to notice. Of crucial significance was Aschoff's claim that this cellular response of the myocardium was unique in rheumatic fever.[81] Carey Coombs, who had studied with Cheadle and Poynton, confirmed Aschoff's finding and labeled the pathological changes "submiliary," or smaller than a millet seed, or about two millimeters. Soon pathologists termed them "Aschoff bodies." Coombs also found similar cellular reactions in the pericardium and endocardium, sparking a debate that raged for decades over whether Aschoff bodies could exist in tissues other than the myocardium.[82]

William Thalhimer and M. A. Rothschild, working at Mount Sinai Hospital in New York City, confirmed the uniqueness of the Aschoff body in rheumatic fever. In every patient dying of rheumatic fever, they found an abundance of Aschoff bodies, especially in the wall of the left ventricle. Additionally, they also found these cellular changes in a patient who died with rheumatic chorea. Significantly, they did not find a single Aschoff body in fourteen patients dying of infectious endocarditis from *streptococcus viridans* in which rheumatic fever was believed not to have been the inciting cause. They also failed to find Aschoff bodies in patients dying of gonococcal, staphylococcal, and pneumococcal endocarditis. Their findings indicated that rheumatic fever left a special mark upon its victim's heart.[83]

The Aschoff body placed an additional burden on laboratory researchers who were attempting to re-create rheumatic carditis in experimental animals. This peculiar cellular reaction became the "gold standard"—perhaps misguidedly and certainly prematurely—against which pathologists judged their success. In 1912 Carey Coombs and Reginald Miller, a pathologist at St. Mary's Hospital, critically surveyed attempts to produce carditis experimentally. They argued that the experimental carditis that Poynton and Paine had produced differed microscopically from what they now considered the pathognomonic Aschoff body, thus falling short.[84] Coombs's affirmation of Aschoff's work and his initial experimental critique were so widely acclaimed that some physicians referred to the myocardial changes as "Coombs' submiliary nodules."[85] Oscar M. Schloss and Nellis B. Foster, working at St. Luke's Hospital in New York City, also failed to produce Aschoff bodies in the hearts of rhesus monkeys injected with *streptococcus pyogenes* isolated from humans with tonsillitis.[86]

Thalhimer and Rothschild followed their autopsy work with experiments in the laboratory. They injected animals intravenously with four varieties of streptococci, including *streptococcus pyogenes* and *streptococcus viridans*. In every instance, they successfully produced focal myocardial inflammation. Significantly, none of these lesions was histologically identical to the complex structure of the Aschoff body. The experimentally induced myocardial changes differed in structure, location, cells involved, and staining characteristics.[87]

It was ironic that researchers, who gave to the Aschoff body such significance, could not always agree on its simple cellular characteristics. Questions abounded. Were Aschoff bodies formed from fibrous tissue, or cardiac muscle, or had so much degeneration occurred that it was impossible to tell origins? Where were they located—in the myocardium alone or in several tissues? If the myocardium was the only site, precisely where within the heart's muscle? Finding Aschoff bodies in the subendocardial region of the myocardium amid the conducting pathways that controlled the heart's rhythm gave a pathological explanation for the disturbance in rhythm clinicians observed in their patients.[88]

### Frustrated Research in 1920

Experimental efforts to reproduce rheumatic fever in laboratory animals were clearly frustrated by 1920. Most workers in the field, Philip Miller of Rockefeller University argued, believed that nonhemolytic *streptococcus viridans* was the leading laboratory contender among bacterial claimants. This widely accepted notion rested on its occasional isolation from dying patients, its ability to produce the closest laboratory approach to the peculiar arthritis in rheumatic fever, and its ability to damage all three tissues of the heart. Yet it was also plainly apparent that rheumatic fever in humans was not a form of bacterial sepsis, that *streptococcus viridans* was not the germ responsible for human tonsillitis, that the experimental arthritis—however similar to the human arthritis in rheumatic fever—differed in key aspects, and that the laboratory carditis was distinctly different from the Aschoff body. Miller's critique went still further. He argued that humans were the only species susceptible to rheumatic fever, a conclusion, if true, which would defeat any laboratory effort. "The transmission of rheumatic fever to laboratory animals is an important problem," he stated, "one which must not be abandoned, for on its solution may rest the elucidation of the etiology of the disease."[89]

Homer Swift concurred, and he asserted that workers needed to go back to square one in thinking about the pathogenesis of the disease. The key, he predicted in a nod to Cheadle, lay in finding the common element connecting the various manifestations of the rheumatic state.[90]

## CHAPTER 5

# Clinical Management, 1890–1925

*W*alter Butler Cheadle's organization of clinical thinking about rheumatic fever largely settled the difficult task of bedside diagnosis. His grouping of the "various manifestations of the rheumatic state" with their several temporal relations was a unique solution for a disease that coursed its way through individuals so differently. Leading physicians quickly adopted Cheadle's scheme, and nearly all discussions at professional meetings and in medical school classrooms—as well as in published scholarly papers—showed clear evidence that his method swiftly reached both practitioners and the prominent researchers in the field.[1] Cheadle's method of diagnosis remained the principal guide for physicians until 1944, when T. Duckett Jones, confronted with the marked decline in morbidity and mortality from rheumatic fever and with a disease that continued to change its biological character, offered his strategy of major and minor diagnostic criteria.[2]

Clinicians did make a few refinements. Continuing a trend that started even before Cheadle, physicians sought to solidify the use of "rheumatic fever." Echoing decades of concern, Carey Coombs, a pathologist in Bristol, declared in 1904 that older terms—still employed by many doctors—such as "rheumatism" or "acute articular rheumatism," constituted a "rubbish-heap" of phrases. By this he meant that many diseases in addition to rheumatic fever were conflated into what physicians had long called "rheumatism." By including the word "articular" clinicians semantically focused attention upon hurting joints, which practitioners in the first years of the twentieth century now believed needed far less emphasis. What had become important to both patient and physician was the search for the bacterial cause of the disease and the identification and treatment for damage done to the heart. Reflecting these changes in focus, English-speaking physicians began to use "rheumatic fever" and "rheumatic heart disease."[3] French and German physicians did not demonstrate this semantic transition, continuing to use *rhumatisme articulaire aigu* and *Gelenkrheumatismus* well into the twentieth century.

## Evolving Rashes

Skin rashes were one aspect of rheumatic fever that showed considerable biological volatility in the first decade of the twentieth century. Cheadle had claimed that several erythemas could be associated with rheumatic fever but that in his experience only erythema marginatum was frequent. Cheadle's observations can be interpreted as a transition. Dramatic rashes that once caught the attention of both patient and physician waned, replaced by a much more visually subtle cutaneous eruption. Despite his observation, other practitioners still believed that erythema multiforme, erythema nodosum, "purpura rheumatica," and erythema papulatum were just as likely to accompany the other manifestations of rheumatic fever.[4] Clinicians were able to separate at least one of these rashes from rheumatic fever, because it mainly occurred in a disease that was different from the one Cheadle described. "Purpura rheumatica" occurred in an illness that shared a few elements with rheumatic fever, such as fever and arthritis. This rash began as a blanching erythema that progressed to frank purpura, or hemorrhages within the skin. Stephen MacKenzie of London Hospital and Murray H. Bass more precisely identified this rash as the "purpura of Schönlein," the skin manifestation of a disease that is now known as Henoch-Schönlein purpura. What led to this refinement was the clear understanding that children with "purpura rheumatica" never developed carditis, nodules, or chorea. But they were at risk for severe gastrointestinal complications, problems that rarely bothered victims of rheumatic fever. Such distinctions were not always so simple. Case histories indicate that patients with certain rheumatic fever developed several different rashes, in particular urticaria (hives), erythema nodosum, scarlatina, and erythema marginatum. Rheumatic fever in the early twentieth century provoked more cutaneous responses than it has since. What linked these rashes was that all were streptococcus-related skin conditions. During the first decades of the twentieth century, erythema marginatum emerged, as Cheadle had predicted, as the rash most specifically related to rheumatic fever. As the streptococcus became less cutaneously provocative, the other rashes ceased to be a part of rheumatic fever.[5] Thus the evolution of rashes in rheumatic fever demonstrated both biological change and shifts in physicians' diagnostic perceptions.

Refinements in the diagnosis and classification of childhood arthritis also defined more precisely the joint ailment in rheumatic fever. Forms of arthritis, which physicians had once included in "rheumatism" but which were clearly not associated with rheumatic fever, were shifted properly to other diseases. For example, in 1896 George Frederick Still described a rare, chronic, deforming arthritis in children that now carries his name. In contrast, arthritis in rheumatic fever was common and never crippled. Still's observation clarified that all arthritis in children did not result from rheumatic fever.[6] With the advent of bacterial culturing in hospital practice, it became possible to sort out those joint problems related to infection with gonococcus, staphylococcus, tubercle bacillus, and pneumococcus.[7] Most—but, as we have seen, not all—physicians thought that the joint fluid in patients with rheumatic fever was sterile.

### Growing Pains

Although the widespread use of salicylate made great strides in the treatment of fever and arthritis, therapeutic humility in the face of rheumatic fever remained pervasive for many practitioners, especially in healing cardiac injury. Most
physicians thought that prompt diagnosis offered the best chance of interrupting
the development of rheumatic manifestations. In the hope of altering the disease
at the earliest possible moment, some parents and doctors singled out "growing
pains" as a likely herald to full-blown rheumatic fever. Always difficult to characterize with precision, growing pains were intermittent and frequently incapacitat-
ing limb aches, localized deeply in the legs or arms, that were seldom confined to
joints and that never led to redness or swelling or to fever. As such, growing pains
were plainly different from the joint distress of rheumatic fever. But might they
be a harbinger? Many children suffered these pains in the early decades of the
twentieth century, as they do in the present day. One British study suggested nearly
one-third of all children complained of growing pains at some point in their childhood;[8] an American study supported their commonness.[9] Practitioners differed
sharply on their significance. Prominent pediatricians, such as Abraham Jacobi,
strongly believed that growing pains not only existed but also led frequently to
rheumatic fever.[10] His dictum was that a child with growing pains needed strict
bed rest to prevent rheumatic fever, advice that many pediatricians and parents
accepted.[11] Not all agreed. One detractor stated in 1894 that growing pains were

> sinking into oblivion in medical literature of the past. As a separate mor-
> bid entity, it exists now principally as an article of faith. The complaint
> still maintains, however, a strong hold on the lay mind and forms an
> extremely common lay diagnosis, which is often the cause of much
> suffering.[12]

It seems likely that physicians conflated worries about two common—but unrelated—limb ailments.

### Myocardial Injury, Disturbances in Heart Rhythm,
### and the Electrocardiogram

The most significant biological change in rheumatic fever in the early twentieth century was the increasing number of victims with myocardial injury. In the
nineteenth century, the initial cardiac target had been the pericardium, joined later
by injury to heart valves, or endocardium. Despite the preponderance of pericardial and endocardial illness, from time to time practitioners would report an isolated case of a patient dying from heart disease in which the autopsy revealed only
a dilated, expended myocardium with unscathed pericardium and heart valves. This
rare observation slowly became the dominant form of heart disease in rheumatic
fever.

Among the first to point out the susceptibility of the myocardium were David
B. Lees and Frederick J. Poynton. In reviewing patients coming to autopsy from

rheumatic fever, they noted in 1897 that 92 of 150 showed marked dilatation of the heart muscle while only 12 had significant pericardial inflammation, a marked change from autopsy findings earlier in the century.[13] Lees and Poynton suggested that myocardial damage predicted poor clinical outcome, a point with which William Osler and Adolf Baginsky concurred.[14] Other clinicians followed suit with additional reports of myocardial damage.[15] In 1904, Aschoff's description of a unique inflammation of the myocardium added pathological confirmation to these earlier clinical reports. After fifteen years of study, David Lees believed that rheumatic fever nearly always injured the muscle of the left ventricle of the heart.[16] His collaborator, Frederick Poynton, was not as adamant, but he concurred that the myocardium was always damaged in fatal cases.[17]

The newly articulated concern for the myocardium presented diagnostic challenges for the clinician. As Frederick Poynton explained, the stethoscope could evaluate pericarditis and endocarditis because those inflammations produced characteristic rubs and murmurs. The diseased myocardium was silent.[18] In 1907 Carey Coombs noted that practitioners could assess severely enlarged hearts only through percussion of the chest wall, giving some measure of myocardial injury during the life of the patient.[19]

Myocardial injury resulted in a new clinical problem: disturbances in the heart's rhythm. Injury to the heart's muscle was often accompanied by damage to the heart's conduction system, which governs heart rate and rhythm. In 1891, I. E. Atkinson, Professor of Materia Medica at the University of Maryland, pointed out that many patients with rheumatic fever suffered from bradycardia, or a slowing of the heart's rate of contraction. Atkinson claimed that sufferers from rheumatic fever had nearly four times the incidence of bradycardia when compared with the general population.[20] After the turn of the century, Pierre Achalme, remembered primarily for his work on the bacteriology of rheumatic fever, pointed out that many patients with rheumatic fever had an irregular heart rate early in the course of the illness. He hoped that prompt use of salicylate would remedy this problem.[21] Were these disturbances in heart rhythm new at the end of the nineteenth century? This is a difficult question to answer. William Charles Wells and others at the beginning of the nineteenth century mentioned a greatly increased heart rate in patients suffering from "rheumatism of the heart." While it is not possible for the historian to relate these observations with certainty to one or another cardiac tissue, it seems likely that pericardial inflammation was responsible, given that chest pain was often present. What these early accounts never described was a slow heart rate.

With the development of the clinical electrocardiogram, physicians were able to confirm these earlier clinical observations with technological precision.[22] In 1914 a British physician claimed that one particular conduction disturbance, atrial flutter, occurred so often in rheumatic fever that its graphic representation served as a valuable diagnostic sign.[23] The following year, another physician demonstrated a common ventricular dysrhythmia in rheumatic fever.[24] Paul Dudley White, the American cardiologist, reported in 1916 that the initial sign in one patient was a prolongation in the conduction time between the atria and ventricles, a finding that became known as "heart block." In other words, the electrocardiogram demonstrated a specific abnormality prior to the development of rash, chorea, or joint involvement.[25] The Aschoff body took on added significance in light of alterations in the electrocardiogram. Physicians interpreted rhythm disturbances as the mechanical disruption of the heart's conduction pathways.

John Parkinson and A. Hope Gosse, physicians at the Cardiac Department of the London Hospital, studied fifty consecutive patients, aged four to thirty-five years in age. Thirty percent developed heart block, which they defined as a prolongation in the "PR" interval of the electrocardiogram of longer than two-tenths of one second. They linked this disturbance in conduction to acute myocarditis, or—more specifically—to the development of Aschoff bodies along the path of the nerve fibers that normally regulated the heart's beating. They predicted that this prolongation, easily measured clinically, would serve as a useful diagnostic tool,[26] a conclusion quickly seconded by Homer Swift and Alfred Cohn at Rockefeller Hospital.[27] Electrocardiographic descriptions of a diseased myocardium thus followed observations of pathologists and clinicians by many years. Even the best hospitals did not own a device to record electrocardiograms until the 1920s. For example, Pennsylvania Hospital purchased an EKG machine in 1921. Only after 1927 was the electrocardiogram considered "routine."[28] As such, the introduction of the electrocardiogram into clinical practice clearly did not "discover" myocarditis. This is not to argue that the electrocardiogram was unimportant. The EKG provided physicians with a technological measure of myocarditis, and significantly—as pericarditis and endocarditis waned—the electrocardiogram was often the only gauge of cardiac injury during a patient's life.

### Laboratory Tests: Opsonin Index and White Blood Cell Count

A few clinicians sought to measure the degree of rheumatic inflammation. In one early attempt, Ruth Tunnicliff tried to apply Almroth Wright's opsonic index to the white blood cells of patients with rheumatic fever. The opsonic index was a diagnostic test—largely confined to the research setting in the first decade of the century—that measured the ability of white blood cells to kill bacteria. To carry out her study, Tunnicliff had to obtain cultures of the "diplococcus rheumaticus" from Beattie and from Poynton and Paine because she, like others before her, had been unable to isolate the germ herself after nearly three years of attempts. She hoped to show that white blood cells from patients with rheumatic fever handled these bacteria differently from similar cells from controls. This study fit nicely with the notion that rheumatic fever was a type of severe bacterial infection. Unfortunately, she failed to detect any differences between the groups.[29]

One laboratory test, widely available to most physicians, was the simple white blood count. By the 1920s this measure was routine in nearly all hospitals. Although generally an indicator of infection, the white blood count can be elevated or depressed by a variety of other types of illnesses, for example, malignancies. At Rockefeller Hospital, Homer Swift, with colleagues C. Philip Miller and Ralph H. Boots—both collaborators with Swift in his animal experiments—explored whether the white blood cell count was an aid in following the course of rheumatic fever.

They found that patients had a persistent elevation in white blood cell count during the active stages of the disease. Of therapeutic value, they noted that the count fell to normal after successful intervention with salicylate, an observation that gave clinicians the first laboratory test to monitor the effectiveness of therapy. Previously most practitioners had measured success or failure through a fall in fever and a cessation of joint pain. But doctors had known that neither indication signaled what was going on with the heart. It was the hope of many physicians that the white blood cell count would help assess cardiac injury.[30]

## Tonsillectomy

Clinical practice reflected concern for bacterial cause with heightened worry about diseased tonsils as the triggering event. To prevent rheumatic fever, physicians sprayed, painted, and scraped tonsils. Those who suffered a bout of rheumatic fever faced certain tonsillectomy during convalescence. Even children who escaped rheumatic fever often underwent surgical removal of diseased tonsils as a preventive measure, a practice that persisted until the 1950s.[31] So popular was tonsillectomy that it became, after circumcision, the most commonly performed operation in the United States.[32]

Naturally there was a spectrum of opinion. Abraham Jacobi exhorted: "Attend to their throats; have hypertrophied tonsils removed."[33] Henry Koplik thought that tonsils needed removal only after the patient recovered from serious heart disease.[34] In contrast, William Osler, while acknowledging Cheadle's "various manifestations," doubted whether any connection existed between tonsillitis and rheumatic fever. To Osler, tonsillitis was so common in childhood that chance alone explained any coincidence.[35]

Nearly all who demanded that the tonsils required some attention cited Poynton and Paine's bacterial hypothesis as the motive for action. Some suggested painting the tonsils with hydrogen peroxide;[36] others urged children to gargle daily;[37] still others brushed salicylate directly on the tonsils. The notion grew that any child who endured a bout of rheumatic fever should have the tonsils removed as a measure to prevent relapses. Initially, most calls for tonsillectomy were based solely on personal experiences. William P. Lucas of San Francisco and Mark H. Wentworth of Boston were early advocates of tonsillectomy;[38] T. H. Halsted of Syracuse and William E. Preble of Boston argued that any site of chronic infection demanded surgical excision.[39]

Some practitioners were more cautious. A physician from Chicago, E. Fletcher Ingalls, did not believe that tonsillectomy prevented relapses,[40] a finding that doctors at Johns Hopkins supported.[41] Physicians at Guy's Hospital provided the most careful analysis of the relationship between tonsillectomy and relapses of rheumatic fever in 1923. In their study of 144 former patients, some with and others without tonsils, they found that surgery provided no advantage. In fact, more who underwent tonsillectomy suffered recurrences. What these physicians did not elaborate was how they had selected cases for operation. Perhaps only the sickest

TABLE 5.1     *Medical inspection of schoolchildren in North Carolina*

| Year | Children examined by public health nurse | Children undergoing tonsillectomy |
|---|---|---|
| 1919–20 | 60,770 | 2,338 |
| 1921–22 | 92,566 | 1,870 |
| 1923–24 | 115,166 | 4,910 |
| 1925–26 | 171,905 | 3,714 |

SOURCE: "Report of the Bureau for Medical Inspection of Schools," *Biennial Report of the North Carolina State Board of Health* (1919–20), 18: 50–52; (1921–22), 19: 33–35; (1923–24), 20: 54–56; (1925–26), 21: 40–41.

patients, those most likely to relapse, received the surgery.[42] Frederick Poynton summarized the argument in 1925 and took a moderate course. Poynton believed that tonsillectomy did not prevent the initial attack, and that removal of apparently healthy tonsils did not lessen relapses. He advocated removing tonsils only if they appeared significantly diseased. The timing of the operation followed a full recovery from rheumatic fever.[43]

Some surgical enthusiasm for tonsillectomy was not nearly so moderate. In North Carolina, the State Board of Health set out to inspect and remove all enlarged tonsils in school-age children in the early 1920s. School teachers examined all throats; county public health nurses confirmed the presence of suspicious tonsils; physicians, in weekend traveling under-the-tent operating theaters, removed thousands of tonsils yearly. Unaccompanied by either bacterial culturing or measure of outcome, this program of tonsillar eradication was nevertheless one of the largest and best-coordinated public health efforts in the state (table 5.1).[44]

### Sera and Vaccines

The bacterial hypothesis also sparked attempts to develop antisera, or antibodies, and vaccines against the germs thought responsible for causing rheumatic fever. During the first decades of the twentieth century, physicians had some success with vaccines and antisera in preventing and treating a few bacterial infections, such as pneumococcal pneumonia.[45] Physicians manufactured antisera by injecting bacteria, either killed or at sublethal doses, into suitable animals, typically horses. So prepared, horse serum, when injected into humans, treated the same bacterial infection but at the risk of serious side effects from serum. Bacterial vaccines, consisting of large numbers of killed bacteria, were injected directly into humans as a preventive measure.

In contrast to tonsillectomy, these efforts with vaccines and antisera did not receive wide clinical trials. Given laboratory work in Paris and London, it is not surprising that initial attempts at producing an antisera were directed at the streptococcus family. In 1897 a French physician injected an antistreptococcal serum into a few patients with rheumatism. Problems abounded with the study: Cheadle's diagnostic rigor was not applied; patients were very close to death; the precise type of streptococcus was not specified. Nevertheless, some of the patients appeared to benefit from the intervention.[46] A similar clinical trial came in Portland, Oregon, five years later. A patient with rheumatic fever lay dying from endocarditis. He received daily injections of antistreptococcal serum (strain also unknown); his symptoms remitted.[47] German physicians reported promising results with similar antistreptococcal sera.[48] In Paris, advocates of the "bacille d'Achalme" produced an antiserum and a vaccine against this germ. Thiroloix and Rosenthal reported some success from both, but their test groups of patients were small.[49]

At Bellevue Hospital in New York, Russell Cecil took a different tack. He suggested that patients with rheumatic fever might benefit from a general goad to the immune system. To accomplish this, he injected his subjects with a foreign protein (typhoid vaccine). Within minutes, most developed shaking chills, fever, and an increased white blood cell count. About one-third of his patients recovered from their bouts with rheumatic fever, but Cecil interpreted this outcome as no real difference from chance alone.[50] By 1925 the consensus emerged that no antibacterial approach—vaccine, antiserum, or immunological stimulant—was clinically helpful.[51]

## Aspirin

The most spirited clinical debate in the years 1890–1925 was the continuation of the controversy surrounding the value of salicylate. One aspect of the debate was over which chemical form of the drug to use. At the beginning of the period there were several rivals in the salicylate family: oil of wintergreen, salicin, and sodium salicylate, among others. By 1925 dozens of minor chemical alterations had appeared, but acetylsalicylic acid, or aspirin, predominantly, because it produced less gastric irritation.[52]

What went uncontested was the widespread use of aspirin in rheumatic fever. Physicians universally agreed that aspirin effectively lowered fever and lessened joint pain. What confounded them was whether aspirin influenced the course of carditis. Early English studies, based on large numbers of hospitalized patients, demonstrated no clear advantage for the heart.[53] One way to assess the acceptance of aspirin between 1890 and 1925 is to ask whether leaders in the field used the drug and, if so, whether they believed that it lessened cardiac damage. Walter Cheadle employed salicylate, but he preferred the older alkaline treatment—therapy he "grew up with"—in difficult cases of heart disease.[54] Frederick Poynton also used salicylate, but he thought that no treatment—including salicylate—was effective in halting damage to the heart, or in combating chorea for that matter.[55] Poynton's colleague, David Lees, disagreed. Not only did he use salicylate, but he believed that it lessened heart disease.[56] Homer Swift used aspirin, but he was not convinced that it altered the course of heart disease.[57] Paul Dudley White also endorsed aspirin for fever and arthritis but withheld support of its effectiveness in heart damage.[58] All considered, leaders in the field used aspirin for patient comfort but doubted its help in preventing or repairing heart disease. One worker bucked the trend in an important way. Reginald Miller, a pharmacologist at St. Mary's Hospital, staked out a middle ground. He argued that the "all-or-nothing" question whether aspirin helped in heart disease might be phrased incorrectly. He argued that the timing of aspirin's use was important, advocating that aspirin be employed during active cardiac inflammation before permanent damage was done.[59]

One unsettled question in the aspirin debate was whether it was a "specific" drug for rheumatic fever (in the way that diphtheria antitoxin worked only against diphtheria) or a nonspecific drug that worked against many different causes of pain and fever. A related—and most important—question was whether a doctor should expect to treat all the manifestations of rheumatic fever with just one drug, or should give each element its own treatment. Thomas Maclagan had hoped that salicin was a "specific" for rheumatic fever, efficacious in treating the whole range of rheumatic complaints. Doubts over its effectiveness in heart disease soon undermined his wish.[60] And aspirin's prompt acceptance as the drug of choice for many illnesses indicated that it had efficacy far beyond rheumatic fever.

From the experimental laboratory came doubts that aspirin even helped in arthritis, contradicting a conclusion that clinicians had reached almost without dissent. David John Davis, a member of the Department of Experimental Medicine at the University of Illinois at Chicago, treated rabbits with aspirin after injecting them with various strains of streptococci. When the animals developed suppurative arthritis, he concluded that aspirin had little value. In his view, aspirin was a failed antibiotic.[61] His colleague Bernard Fantus accepted Davis's proposal that aspirin was a weakly antibacterial drug, but he criticized Davis for not using enough of the drug to suppress inflammation. He repeated the experiment using frequent doses of aspirin—much like clinicians when treating human patients—after injecting rabbits with *streptococcus pyogenes*. Despite the alteration in dosing, the rabbits received no protection from the development of suppurative arthritis.[62]

These experiments did not sit well with Homer Swift. He pointed out that the experimental method of producing arthritis with *streptococcus pyogenes* had been rejected by most other workers in the field. When Swift gave aspirin to animals in which he had induced arthritis with his usual method (intravenous injection or multiple subcutaneous injections with *streptococcus viridans*), he found that all joints suffered less inflammation. This finding suggested to Swift that the action of aspirin in rheumatic fever was to lessen the immunological response, or as he phrased it, to "depress the susceptibility of the animal to antigenic stimulus." This observation had clinical significance for Swift. He argued that doctors were stopping the use of aspirin too early, normally when the patient ceased complaining of joint symptoms. Swift speculated whether a more prudent policy would be to continue aspirin as long as the patient remained in an immunologically altered state.[63]

## Homer Swift's Management of Rheumatic Fever in the 1920s

In the early 1920s, Homer Swift emerged not only as a leading experimentalist in the field but also as a prominent clinician. Examination of his case reports yields clues about how practitioners managed patients who suffered from rheumatic fever. Diagnosis rested firmly on Cheadle's "various manifestations." The clinician in 1925 would invariably support the diagnosis with laboratory tests that were not available to Cheadle. Most patients received an electrocardiogram; serious cases had cultures taken of blood and joint fluid, and all had serial white blood cell counts. Therapy consisted of bed rest and aspirin. Swift advocated aspirin as a "specific" remedy in rheumatic fever. He noted that other antipyretics did not work as well in rheumatic fever and that other painkillers failed to provide the relief that aspirin provided. To Swift, aspirin was a special drug for the disease. To prevent relapses, Swift, despite evidence to the contrary from Johns Hopkins Hospital and Guy's Hospital, routinely sent his patients to a surgeon for tonsillectomy.

# Allergy, Heredity, Environment, and the Emergence of the Streptococcus, 1925–1945

⊹⊨

$B$y the early 1920s clinical and laboratory efforts to link rheumatic fever to bacterial sepsis had failed, a frustration that propelled researchers in other directions. Nevertheless, the conviction remained strong that some member of the streptococcus family was intimately involved with causing and transmitting the illness. In the interwar years four research strategies emerged, each with extensive historical roots and each with a recognized leader: bacterial allergy or hypersensitization (Homer F. Swift), heredity (May G. Wilson), environment (John R. Paul), and infection with Group A beta-hemolytic streptococcus (Alvin F. Coburn). Each camp had its articulate proponents, and, with much of the work carried out in New York City, each group intimately knew the achievements of the other researchers. Each camp soon recognized how difficult it was to sort out these closely related factors in human populations, a task confounded by the failure to find a suitable animal model. Those who argued for heredity, environment, allergy, and infection all conducted large, innovative clinical studies. Their special populations were normally drawn from heart clinics conducted at children's hospitals, or from that unfortunate subset of children who resided in convalescent homes established to provide extended care for youngsters recovering from a serious bout of rheumatic fever. Sorting out conflicting ideas often required researchers to leave the hospital setting and visit the patient's home or school.

The problem of sorting out infection, heredity, and environment was this: if two family members contracted rheumatic fever in the same house, was their common affliction the result of being related, of exposure to some environmental pollutant, of infection caused by a common germ, or of some combination of factors? At the beginning of this period, most researchers argued that some combination of factors led to rheumatic fever; by the end, infection with Group A beta-hemolytic streptococcus was clearly thought to be the trigger. But infection with the germ was not enough. Victims also required genetic susceptibility and appropriate living arrangements that enhanced the spread of the germ. As it turned out, the disease was not only a simple infection but also a cascade of immunological mischief that resulted in clinical signs and symptoms that doctors and patients recognized as rheumatic fever. A few short years later, in 1950, after the introduction of penicillin, many physicians focused their attention so tightly on the triggering germ that genetic and environmental factors slipped almost imperceptibly offstage.[1]

## Homer F. Swift and Hypersensitization

Assessing the array of views about the cause of rheumatic fever in 1925, Homer Swift was struck with the analogy he saw between rheumatic fever and tuberculosis and the later stages of syphilis. Both tuberculosis and syphilis were sparked by specific microorganisms, but significantly the real bodily damage came from the victim's immunological "overreaction" to the germs. For example, the cause of death in tuberculosis came not from the tubercle bacillus as such but from massive tubers replacing lung tissue that eroded into the lung's blood vessels, causing hemorrhage. Similarly, death from syphilis resulted not from the spirochete but from the victim's generation of gummas that wreaked havoc in the brain or aorta. For Swift, the examples of tuberculosis and syphilis provided the nidus around which the varied elements of rheumatic fever crystallized.[2] Heart disease, arthritis, chorea, rashes, and nodules were the result of not simply infection, but, rather, the body's "allergic" overreaction or "hypersensitization" to some provocation.[3]

For Swift, allergy solved several of rheumatic fever's puzzles. The development of an allergy took time, which accounted for the absence of rheumatic fever among infants and toddlers. The tendency of allergies to worsen over time helped to explain the nature of rheumatic fever to relapse. The affinity of some allergies for certain families accounted for the domestic pattern of rheumatic fever. The often-observed characteristic of allergies to worsen in specific surroundings provided Swift with an environmental link.[4] Sensitization over time to some member of the streptococcus family laid the groundwork; rheumatic fever then followed a subsequent specific infection.[5]

Swift's first task was to make laboratory animals hypersensitive to streptococci. Drawing upon his earlier experimental work, he employed the nonhemolytic streptococcus, or *streptococcus viridans.* Repeated inoculations, either subcutaneously or intravenously, over the course of days or weeks, produced animals that were acutely sensitive to further provocations with the streptococcus.[6] Swift then challenged the susceptible animals with a subcutaneous injection of *streptococcus viridans,* frequently producing a nonsuppurating arthritis, endocarditis, and myocarditis (although a different inflammatory pattern than the cardinal Aschoff body).[7] With a similar method, other researchers produced subcutaneous nodules.[8] Although Swift achieved considerable laboratory success with hypersensitization, he understood that the bacterium he used differed from the one associated with rheumatic fever in humans.

To Swift, desensitization offered a potential therapeutic strategy. To accomplish this, he "vaccinated" hypersensitized animals with intravenous doses of strep-tococci. When he did this, his laboratory animals lost their irritability to the strep-tococcus that previously resulted in arthritis and carditis.[9] The success of this line of experiment suggested immediate clinical value for patients. Homer Swift joined forces with May Wilson at the Heart Clinic of New York Nursery and Child's Hospital. They vaccinated 172 children with increasing doses of killed hemolytic strep-tococci in an effort to prevent relapses of rheumatic fever. Initial results looked promising, but careful analysis of outcomes over time showed no value to this therapy in human cases.[10] The failure of this line of experimentation had the incidental effect of convincing May Wilson, early in her career, that infection played only a small role in rheumatic fever, a conclusion that Swift never shared.

Skin testing was a time-honored means of demonstrating allergy. In this technique, a small amount of pulverized streptococci was injected under the skin. A person with prior sensitivity reacted dramatically with redness, swelling, and itching at the injection site. In 1929 Swift, Wilson, and E. W. Todd, who was then a fellow at Rockefeller University and would later gain fame for describing antistrep-tolysin, found that children with rheumatic fever reacted far more vigorously to skin tests with streptococci than did controls, an observation that was repeated over and over again.[11]

Swift's laboratory strove to attain the elusive goal of re-creating the Aschoff body in animals. Decades later, in the late 1940s, Swift and George Murphy revived Swift's method of sensitizing animals with repeated subcutaneous injections with streptococci. The heart lesions which they induced after World War II were the closest yet to the gold standard. A research team at Washington University improved on the results still further with sensitization produced by repeated pharyngeal applications of streptococci.[12]

By the time of these last myocardial experiments, Swift quickly conceded that rheumatic fever required a prior throat infection with Group A beta-hemolytic streptococcus. But he took issue with those who claimed that rheumatic fever was merely the aftermath of a sore throat. He noted that virtually all people were infected with streptococci at one time or another but that only some developed rheumatic fever—those, Swift believed, who had inherited the ability to overreact to streptococcal infections. Similarly he argued that the destructive means in which humans manifested the various symptoms of rheumatic fever were mediated through the allergic mechanisms he had outlined.[13]

## May G. Wilson and Heredity

The clustering of rheumatic fever in several members of the same family had raised issues of hereditary passage as early as the middle of the nineteenth century. In 1926 one study, summarizing several of the better previous works assessing heredity—those by Garrod, Cheadle, Coombs, and Faulkner and White—claimed that family members of a child with rheumatic fever had over twice the chance of coming down with the disease as selected control groups.[14] After World War I, the traditional method of enumerating additional afflicted family members through historical recollection and then comparing these memories with a control family gave way to newer methods that included longitudinal family studies—spanning decades—analyzed by statistical tools to assess the relevance of conclusions.

May Wilson, a physician at Nursery and Child's Heart Clinic (later the Department of Pediatrics at New York Hospital), pioneered prospective family studies in rheumatic fever in her quest to establish a genetic link. Intending to sort out heredity, environment, and communicability, Wilson, beginning in 1916, enrolled 112 "rheumatic" families with roughly 500 children. She followed many of them for decades. Her evaluations were frequent, often monthly, at home as well as in the hospital. Wilson explained that poor human memory necessitated prospective studies of entire families. In one early pilot series, only sixteen parents could recall whether they had suffered from rheumatic fever as children, while medical personnel could document the disease in an additional twenty-three. Good data, then, enhanced the genetic link. Wilson created a linear temporal chart for each family member that showed the coming and going of each of the most conspicuous of Cheadle's "various manifestations": arthritis, carditis, nodules, and chorea. She did not record episodes of colds, rashes, or tonsillitis because, Wilson argued, these minor illnesses occurred virtually all the time in children. Given the course of subsequent research on rheumatic fever that centered on throat infections with Group A beta-hemolytic streptococcus, this omission was regrettable. In essence, Wilson's nearly 600 charts followed in the graphical tradition of Cheadle's "series," now carried out in far greater detail.[15]

Illustration 2 gives a flavor of Wilson's achievement. This graph, one of hundreds, contains an enormous amount of information about twenty patients over twenty-five years, from onset of disease until death. Consider patient "F": She was initially hospitalized at four years of age with polyarthritis. She relapsed with chorea at five, six, and seven years. With this last bout of chorea, she suffered for the first time with mitral valve disease. At ten, she had another relapse with polyarthritis. At this point her heart disease worsened. At eleven, another relapse with chorea. At thirteen, she had chorea again, now accompanied by severe mitral valve stenosis. At fifteen, she relapsed still again with polyarthritis and chorea. The next year, another similar relapse, but this time she developed infectious endocarditis on her mitral valve and died shortly afterward.[16] Such charting gave a clear picture of chronic suffering. In other words, Wilson augmented Cheadle's ten series studying rheumatic fever in many children over a far longer period of time.

In New Haven, Connecticut, John R. Paul and Robert Salinger also began collecting life charts on the families of two hundred children with rheumatic fever seen in their cardiac clinic at Yale. Like Wilson, Paul and Salinger could depict in graphic detail that "acute" rheumatic fever was actually a chronic disease. With additional merit, they grouped all members of the same family living together in the same chart. Illustration 3a (key) and b portrays the experience of Family no. 12 with rheumatic fever. Note that illustration 3b provides forty years of data about both parents and four children. The "side-by-side" presentation allowed for striking observations. In early 1922, Lester, one of the children, was the first family

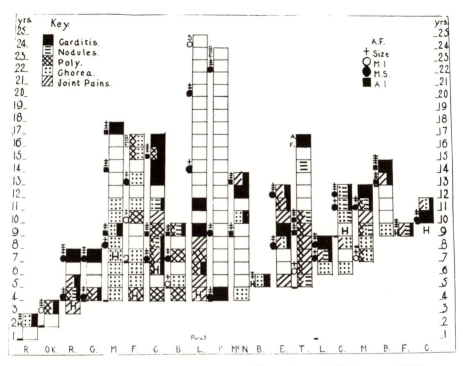

ILLUSTRATION 2. Family study. Reprinted from May Wilson, *Journal of Pediatrics* (1937), 10: 459. Reprinted with permission of Mosby, Inc., St. Louis, MO.

member with obvious signs of rheumatic fever. He suffered from arthritis, chorea, and the suspicion of heart disease. Shortly later, Pauline, his sister, developed definite carditis; Helen, a second sister, then developed arthritis, and Ola, the third sister, a case of chorea. Ola went on to experience three bouts of arthritis between 1924 and 1925, the last accompanied by heart disease, about the same time Helen endured another bout of arthritis.[17]

Wilson's painstaking collection of family data led her to conclude that heredity was the key factor in rheumatic fever. Despite frequent home visits, she could ferret out no common environmental influence. Her division of families into social groupings according to type of housing, clothing, quality of food, and warmth of maternal care failed to yield distinctions.[18] Wilson did not think that exposure to a family member with rheumatic fever resulted in added risk of developing either a first attack or a relapse in the remaining members. With hindsight, it is possible to see how she reached her conclusions. First, Wilson tracked only arthritis, carditis, chorea, and nodules. These afflictions could last months, and in the case of carditis, years. In other words, it was hard for her to sort out "active" from "inactive" phases of the disease; first attacks and relapses blended, obscuring periods of enhanced susceptibility. In Wilson's view, it was just as likely for a second

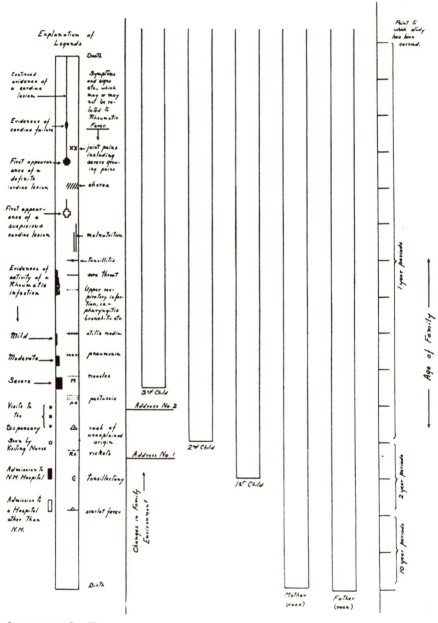

ILLUSTRATION 3a. Key

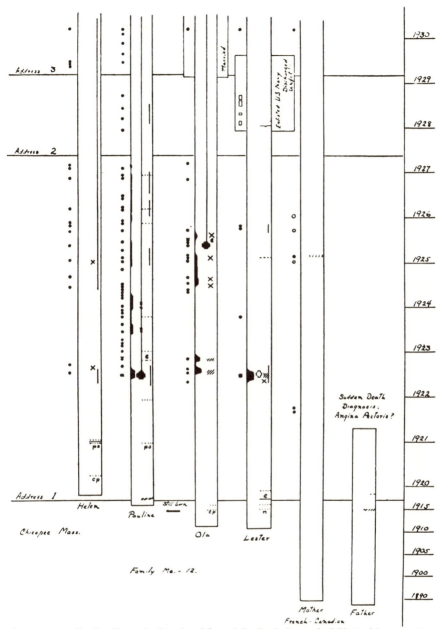

ILLUSTRATION 3b. Family study. Reprinted from John Paul, *Journal of Clinical Investigation* (1931), 10: 33–51. Reprinted with permission of The Rockefeller University Press, New York, NY.

family member to come down with rheumatic fever during the active or inactive phase of the illness. Second, she unfortunately abandoned one of Cheadle's manifestations, tonsillitis, electing not to culture for bacteria.[19] In so doing, Wilson overlooked streptococcal infections which placed family members at risk.

Wilson's genetic pedigrees pushed her to conclude that the expression of the disease followed a pattern that suggested autosomal recessive transmission. For example, if neither parent had ever contracted rheumatic fever, a child had a 40 percent chance of developing rheumatic fever; one parent with a history of the disease increased the risk to over 60 percent; two parents raised the risk to 100 percent.[20] So convinced was Wilson that heredity explained everything that she did not believe that any therapy was helpful: rheumatic fever ran its course benignly or malignantly depending on the genetic makeup of the individual. Studies with twins, a classic way to separate genetic from environmental influences, also seemed to support Wilson's claims. In her experience, identical twins shared similar histories: either both twins contracted rheumatic fever or neither twin did. Fraternal twins were as likely to have similar or dissimilar experiences.[21]

Wilson understood that her calculations did not jibe precisely with expected Mendelian distributions. Early in the 1940s, Wilson addressed this issue and improved still further on her predictive ability by adding the extra factor that risk of contracting rheumatic fever declined with age. Age-susceptibility plus autosomal recessive inheritance predicted the experience of her cohort of patients almost perfectly.[22]

May Wilson never shrank from her opinion that heredity held the key to transmission of rheumatic fever. Even after most researchers in the field believed that the Group A beta-hemolytic streptococcus was the instigator, Wilson demurred, most likely because of the design of her study, which omitted bacterial investigations, and because of her initial unsuccessful studies of streptococcal vaccines with Homer Swift. Others, however, appreciated that Wilson demonstrated how rheumatic fever struck some families but avoided others.[23]

### John R. Paul and the Environment

The special role of the environment intrigued workers during the interwar period. The environmental parameters most commonly explored were poverty, crowding, diet, geography, and dampness. John R. Paul, who played a leading role in family studies, was among the first to tackle the problem of poverty. Starting at home in New Haven, Paul identified Yale University undergraduate students who had evidence of residual rheumatic heart disease and then investigated the type of secondary school each had attended: private preparatory school or public high school. His assumption, of course, was that students attending private schools came from more privileged backgrounds. For his measure of rheumatic heart disease, Paul counted only heart murmurs, which signaled endocardial damage: injury to either mitral or aortic valves. What he found was that public high school graduates had more than twice the incidence of rheumatic heart disease. In a similar study, Paul found that Yale graduate students, who came from less wealthy backgrounds than undergraduates, demonstrated about one and one-half times more rheumatic heart disease.[24] Care should be taken in evaluating these studies, because Paul used endocardial damage as his measure of heart disease in a period when myocardial damage was emerging. Paul understood this limitation, but he argued that it was far easier to appreciate endocardial damage in the setting of a high school or college student health clinic.

Paul next turned his attention to schoolchildren in New Haven, comparing the rates of rheumatic heart disease among those who attended "better," or private, schools and "poorer," or public, schools. Again his yardstick for rheumatic heart disease was "organic-sounding" heart murmurs—endocardial not myocardial findings. Paul found that public school children had one and one-half as many heart murmurs as those attending private schools. From these studies, Paul concluded that poverty most likely was a factor in the expression of rheumatic heart disease.[25] In neither investigation did Paul actually obtain financial data from the students, relying instead on school enrollment as the measure of the families' wealth. A house-to-house survey, which he published in 1940, reinforced Paul's view that poverty played a role.[26]

In Bristol, England, G. H. Daniel attempted to assay the influence of family income on the prevalence of rheumatic fever. His results were striking: families earning twice the income necessary to cover "minimal" needs suffered half the incidence of rheumatic fever. In addition to earnings, Daniel thought crowding, another measure of poverty, was a critical determinant in its own right. He found that Bristol families living in flats with one room per person had twice the incidence of rheumatic fever of families living in larger apartments. Of note, Daniel did not measure actual area or volume of living space.[27]

The collected wisdom of workers in the field held that people living in cities were more likely to succumb to rheumatic fever. Sorting out the ingredients that accompanied urban life—poverty, crowding, malnutrition, garbage, sewage, air pollution—proved difficult.[28] Arnold and Bernice Wedum chose Cincinnati to sift through some of the variables. The Wedums began by locating on a city map the home of every person admitted to a hospital with rheumatic fever. Once the locations were pinpointed, they analyzed rents, race, and crowding. Only crowding passed the statistical test.[29] In Iowa, the Crippled Children's Rheumatic Fever Program was so convinced that packed environments enhanced the spread of rheumatic fever that managers budgeted extra funds to provide each convalescing child with her own room.[30]

Were specific locations within a city more likely to bolster rheumatic fever? The traditional view, of course, was that rheumatic fever followed exposure to cold and damp places. In Birmingham, England, A. P. Thomson mapped the location of eight hundred people with rheumatic fever. Like the Wedums, Thomson found that most cases occurred in the densest ward of the city. Within these packed areas, the greatest proportion of cases occurred in families living closest to the rivers. This suggested to Thomson that cold and dampness were additional factors.[31] Illustration 4 details a similar set of observations for Philadelphia in the early 1930s. Reviving views that August Hirsch and Arthur Newsholme had

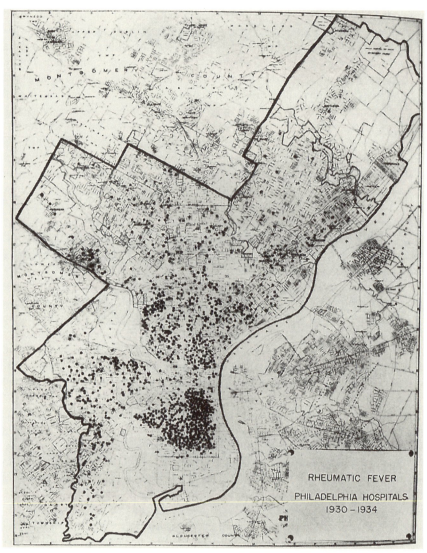

ILLUSTRATION 4.  Home location at time of death of 603 fatal cases of rheumatic fever admitted to Philadelphia hospitals from January 1, 1930, to December 31, 1934. Reprinted from *Public Health Reports* (1940), 55: opp. p. 1859.

explored at the end of the nineteenth century, Matthew Young found that a cold and wet climate did predict the onset of rheumatic fever for England and Wales.[32] In contrast, Theodore Thompson and M. Greenwood analyzed admission statistics at London Hospital for the years 1873 to 1903. They found that rain, low barometric pressure, and colder temperatures predicted most, but not every, admission for rheumatic fever, a conclusion that squared with Newsholme's observations.[33] In 1924 James Faulkner and Paul Dudley White extended the analysis globally, gathering published statistics from twenty-eight hospitals around the world. Those with the coldest and wettest climates reported the most rheumatic fever.[34]

Geography also appeared to play a role. Faulkner and White demonstrated that a gradient of hospital admissions existed, with northern hospitals hosting more patients with rheumatic fever than southern hospitals.[35] Tinsley Harrison and S. A. Levine confirmed this geographic variation. They found that Peter Bent Brigham Hospital in Boston had twice the rate of admissions for rheumatic fever when compared with Johns Hopkins Hospital in Baltimore and six times the rate at Charity Hospital in New Orleans.[36] These and other studies in 1924 convinced Frederick Poynton, the champion of his "diplococcus rheumaticus" for a quarter century, to conclude that climate, environment, and geography had to be taken into account in the epidemiological expression of the disease.[37]

When John Paul began his investigations, the conventional view of the role of geography was that the prevalence of rheumatic fever increased as one moved toward either pole. The Wedums investigated the common wisdom with a comparison of Cincinnati and Philadelphia. Their hypothesis was that these cities—both at 39 degrees latitude, with similar climates, both located along rivers, with roughly the same economic and racial mix—would have virtually the same experience with rheumatic fever. Indeed this proved to be the case.[38] From Australia and New Zealand came analysis that confirmed a striking differential in mortality from rheumatic fever as one moved toward the southern pole.[39] A survey from twenty-four hospitals in the United States and Canada confirmed that hospital admissions for rheumatic fever declined as one migrated south.[40] So rare was rheumatic fever in Florida that several investigators claimed that they could scarcely find mention of it from records of hospital admissions, autopsy reports, or state death certificates.[41] A comparison of hospital admissions between San Francisco and Los Angeles confirmed the geographical bias: San Francisco hospitals reported an astonishing seven times as many admissions as hospitals in Los Angeles.[42]

John Paul conducted the most sophisticated geographical study. He compared the incidence of rheumatic heart disease among American Indians living in different locations. He chose Native Americans because of the close genetic similarities among Indian groups and because living conditions, while poor, were uniformly so. Thus he controlled for hereditary and environmental factors. Paul found that there was an increasing gradient of rheumatic heart disease from south to north.[43]

When August Hirsch surveyed rheumatic fever and geography in 1886, he had concluded that rheumatic fever could exist anywhere, but that it was rare in the Tropics. Some later observers were more emphatic. In an analysis of the tropical regions of Africa, the South Pacific, and Central America, J. Tertius Clarke found virtually no report of rheumatic fever, mitral stenosis, or chorea.[44] Some claimed that rheumatic fever simply did not exist in Puerto Rico.[45] More careful studies—some based for the first time on autopsy data or on admissions to European- or American-run hospitals in the Tropics—tended to support Hirsch's original conclusion. At the Hospital San Juan de Dios in Costa Rica, there were 22 bona fide admissions for rheumatic fever (out of a total of 3,771 admissions); a survey of 1,000 autopsies showed about 1 percent with mitral or aortic valve disease.[46]

Reports from Curaçao, New Guinea, Mexico, and Panama demonstrated a small number of documented cases in the Tropics.[47]

Taken together, these studies indicated that geography had a part to play in the expression of rheumatic fever, but the part was not fleshed out until the Group A beta-hemolytic streptococcus assumed its starring role.

Just how to sort out environment from heredity was a difficult problem in human disease with so many variables to control. At Johns Hopkins, Ross Gauld and Frances Read, after affirming May Wilson's genetic link, set out to see whether there was an additional environmental connection. In their view, a disease solely influenced by heredity would have a random temporal sequence, but a disease influenced by surroundings would cluster around the environmental precipitant. With this in mind, they looked at the pattern of cases in their heart clinic at the Harriet Lane Home. They found that the rate of cases doubled in families after an acute case of rheumatic fever occurred—an observation that conflicted with May Wilson's work—thus suggesting to them that there was an environmental influence, an observation that bore fruit with the enthroning of the Group A beta-hemolytic streptococcus.[48]

## Infection

Despite the careful refutation of the sepsis model, many prominent researchers persisted in the view that rheumatic fever was a type of blood-borne infection. As late as 1928 James Small of Philadelphia, in a manner reminiscent of Poynton and Paine nearly three decades earlier, obtained blood cultures from patients with rheumatic fever, and he identified a nonhemolytic streptococcus that he picturesquely called "streptococcus cardioarthritidis."[49] Injecting this germ into animals produced arthritis and myocarditis. In a remarkable series of cases, Small found that injecting antiserum to this bacteria into the victims of rheumatic fever seemed to lessen symptoms. Contemporary observers did not know what to make of these seemingly careful experiments. Hans Zinnser, a renowned bacteriologist, noted that earlier attempts along analogous lines by Poynton and Paine had generally been refuted.[50] With the benefit of hindsight, it is certain that Small repeated Poynton and Paine's error of culturing only the sickest patients, those with infectious endocarditis. That this older notion, thoroughly disproved more than a decade earlier, could be revived in the late 1920s, gives credence to the power of the idea. Even a scientist as prominent as Russell Cecil of Cornell as late as 1942 was still obtaining blood cultures in the hope of identifying the bacterial culprit.[51]

The science of bacteriology had changed drastically since the days of Poynton, Paine, and Rufus Cole at the turn of the century. In just the world of the streptococcus, scientists in 1930 recognized thirty-five separate species divided by differences in morphology, staining characteristics, and chemistry. Bacteriologists understood that various species of streptococcus were found on bodily surfaces, inside and out, of many animals, including mice, guinea pigs, rabbits, cats, and chickens. But in only a few instances did the presence of streptococci result in disease. In humans, most disease was caused by streptococci that produced beta-

TABLE 6.1   *Results of bacterial culture of surgically removed tonsils*

|  | Rheumatic fever | Controls |
|---|---|---|
| Number | 50 | 48 |
| Hemolytic streptococci | 14% | 14% |
| Nonhemolytic streptococci | 86% | 86% |

SOURCE: David Nabarro and R. A. MacDonald, "Bacteriology of the Tonsils in Relation to Rheumatism in Children," *British Medical Journal* (1929), 2: 758–759.

hemolysis on blood agar plates in the laboratory, for example, scarlet fever, puerperal fever, erysipelas and subsequent skin abscesses, and respiratory tract diseases such as otitis media, sinusitis, mastoiditis, and septic sore throat (pharyngitis).[52] Rebecca Lancefield further divided the streptococci into groups—according to differing polysaccharides in the bacterial cell wall—with Group A receiving the designation for streptococci responsible for human disease.[53] The complete designation of the germ responsible for human disease thus became *Group A b*eta-hemolytic *s*treptococcus, often abbreviated in scientific publications as GABS. A decade later, Lancefield further subdivided Group A streptococci into types, based upon the existence of proteins in the cell wall, designated M proteins, because of the ability to produce mucoid colonies on agar plates.[54]

Walter Cheadle had affirmed that inflamed tonsils were a cardinal manifestation of rheumatic fever. The tonsils, it turned out, were normally loaded with many different types of bacteria, including several kinds of streptococci. The question posed to physicians: was a germ isolated from the throat a normal resident, a regular occupant turned suddenly pathogenic, or a nonresident invading to cause illness? By the twenties, many researchers believed that the hemolytic streptococcus was somehow related to rheumatic fever. Into this certainty came a somewhat puzzling bacterial analysis of tonsils removed from patients with rheumatic fever compared with patients who had tonsils removed for other reasons (table 6.1). One reading of these data argued that streptococci of any kind were of no importance. Another interpretation was that the hemolytic streptococcus infected the entire population similarly but that it triggered rheumatic fever only in certain people. This latter reading would strengthen May Wilson's view of the importance of heredity or John Paul's on environment. What was particularly striking was that so few patients with active rheumatic fever had hemolytic streptococci cultured from their tonsils.[55]

Proving that the hemolytic streptococcus was essential to the development of rheumatic fever, in the absence of an experimental animal model, would have to rely on circumstantial evidence.[56] Although researchers in the bacteriological laboratory had been unable to cement the relationship between any member of the streptococcus family and rheumatic fever, epidemiologists were reaching the conclusion that a throat infection with the hemolytic-streptococcus preceded rheumatic

TABLE 6.2    *Analysis of throat cultures during 1928 epidemic*

| | |
|---|---|
| Relapse AND hemolytic streptococci | 11 |
| Relapse WITHOUT hemolytic streptococci | 1 |
| No Relapse AND hemolytic streptococci | 16 |
| No Relapse WITHOUT hemolytic streptococci | 9 |

SOURCE: Alvin F. Coburn, *The Factor of Infection in the Rheumatic State* (Baltimore: Williams and Wilkins, 1931), 195.

fever. In 1923 Arthur Bloomfield, then on the faculty of Johns Hopkins Medical School,[57] and Augustus Felty demonstrated that *streptococcus pyogenes* was often responsible for human tonsillitis.[58] Alison Glover, who served in the Epidemiology Branch of the British Ministry of Health between 1920 and 1934 before moving to the Board of Education where he would later document the accelerating decline of rheumatic fever, offered an additional clue. In army barracks and boarding schools, Glover observed that rheumatic fever followed tonsillitis roughly two weeks later in a pattern very similar to the way that meningococcal meningitis followed upper respiratory illnesses. This comparison suggested to Glover that coughing and sneezing spread rheumatic fever through droplets.[59] In 1931, W.R.F. Collis claimed that over one-half of children admitted with rheumatic fever to the Hospital for Sick Children, Great Ormond Street, had *streptococcus pyogenes* cultured from their throats. Additionally, Collis reported that nine of eleven children who suffered relapses had contracted a streptococcal sore throat about ten days earlier.[60]

## Alvin Coburn, Group A Beta-Hemolytic Streptococcus, and Rheumatic Fever

Alvin Coburn, physician at Presbyterian Hospital in New York City, cemented the relationship between the hemolytic streptococcus and rheumatic fever in a fashion that stuck. Coburn began his studies with a bow to Cheadle.[61] Sensing the continuing power of the sepsis model, Coburn consulted the extensive case records at Presbyterian Hospital to add yet another refutation of this discredited idea. Reviewing the charts of 463 patients on medical wards who had blood cultures drawn that grew bacteria, Coburn found that physicians had isolated fifteen different species of bacteria. Close reading of the charts demonstrated that no patient suffered with the symptoms of acute rheumatic fever.[62] In Coburn's view, the scientific reports that claimed a role for the nonhemolytic streptococcus "represent[ed] only an accidental implantation of this organism in the endocardium."[63]

Coburn's evidence justifying the pivotal role of the Group A beta-hemolytic streptococcus came from four sets of observations. Student nurses provided the initial set of data. Coburn understood that student nurses were exposed to much illness and that many fell sick during their years of training. Beginning in 1928, he followed a cohort of student nurses and found that upper respiratory tract illnesses (tonsillitis, pharyngitis, sinusitis, otitis media, and mastoiditis) accounted for more than one-half of all disability. In this particular year, nearly 10 percent of the class developed rheumatic fever, each after suffering an upper respiratory tract infection.[64] In all but two cases, Coburn was able to culture the Group A beta-hemolytic streptococcus from the pharynx or nose of the students.[65]

A second set of data came from studying relapses in children convalescing from serious bouts of rheumatic fever at the Pelham Home. For over a year, Coburn cultured the throats of all patients frequently, observing the changing patterns of mouth flora at the hospital. In December 1928 an epidemic of relapses of rheumatic fever occurred (table 6.2). Striking was the susceptibility of these children to streptococcal outbreaks. Intriguing was the observation that infected children did not automatically relapse. Inescapable was that infection preceded relapse.[66]

The third set of data came from the experience of chronically relapsing patients who were sent to Puerto Rico in the hope that a change in environment would interrupt the downhill course of the disease. The selection of Puerto Rico stemmed from the repeated observation that rheumatic fever scarcely occurred on the tropical island. In New York City, all selected patients were sick with rheumatic fever; in San Juan all improved. When they returned to New York City, nearly all sickened immediately. In analyzing the throat cultures from this unfortunate group, Coburn found that eight of eleven had Group A beta-hemolytic streptococcus in their throats when they left New York. In Puerto Rico, the throat flora changed dramatically so that only one child had persistent streptococcus. When the group returned to New York City, nearly all were recolonized with Group A beta-hemolytic streptococci, some in fewer than twenty-four hours.[67] This observation had key geographical implications: the geography of rheumatic fever coincided precisely with the geography of streptococcal infection.

Coburn drew the fourth set of data from the results of Homer Swift and others in skin testing patients with various components of the streptococcus. Sufferers of rheumatic fever mounted the most dramatic skin responses, suggesting to Coburn a peculiar sensitivity to the streptococcus.[68] Swift and his colleague Charles H. Hitchcock added further evidence by demonstrating that fluids from the joints, pleurae, and pericardia of patients with rheumatic fever contained a substance that clumped Group A beta-hemolytic streptococci, implying an immunological connection.[69]

Summing up these four lines of evidence, Coburn believed he had shown that the Group A beta-hemolytic streptococcus acted as a stimulus for rheumatic fever. He realized that the evidence was all circumstantial, but he argued that in the absence of an animal model or more precise immunological markers for streptococcal infection—one was to come within the year—this proof would have to suffice.[70] In clear recognition of other workers in the field, Coburn concluded that "at least these four patient factors—susceptibility, age, environment, and infection" were imperative to the development of rheumatic fever.[71] No less important was the "silent" period of several weeks that followed infection. During the next decade, researchers placed considerable attention on just what happened during the time between infection and the unfolding of symptoms.[72]

Support for Coburn's streptococcal hypothesis came from a number of sources. A streptococcal epidemic on a convalescent ward in England provided an opportunity to check the linkage between throat infection and relapse. Careful bacteriological investigation demonstrated that of thirty-two children with hemolytic streptococcal pharyngitis, twenty-four experienced a relapse about two weeks after the throat infection. All of the children on the convalescent ward demonstrated marked sensitivity to skin testing with streptococcal exotoxins, suggesting a particular receptiveness to streptococcal infection.[73] In similar studies from Cambridge and Edinburgh, physicians concluded that relapses could not occur without a preceding infection with hemolytic streptococcus. As with the experience at other hospitals, infection did not automatically lead to relapse; rather, it was a precondition to relapse for a sizable proportion of vulnerable children.[74] From the Illinois Soldiers' and Sailors' Children's School came another confirmation. An epidemic of streptococcal disease infected 241 of 501 students. Eighty-eight subsequently developed acute rheumatic fever.[75]

In 1932, E. W. Todd provided Coburn with an immunological confirmation of streptococcal infection. To back up a moment, until then physicians could document a streptococcal throat infection only by culturing the tonsils and then identifying the beta-hemolytic streptococcus from the array of bacteria that grew out on a blood agar plate. It was a painstaking process and very unlike the "rapid" enzyme analysis that patients have come to expect in the doctor's office in recent years. In 1930 throat culturing was largely a test available for clinical use in only a few hospitals. It had a serious limitation for aid in rheumatic fever. The culture was only of value if the streptococcus still resided on the tonsils. If the body had cleared the germ through its own immunological surveillance, the culture would not grow streptococci and the physician would not know that the suspected streptococcus had recently been present. What Todd described was a substance in the blood, antistreptolysin, that greatly increased after a hemolytic streptococcal infection. The streptococcus could be gone from the tonsils, but antistreptolysin remained in the blood. In the usual scheme of events with rheumatic fever, the patient sought out a doctor when afflicted with the symptoms of arthritis, chorea, rash, or carditis—weeks after the preceding throat infection. A simple culture would frequently fail to yield streptococci. In contrast, Todd's antistreptolysin demonstrated the recent infection. Antistreptolysin, of course, was not a means of diagnosing rheumatic fever; that remained a task based on symptoms. But antistreptolysin provided a crucial constituent of the glue that cemented the preceding streptococcal infection with the subsequent disease.[76]

Confirmation of the value of antistreptolysin came over the next several years. As with any test, normal values needed to be ascertained; investigators had to be assured that the test was accurate only in hemolytic streptococcal infections; rapid and reliable means needed to be developed for clinical application. Alvin Coburn was quick to seize upon the test's worth as a reliable way to document recent streptococcal disease. For Coburn, antistreptolysin took on an added meaning. A simple tonsillar culture indicated only that streptococci resided in the throat. Antistreptolysin indicated that the body was reacting, perhaps even overreacting, to the presence of streptococci.[77] Working together, Todd and Coburn came to understand that there were two components to antistreptolysin: "O" that was sensitive to oxygen, and "S" that was soluble in serum. Only antistreptolysin O, or "ASO" as it quickly became known, proved serviceable clinically.[78]

Other immunological markers followed. Cultures of hemolytic streptococci are able to lyse, or dissolve, a fibrin clot. The serum from patients with recent hemolytic streptococcal infection contains a substance that blocks this lysis. Detection of "streptococcal antifibrinolysin" was both an indication of recent infection and a demonstration that the body was reacting, maybe overreacting in Coburn's view, to the infection. Unlike the ASO titer, antifibrinolysin remained largely a research tool.[79] Homer Swift investigated the reaction to specific hemolytic streptococcal "M" proteins, demonstrating a precipitin reaction in the serum of patients with rheumatic fever. "M" proteins also served as a provocative skin test of streptococcal reactivity.[80] Years later, after World War II, another substance, antihyaluronidase, was also found in the serum of patients after streptococcal infection, serving as an additional marker of bodily response.[81] In 1941 T. Duckett Jones, who would be at the center of the study of rheumatic fever in the forties, sorted out the clinical merit of the several immunological indicators of streptococcal infection among Boston clinic patients and residents of the House of the Good Samaritan. For Jones, the antistreptolysin O titer proved most useful in the clinical setting.[82]

Another laboratory test that was making headway as a clinical tool, the erythrocyte sedimentation rate, found its way into the assessment of patients with rheumatic fever. Originally described in 1918, the erythrocyte sedimentation rate, often shortened to sedimentation rate or ESR, measured the gradual settling of red blood cells which occurs in an undisturbed sample of whole blood. In diseases marked by considerable inflammation, such as rheumatic fever, the rate of sinking is increased: the more "active" the disease, the higher rate of fall of the red blood cells. An elevated sedimentation rate was a rough indication of an active inflammatory response. Like the measurement of temperature, the sedimentation rate did not single out the cause of illness, only serving as a guide to current disease.[83] In rheumatic fever, the sedimentation rate was greatly raised during the symptomatic phase of the illness, gradually returning to normal as the patient recovered.[84] Like others, Alvin Coburn quickly grasped the value of the new test for rheumatic fever, but for him, the sedimentation rate took on added significance. Coburn interpreted the sedimentation rate to be an indicator of the body's exaggerated reactivity following a hemolytic streptococcal infection, in essence a laboratory summation of the various immunological repercussions. Coburn thought the sedimentation rate could serve as a critical guide to the period of vulnerability of the heart in rheumatic fever, and he thought it crucial in determining the length of any treatment.[85]

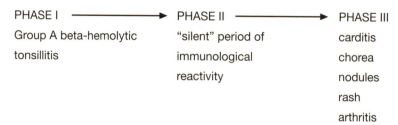

FIGURE 6.1. Coburn's theory of rheumatic fever

In the mid-thirties, Coburn formulated a model of the pathogenesis of rheumatic fever that took into account much of the research since World War I. In doing so, he incorporated the emerging immunology of the streptococcus. For Coburn, these streptococcal markers were both diagnostic tools and potential pathological agents. He speculated that these antibodies, such as antistreptolysin, were somehow responsible for damaging the heart, inducing chorea, or producing arthritis. What Coburn hypothesized was an illness in three phases.

*Phase I* consisted of a relatively innocuous upper respiratory infection with beta-hemolytic streptococcus, now more precisely identified as a member of Lancefield Group A.

*Phase II* was the "silent" period of about two weeks during which the body mounted an immunological response characterized by the rise of antistreptolysin O and S in the serum, the appearance of precipitin to the M protein, the ability to react to various streptococcal skin tests, and the elevation of the sedimentation rate.

*Phase III* was Cheadle's "various manifestations," with one exception. Tonsillitis was now limited to throat disease produced by GABS (figure 6.1).[86]

A further piece of evidence strengthening the streptococcal connection was the response of patients to antibiotics. Very shortly after the introduction of sulfonamide, several attempts were made to see whether this drug would halt the symptoms of rheumatic fever. While much controversy came in interpreting the results of these early tests, most researchers were disappointed that sulfonamide did not abort rheumatic fever once the streptococcal illness had commenced. Despite this initial failure, researchers pressed on, led by Coburn and Caroline Bedell Thomas at Johns Hopkins. They developed a more fruitful line of research, the daily use of sulfonamide to prevent relapses in hospitalized children. These experiments with prophylaxis were clouded with controversy—over study designs, side effects of the drug—but the conclusion reached was that sulfonamide worked to prevent relapses by eradicating streptococci from the pharynx. The antibiotic trickle of the thirties became a flood during the war.[87]

## Conclusion

Looking back at research during the interwar years, John R. Paul, champion for environmental influences, concluded in 1943 that "the circumstances under which rheumatic fever occurs are similar to the circumstances under which streptococcal infection occurs; the similarity is due to a common cause."[88] This contrasted sharply from the judgment he had reached in 1930: "We do not know the causative agent for rheumatic fever."[89] For Paul, the geographical, climatic, and social dimensions of rheumatic fever had become aspects of the ecology of streptococcal infections. Rheumatic fever occurred in cold, wet, crowded, northern regions, because these were the environments preferred by the Group A beta-hemolytic streptococcus. Drawing on a metaphor fit for a world on the brink of another war, Homer Swift agreed. The Group A beta-hemolytic streptococcus was the "detonator" that led to rheumatic explosion.[90] Swift's choice of metaphor was apt: a detonator was not the same as a bomb; the streptococcus required proper powder and shot to wreak its damage.

Paul and Swift joined all prominent workers in the field in drawing elements from each of the lines of research in explaining rheumatic fever. As early as 1925, Homer Swift suggested that heredity, environment, and infection were crucial. Given these prerequisites, Swift believed that an allergic overreaction best explained the disease.[91] Frustrated by his inability to produce rheumatic fever in animals, Swift thought the key might lie with careful analogy to syphilis and tuberculosis.[92] But rheumatic fever differed in key respects. Of these, the most important was that the streptococcus could not be found at the site of inflammation, unlike the mycobacterium in tuberculosis or the spirochete in syphilis. Rather, the streptococcus provoked the body to overreact. Shortly after Coburn put forth his scheme, T. Duckett Jones accepted his hypothesis. Yet Jones was convinced that environment and heredity also played important roles, largely because only a few people who suffered the commonplace infection with Group A beta-hemolytic streptococcus later developed rheumatic fever.[93] May Wilson convinced John Paul that heredity was crucial in determining who would react to the streptococcus, which for him became the key environmental determinant. The hemolytic streptococcus flourished in crowded, cold, and wet environments. With this understanding, Paul also accepted Coburn's synthesis.[94] Coburn, too, saw the merit of other positions. In 1943 he argued that to contract rheumatic fever one had to be a member of the population with a genetic vulnerability (about 5 per cent of the population, according to May Wilson), be living in a conducive environment, and be infected with Group A beta-hemolytic streptococci. What genetic susceptibility entailed was the capacity to produce a destructive immunological response.[95]

# PART III

# The Disappearance of Rheumatic Fever in the Twentieth Century

*I*n the twentieth century, biological changes drove rheumatic fever into extinction. Each element of the illness—chorea, heart disease, arthritis, rashes, and nodules—lessened in severity and eventually disappeared. Before extinction occurred, the amelioration of symptoms greatly lessened mortality, but—in permitting victims to live longer, if handicapped, existences—rheumatic fever paradoxically evolved into a chronic disease.

Biological disappearance did not signify that physicians and public health workers simply sat on their hands and watched rheumatic fever vanish. With gusto, they attacked the streptococcal "detonator" first with sulfonamide and later, more effectively, with penicillin. Physicians redefined a streptococcal sore throat from a benign experience of childhood into a menace, and public health officials mounted massive programs targeting the detection and treatment of streptococcal illness. For those who still contracted rheumatic fever, doctors employed powerful new drugs aimed at preventing permanent injury to the heart, and surgeons developed operations to repair or replace damaged heart valves.

Clinical zeal did not obscure that rheumatic fever was a rapidly evolving disease. Insights gained from the emerging science of molecular biology—years after rheumatic fever ceased to be a major plague—pointed to the fluid structural makeup of the streptococcus as the prime reason for the disappearance of the disease. To be sure, the efforts of physicians to detect, prevent, and treat streptococcal infections benefited patients, but the streptococcus had changed so drastically that even untreated children rarely suffered from rheumatic fever.

## CHAPTER 7

# *From Acute to Chronic, 1925–1945*

*W*hat strikes the historian's eye about rheumatic fever between 1925 and 1945 is that the disease nearly vanished (illustration 5). Once part of every physician's practice—in the office or hospital—rheumatic fever declined at an astonishing rate. Shifts in the incidence of a disease can often be appreciated only with the benefit of hindsight. In the case of rheumatic fever, the decline was sufficiently rapid that all students of the disease were vitally aware of its disappearance while it occurred. Only in children did new cases of rheumatic fever remain a significant problem. In the pediatrician's office or on the children's hospital ward, one could still find a fair number of patients with rheumatic fever. Even in these settings, the prevalence was much less than in prior decades.

As the number of new sufferers from rheumatic fever diminished, physicians realized more than ever that what was important about this disease was the permanent damage left on its declining number of victims. These between-the-wars years saw rheumatic fever emerge as a "chronic" illness, specifically "chronic rheumatic heart disease," continuing emphasis on the heart as the most prognostically significant aspect of the disease. "Acute" returned to rheumatic fever's lexicon, now limited to initial bouts with the disease. In part this shift in emphasis from "acute" to "chronic" stemmed from the publication of excellent longitudinal, community-based studies: May G. Wilson's study in New York City, John R. Paul's in New Haven, and O. F. Hedley's in Philadelphia. To be fair, these studies painted a picture of exacerbations and remissions in patients that ran in some cases a course of decades. But the dramatic, acute aspects of this illness—whether on initial presentation or on relapse—took a back seat to the chronic damage. New questions about the nature of the heart injury in rheumatic fever also helped to shift attention toward the permanent aspects of the disease. In the nineteenth century, most victims had died shortly after contracting the disease or just after a relapse, most often as a result of pericarditis or endocarditis. In the twentieth century, most who died from rheumatic fever succumbed to congestive heart failure—a myocardial

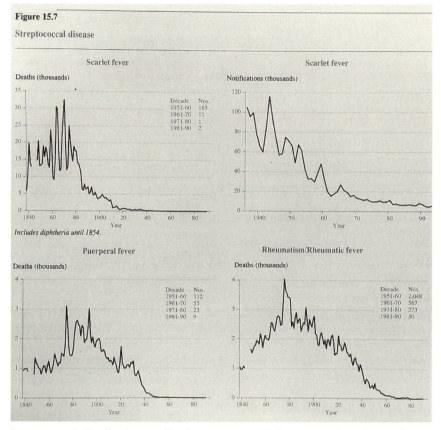

ILLUSTRATION 5. Decline in mortality from streptococcal disease. Reprinted from Office of National Statistics, *The Health of Adult Britain 1841–1994,* vol. 2 (London: Stationery Office, 1997), figure 15.7.

problem—that came decades after the first attack. One British physician observed: "We are now inclined to consider [rheumatic fever] rather as a chronic disease with acute exacerbations than as the reverse."[1]

Between the world wars, physicians attempted to put rheumatic fever on the public health agenda of Britain and the United States. To some extent, the appreciation that rheumatic fever was now a chronic disease forced it on public health officers. An illness that affected 2 percent of all children and that required, by one estimate, one rehabilitation bed for every 550 children necessitated planning and the marshaling of resources by professional and governmental bodies. Comparative studies, pitting rheumatic fever's morbidity and mortality against other recognized public health menaces, clearly showed that rheumatic fever led all but tuberculosis and perhaps pneumonia as infections confronting the nation's health. The irony, of course, was that rheumatic fever achieved the "status" of a public health problem precisely when its acute phase was about to become extinct.

Problems with health statistics tended to camouflage the decline of rheumatic fever. Only after 1920 did the U.S. Census create a special category for "rheumatic fever," replacing the older "acute articular rheumatism." Even in more medically sophisticated circles, the shift to modern nomenclature came relatively late. For example, *Index Medicus* shifted to "rheumatic fever" from "rheumatism" in 1903.[2] As late as the 1930s, epidemiologists complained that American statistics obscured trends because deaths from heart diseases were listed by tissue type (pericardium, endocardium, and myocardium) instead of by etiology. There were suspicions that all appropriate deaths were not being attributed to rheumatic fever. For example, a patient might die from infectious endocarditis or from congestive heart failure decades after a bout with rheumatic fever. In the manner that statistics were kept, this death almost certainly would not be listed under rheumatic fever. Deaths where rheumatic fever played a significant, but temporally distant, role thus tended to get lost.[3] In spite of such difficulties, physicians could still conclude that rheumatic fever remained a serious health problem. In 1925 one estimate was that 30,000 people died each year from rheumatic heart disease in England and Wales alone.[4]

## Rheumatic Fever Declines in Mortality and Morbidity

Nearly all epidemiologists believed that rheumatic fever was declining both in incidence and in its ability to provoke injury to any cardiac tissue. These observations had been lurking for years. In the same year as Cheadle's lectures, W. S. Church at St. Bartholomew's Hospital claimed, "I have for some years had the impression that acute rheumatism, as we meet it now in hospital practice, is less severe and less frequently accompanied by pericarditis than it was twenty years ago."[5] Church compared his experience with that of Philip Pye-Smith from Guy's Hospital, published in 1871. Ten percent of Church's patients developed pericarditis (compared with 24 percent for Pye-Smith); just over 1 percent of Church's patients died (compared with nearly 5 percent for Pye-Smith). Thomas McCrae, analyzing the experience at Johns Hopkins Hospital in 1903, noted that 2 percent of all admissions were attributed to rheumatic fever, confirming his suspicion that rheumatic fever was a less common reason for hospitalization in Baltimore than in London. Similar admission statistics for St. Thomas's Hospital showed over 5 percent due to rheumatic fever; at St. Bartholomew's Hospital the number was 4 percent.[6]

When Alexander Lambert returned to Bellevue Hospital in New York City after a stint in the U.S. Army in World War I, he "was struck by the fact that there were no cases of acute rheumatism on the service." He reviewed admissions at Bellevue from 1906 to 1919 and demonstrated a steady drop from 2.5 percent in 1907 to 0.5 percent in 1919.[7] Reginald Atwater carefully evaluated American trends in 1927. He claimed that the rate of contracting rheumatic fever had fallen from over 9 per 100,000 in 1907 to 3 per 100,000 twenty years later, matching a similar drop in Britain. Atwater noted that the plunge paralleled declines in the incidence of erysipelas, scarlet fever, and childbed fever, other streptococcus-related illnesses. He counted 157,000 American deaths from rheumatic fever in 1923 compared with

Table 7.1    *Mortality from rheumatic fever in England and Wales*

| Year | Deaths/100,000 population/year |
|------|--------------------------------|
| 1852–1892 (40-year average) | 8.7 |
| 1901 | 6.7 |
| 1913 | 4.8 |
| War years | 5.6–6.0 |
| 1919 | 4.2 |
| 1928 | 3.8 |
| 1937 | 2.2 |
| 1940 | 2.0 |
| 1942 | 1.2 |

SOURCE: (composite) J. Alison Glover, "Milroy Lectures on the Incidence of Rheumatic Diseases," *Lancet* (1930), 1: 499–505; Glover, "Rheumatic Fever," *Lancet* (1939), 1: 465–468; Glover, "War-time Decline of Acute Rheumatism," *Lancet* (1943), 2: 51–52; and Glover, "The Decline of Mortality from Rheumatic Fever," *Monthly Bulletin of the Ministry of Health and the Emergency Public Health Services* (1946), 5: 222–229.

167,000 in 1916.[8] Homer Swift demonstrated a similar decline using statistics for New York State.[9]

The British epidemiologist J. Alison Glover, who had postulated that epidemics of rheumatic fever in barracks or boarding schools followed a pattern of droplet infection, was primarily responsible for documenting the decline in rheumatic fever in England and Wales, a trend that Arthur Newsholme had detected thirty-five years earlier.[10] Initially, Glover chose to look at mortality data. He calculated that mortality from rheumatic fever in England had fallen precipitously (table 7.1).

Morbidity data also startled. Glover calculated that rheumatic fever had caused 11 percent of all admissions to London's hospitals in 1852. In 1914 rheumatic fever was responsible for only 5 percent of admissions at St. Bartholomew's Hospital and Guy's Hospital. In 1926, the rate was only 1 percent. Even in the British Army, with its ease of spreading disease owing to close living quarters, cases of rheumatic fever fell from 430 per 100,000 troops per year in 1913 to 170 per 100,000 troops per year in 1927.

Glover concluded that rheumatic fever was moving into its "obsolescence," with its mortality and morbidity rates declining in each age category. Only in children from ten to fifteen years of age did rheumatic fever account for many deaths. Glover also noted a striking social dimension. Among poor children, rheumatic fever struck much more frequently.[11]

In the 1940s, Glover elaborated on morbidity data. School heart examinations provided compelling evidence for the decline in rheumatic heart disease. For example, the London County Council program screened 292,202 children in 1927, finding 5,629, or 1.9 percent, with cardiac disease from rheumatic fever. A decade later, school health doctors screened 314,959 children; only 2,431 had heart disease, or 0.77 percent.[12] Glover observed a similar trend for Britain as a whole.

Table 7.2   *Admissions for rheumatic fever in the Crimean War and in World War I*

|  | Crimean War | World War I |
| --- | --- | --- |
| Percent of total admissions to military hospitals | 3.2 | 0.84 |
| Deaths/1000 troops | 1.16 | 0.15 |
| Deaths/100 cases of rheumatic fever | 4.7 | 0.26 |

SOURCE: J. Alison Glover, "Acute Rheumatism in Military History," *Proceedings of the Royal Society of Medicine* (1946), 39: 113–118.

The proportion of British schoolchildren with detectable heart disease fell to 0.68 percent in 1938 from 2.1 percent only fifteen years earlier. Glover concluded that "it is now hard to realize the scourge that rheumatic fever was within living memory."[13] Similarly, Glover found marked reductions in rheumatic fever when comparing military data from the Crimean War with that from World War I (table 7.2).

### Children Still at Risk

Glover based his conclusion that children and young adults were now the main victims of rheumatic fever on several lines of evidence. Examination of schoolchildren gave an idea of the prevalence of permanent cardiac damage.[14] In London, Frederick Poynton reported that over 2 percent of 200,000 London schoolchildren examined in 1911, or 4,679 pupils, had a cardiac injury.[15] In Bristol, Carey Coombs described similar results among schoolchildren.[16] On a smaller scale, a survey in New York City yielded roughly the same figure of 2 percent of children with residual rheumatic heart disease. Induction examinations among recruits during the mobilization for World War I confirmed that about 2 percent of adolescent males had signs of rheumatic heart disease.[17] One reason for the persistence of rheumatic fever among children and adolescents was that their social environments—at school or in barracks—placed them in ideal settings for the spread of streptococcal infections.

Although 2 percent was the composite figure for cardiac morbidity in the school-age population, some areas reported far higher numbers. For example, in 1912 physicians found that a surprising 25 percent of Middlesex children between five and thirteen years of age had signs of rheumatic heart disease; in Lancashire in 1919 the finding was an astonishing 29 percent.[18] It is important to emphasize that only a few of these children had overt symptoms from their heart disease. The majority had recovered from acute rheumatic fever years earlier. School physicians detected previously undiscovered heart murmurs or disturbances in heart rhythm which were picked up on screening examinations. For Britain as a whole, one estimate in 1930 gauged the extent of rheumatic heart disease at 5 percent or 250,000 schoolchildren. Of these, examining physicians thought that 40,000, or about 1 percent, had serious cardiac illness, leading to 25,000 deaths each year.

Table 7.3    *Rheumatic heart disease in Minnesota, 1923–1936*

| | |
|---|---|
| Initial abnormal heart examinations | 1,791 |
| Normal heart on second examination | 677 |
| Abnormal heart on second examination, attributed to causes other than rheumatic fever | 401 |
| Rheumatic heart disease on second examination | 713 |

SOURCE: M. J. Shapiro, "The Natural History of Childhood Rheumatism in Minnesota," *Journal of Laboratory and Clinical Medicine* (1936), 21: 564–573.

This survey pointed out that poor children attending dispensaries for health care had a far greater chance of suffering from serious heart complications of rheumatic fever.[19]

Heart examinations in a schoolroom setting, while adequate for screening purposes, were far from ideal for precise diagnosis. In Minnesota, public health officials relied on an initial screening examination followed by a second, confirmatory examination performed by a more experienced physician before labeling a child with rheumatic heart disease. This two-step process gave a more refined estimate of permanent cardiac damage (table 7.3).[20]

In 1938 one survey estimated the number of American college freshmen who had evidence of rheumatic heart disease. O. F. Hedley sent questionnaires to health officials at 213 colleges; 87 replied. From this response he found that just over 1 percent of entering college students had cardiac damage, somewhat less than the 2 percent figure reached for younger children.[21]

What happened to these children with signs of persistent heart damage? In Minnesota, about 5 percent of children with confirmed heart disease died during the thirteen-year period of the survey.[22] Children followed in special cardiac clinics fared worse. These children, in contrast to those identified during school examinations, were often considerably troubled by their cardiac disease. In Philadelphia, 22 percent of the more than four hundred children followed in the rheumatic heart disease clinic at Children's Hospital died. Of note, over one-half of them died of acute pericarditis, a manifestation not commonly seen in the twentieth century.[23] Physicians at King's County Hospital in New York uncovered a much lower mortality rate. During a two-year observation period of 107 children, doctors found that 3 percent died. The lower death rate was almost certainly due to the short duration of the study.[24] Rheumatic fever, while diminishing in the population as a whole, still ravaged some young hearts.[25]

Rheumatic fever also emerged as an obstacle for recruits during World War II. Epidemics, an event that was virtually unknown in civilian life by 1940, occurred in crowded training camps, usually among men in their late teens.[26] The epidemic form of rheumatic fever yielded some of the most crippling cases of heart disease. So concerned was the American military about the risk of contagion with Group A beta-hemolytic streptococci and the debility following infection that examining physicians rejected applicants with any suspicious heart murmur. For healthy recruits, the period of greatest risk proved to be the first month after induction.[27] In Britain, the incidence of acute rheumatic fever was nearly five times greater among trainees than among all members of the Royal Air Force.[28] One British estimate blamed rheumatic fever for three-quarters of all rejections from the military.[29]

### Rheumatic Fever: Declining but Far from Gone

The incidence of rheumatic fever had declined sharply, but the disease was far from gone. Admissions to general hospitals gave one measure of rheumatic fever in the interwar years. These demonstrated that rheumatic fever, despite the epidemiological downturn, remained a serious health problem. At St. Luke's Hospital in New York City (where Lambert's study had detailed a decline in admissions in the years before 1919), the registrar recorded a slight increase between 1919 and 1931.[30] In New Haven, John Paul and Lucille Farquhar found that rheumatic fever ranked third among reasons for admission, after tuberculosis and syphilis.[31] In a detailed urban study, O. F. Hedley surveyed thirty-six hospitals in Philadelphia between 1930 and 1934. Patients with rheumatic fever accounted for 0.7 percent of all admissions, with the rate of pediatric admissions twice the overall number. The average admission lasted forty-one days. Hedley calculated that rheumatic fever patients occupied over 2 percent of the city's total "bed-days." During the period of his study, 1,020 people died from rheumatic fever while hospitalized.[32]

Hedley realized that hospital admissions were only a poor reflection of the scope of rheumatic fever. In 1935 he contacted all physicians, coroners, and members of the Philadelphia County Medical Society, asking to be informed of deaths from rheumatic fever in 1936. These sources reported a total of 552 deaths, nearly all from heart disease, or a rate of 27.2 per 100,000 population, a much higher figure than rates tabulated just from counting deaths in hospitals. In Philadelphia, rheumatic fever ranked fourth as a cause of death for all age groups after tuberculosis, pneumonia, and syphilis; and second for children after only tuberculosis.[33]

### Rheumatic Fever as a Chronic Disease: A Public Health Priority

Mortality rates told only part of the story. What became clear in the interwar years was that rheumatic fever more often crippled than killed. This change in perception stemmed in part from the findings of longitudinal studies. At New York Hospital, as we have seen, May Wilson followed 112 families with nearly 500 children with rheumatic fever. Similarly, John Paul followed families in New Haven. Although these studies took decades to complete, preliminary reports showed that victims of rheumatic fever could expect exacerbations and remissions over many years, even decades.[34] Rheumatic heart disease was a chronic ailment.

Homer Swift came to view rheumatic fever as a chronic problem from another vantage. Swift interpreted the various pathological changes of the disease—

the myocardial Aschoff body, scarred heart valves, and subcutaneous tendinous nodules—as signs of chronic inflammation. To Swift's eye, these cellular changes were microscopically closer to the inflammatory responses in tuberculosis and syphilis—both chronic diseases in the interwar period—than to microscopic changes in acute illnesses.[35]

What was the measure of this chronic disease? In Denmark, researchers found that nearly 17 percent of patients continued to endure cardiac problems one and even two decades after contracting the disease.[36] An analysis of one thousand patients at Convalescent Heart Hospital in West Wickham, England, showed that nearly 20 percent either had died or were left with chronic heart ailments.[37] Of 685 children cared for at the Children's Heart Hospital of Philadelphia between 1922 and 1937, 20 percent died and roughly 10 percent were left incapacitated.[38] Similarly, T. Duckett Jones compiled the long-term experience of one thousand children at the House of the Good Samaritan between 1921 and 1931. He found that 208 had died; 135 continued with severe restrictions placed on activities because of heart disease.[39] Many survivors could expect to become "cardiac cripples."

The realization that rheumatic fever was now a chronic illness lent support to the cry that care for victims should be a public health priority. In New York, Homer Swift pointed out that of major cities only London had adequately planned for enough hospital beds to care for children convalescing from rheumatic fever. In London, one bed was set aside for every 550 children under sixteen years of age. In contrast, New York City had only 300 "chronic" beds, less than one-fifth the recommended number. Swift also used mortality statistics to get the attention of public health leaders. He claimed that rheumatic fever killed more children than many of the diseases that had already caught the public's eye, such as whooping cough (pertussis), meningitis, measles, diphtheria, or scarlet fever. In New York City, more children died from rheumatic fever in a single year than from polio in a decade.[40]

One tactic aimed at convincing public health workers of the relative importance of rheumatic fever involved comparing deaths from rheumatic heart disease with deaths from other diseases by age-specific categories. This more sophisticated statistical approach yielded several insights. Among them was that rheumatic fever trailed only tuberculosis among infections as a cause of death in children. Only in children under five years of age did deaths from whooping cough and polio exceed the mortality rate from rheumatic heart disease, not surprising given that rheumatic fever normally spared the youngest children. Age-specific analysis also reinforced that rheumatic fever was a chronic disease. While nearly all victims were stricken in the first or second decade of life, mortality from the disease actually increased in each decade. Of all childhood infections only rheumatic fever and polio commonly left a lifelong scar.[41]

Public health organizations, at first on the local and state level, responded to the challenge imposed by what became known as the "cardiac cripple." Britain's London Council on Rheumatism provided the model for many American communities in forming organizations such as New York City's Association for the Prevention and Relief of Heart Disease (1915), which later became the New York Heart

Association.[42] Initially, the purpose of these local organizations was to educate the public and to lobby for specific services, such as adequate diagnosis for poor children and consultative support to school nurses. Each community also needed hospital beds for acutely ill patients in order to manage problems during the first weeks of illness. More pressing was the necessity of convalescent hospital beds and foster homes for children left severely handicapped. Children often lived in these facilities for months, even years. Once discharged, most children required regular monitoring in specialized heart clinics that were usually attached to children's hospitals. In Boston, Richard Cabot persuaded the Children's Mission (founded in 1849) to add victims of rheumatic fever to its list of charitable concerns. Fritz Talbot began the Children's Cardiac Clinic at Massachusetts General Hospital in 1912, and his wife founded a philanthropic association, the Committee for the Care of Children with Heart Disease. The convalescent hospital for the Boston area was the House of the Good Samaritan.[43]

Acutely ill patients found their way to children's hospitals or the pediatric wards of general hospitals, often occupying a large number of beds. Harder to provide were the convalescent beds for the chronically handicapped. How many beds were needed? The London County Council on Rheumatism estimated that a community required 1 convalescent bed for each 550 elementary school children, based on its assumption that a victim required six to twelve months of bed rest. Alternatively, Bernice and Arnold Wedum, on the basis of their experience in Cincinnati, projected the need for convalescent beds at roughly twice the number required to handle acute admissions for rheumatic fever. In his study of Philadelphia, Hedley offered a third calculation: a community required 7 convalescent beds for each 100,000 population. These estimates suggested very different public health goals (table 7.4).[44] No matter what estimate public health officials used, the United States fell far short. In 1941 Hedley surveyed the nation's facilities for rheumatic fever and concluded that the country had fewer than 2,000 convalescent beds (illustrations 6–9).[45]

The federal government aided state efforts. The Social Security Act of 1935 created the Crippled Children's Program as part of the Children's Bureau. Three years later, at the urging of the American Academy of Pediatrics, this federal program accepted the concept of the "cardiac cripple." An advisory board, which included T. Duckett Jones and John R. Paul, recommended funding programs that covered the full medical needs of the disease: diagnosis, acute care, and convalescence.[46] Congress approved funding in 1939, and Oklahoma organized the first federally funded program the following year. The number grew to sixteen state programs by 1945.[47] That year the Children's Bureau distributed $475,000 to programs in Oklahoma, California, Connecticut, the District of Columbia, Idaho, Iowa, Maine, Maryland, Michigan, Minnesota, Missouri, Montana, Nebraska, Rhode Island, South Carolina, Utah, Virginia, Washington, and Wisconsin.

The initial program in Oklahoma supported a director (who was also the chief of the pediatric service at the Oklahoma Hospital for Crippled Children), a part-time pediatrician, a consultant cardiologist, a social worker, and a pediatric resident. These professionals conducted one home-based clinic and one "itinerant"

Table 7.4    *Projections of the number of convalescent beds for rheumatic fever*

|  | London estimate | Wedum's estimate | Hedley's estimate |
|---|---|---|---|
| New York City | 1,886 beds | 1,558 beds | 522 beds |
| Philadelphia | 555 | 192 | 200 |
| Cincinnati | 108 | 33 | 55 |

SOURCE: Bernice G. Wedum and Arnold G. Wedum, "A Method for Determining the Number of Beds Required for Convalescent Care of Rheumatic Infections," *American Journal of Public Health* (1942), 32: 1237–1241.

clinic each week.[48] In Virginia's program, a nutritionist, a public health nurse, and a visiting teacher joined the "core" group of pediatrician, cardiologist, and social worker. The group conducted two weekly cardiac clinics at the Medical College of Virginia, whose beds also served children who were acutely stricken. The Instructive Visiting Nurses' Association supervised the convalescent care.[49]

### Rheumatic Fever as a Chronic Disease: The View from Pathology

While politicians and public health workers struggled with providing enough services for sufferers of rheumatic fever, pathologists attempted to define more precisely what constituted the chronic cardiac insult that necessitated prolonged care. Public health and pathology, not often so closely linked, forged an alliance that squarely confronted the chronicity of the disease.

By the mid-1920s, most pathologists described Aschoff bodies as barely-visible-to-the-naked-eye areas of damage to the myocardium. The precise cellular origin and natural history were not entirely agreed upon, largely because autopsies necessarily occurred long after the initial insult to the heart. Questions abounded. Were Aschoff bodies composed solely from the degeneration of myocardial cells, or did other types of cardiac cells form part of the structure? How precisely did Aschoff bodies lead to congestive heart failure? Was it because they replaced too much of the functioning myocardium with noncontracting cells? What was without doubt was that Aschoff bodies disrupted and slowed normal electrical impulses through the heart, prolonging the time between the contraction of atria and the contraction of the ventricles, when measured by the electrocardiogram. Debate also centered on collections of altered cells that pathologists discovered in organs other than the heart. Was the myocardium the only tissue afflicted with Aschoff bodies, or could other organs, such as blood vessels or the kidney, play host to Aschoff bodies? Some physicians argued that Aschoff bodies were the proliferation of connective tissue which could form almost anywhere in the body. More was at stake here than hairsplitting among pathologists. If one argued, as Aschoff had, that these bodies originated in myocardial cells, then there was no plausible reason to connect them with cellular changes in other organs. Some pathologists, such as Benjamin Sacks, maintained that changes he saw in the endocardium, pericardium,

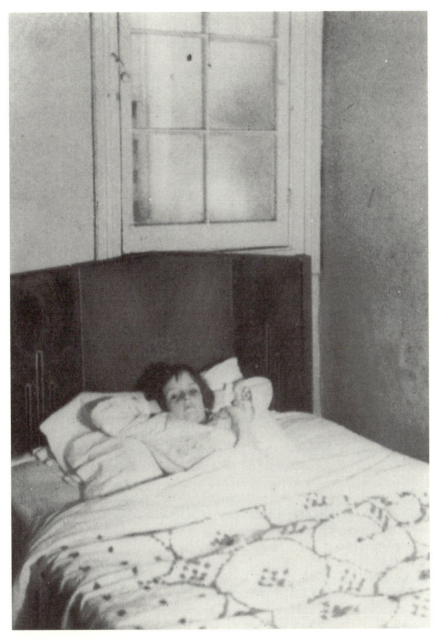

ILLUSTRATION 6. Patient convalescing in a tenement home. Reprinted from May Wilson, *Rheumatic Fever* (New York: Commonwealth Fund, 1940). Reprinted with permission of The Commonwealth Fund, New York, NY.

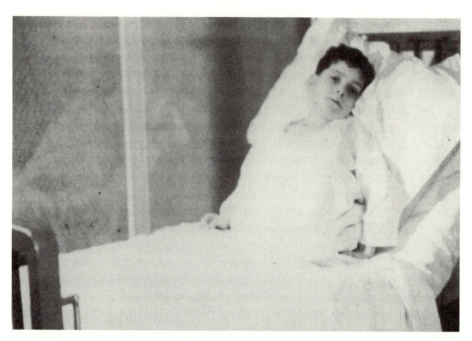

ILLUSTRATION 7. Child with congestive cardiac failure in hospital. Reprinted from May Wilson, *Rheumatic Fever* (New York: Commonwealth Fund, 1940).

and distant blood vessels, despite structural similarities, differed from Aschoff bodies in key details. Sacks thus defended the idea of a unique myocardial injury.[50] Other pathologists disagreed. Alwin Pappenheimer and William von Glahn at New York's Presbyterian Hospital, where Alvin Coburn also worked, interpreted inflammatory changes in the endocardium, aorta, vasa vasorum, lungs, kidneys, adrenal glands, colon, testes, and ovaries as Aschoff bodies, undermining myocardial uniqueness.[51] In 1939 Ludwig Aschoff, carefully reviewing the "bodies" that carried his name and their history and histology, adamantly maintained that they were unique to rheumatic fever and occurred only in the myocardium.[52]

Homer Swift, who so often summarized complicated issues, concluded that Aschoff bodies occurred only in the myocardium, but he argued that similar, if less regularly organized, cellular reactions were found in other tissues. In Swift's view, these widespread pathological changes simply added fuel to the notion that rheumatic fever was a chronic disease.[53]

In his analysis of Aschoff bodies, Swift made a crucial additional observation. He divided the process of myocardial damage into an initial "exudative" phase, when inflammatory fluid and white blood cells amassed at the area of subsequent formation of Aschoff bodies, and a later "proliferative" phase, when fibrous cells mounted up, leading to the actual construction of the Aschoff body. Swift also believed this biphasic inflammatory sequence accounted for other inflammatory

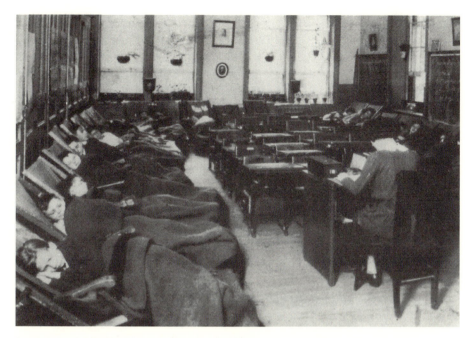

ILLUSTRATION 8. Children in special cardiac class in public school during rest period. Reprinted from May Wilson, *Rheumatic Fever* (New York: Commonwealth Fund, 1940).

changes in rheumatic fever, such as pericarditis and arthritis. Swift's conception of how damage occurred in rheumatic fever had significant ramifications for therapy. Aspirin diminished the exudative, but not the proliferative, phase of the pathological response. To be effective, aspirin needed to be given early in the course of rheumatic fever.[54]

Physicians also debated the cause of death in patients who succumbed from rheumatic fever in the twentieth century. In the nineteenth century, restrictive pericarditis or infectious endocarditis on damaged heart valves provided doctors with ready explanations. In the twentieth century, the pericardium and endocardium were involved less often. Patients died from congestive heart failure often years or decades after the initial bout of rheumatic fever. This raised the question: was heart failure the result of prolonged weakening of the myocardium, an insult that actively continued long after the cessation of fever, joint pains, and chorea?

William von Glahn, now working with Alvin Coburn, studied the hearts of 320 people who died of rheumatic fever. Forty-nine died of infectious endocarditis on old damaged heart valves; and 74 died of congestive heart failure from old myocardial injury. Surprisingly, 100 had evidence of active myocarditis at the time of death.[55] Between 1913 and 1932, when Clarence Laws and Samuel Levine at Peter Bent Brigham Hospital in Boston reviewed autopsies of those who had had rheumatic fever at some point in their lives, they concluded that most had active

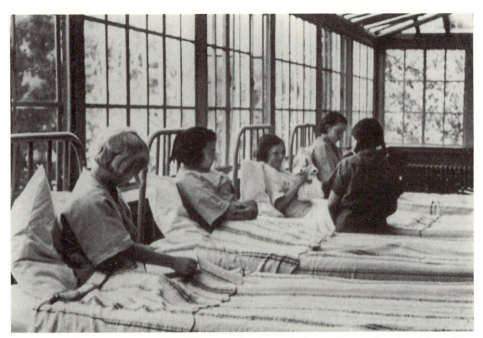

ILLUSTRATION 9. Cardiac patients convalescing at Irvington House. Reprinted from May Wilson, *Rheumatic Fever* (New York: Commonwealth Fund, 1940).

myocarditis at the time of death.[56] At Mount Sinai Hospital in New York City, physicians reached a similar conclusion when they reviewed 3,000 autopsies. At the time of death, most had fresh Aschoff bodies. In 1947 William von Glahn reported the case of a patient who had active Aschoff bodies in the myocardium 44 years after surviving a bout of acute rheumatic fever. Far from being a transient, acute illness, rheumatic fever smoldered, doing its damage as time went on.[57]

## Conclusion

All workers in the field were quite aware of the diminishing mortality and morbidity from rheumatic fever, the emergence of rheumatic heart disease as a chronic disease, and the triggering role of the streptococcal "detonator." The question that puzzled was: were these observations related? During World War II, J. Alison Glover reached a startling conclusion. He gave scant credit to preventive measures or therapy, to public health programs, better diet, or the generally improving standard of living. Instead, Glover argued, "it seems probable that the main cause of the decline is of a more subtle kind, a change in the relationship between man and the *streptococcus pyogenes*."[58]

Demographers, analyzing the profound changes in mortality patterns in the twentieth century, have pointed to the transition in the causes of death from infectious diseases, such as tuberculosis and pneumonia, to chronic diseases, such as stroke, cancer, and heart disease.[59] Rheumatic fever provided the unique example of this transition occurring in a single disease over the span of a few short decades. In the biological shift to myocarditis, rheumatic fever largely ceased being an acute infectious scourge that plagued children. In its stead, rheumatic heart disease joined other chronic illnesses.

## CHAPTER 8

# At the Bedside, 1925–1945

$\mathcal{A}$lvin Coburn's "tri-phasic" theory of rheumatic fever, so important for laboratory scientists and epidemiologists, had prompt and far-reaching ramifications for clinical medicine. Disease (Phase III) required a triggering bout with Group A beta-hemolytic streptococcal (GABS) tonsillitis (Phase I) and a destructive immunological response (Phase II). Clear, sequential ordering permitted clinicians to focus their attack. Tonsillitis, which for Cheadle had been the least crucial of his "manifestations," became central. Doctors and patients, long accustomed to playing down the significance of minor throat infections unless they resulted in a rare tonsillar abscess, had to reorient fundamentally. A sore throat, once thought trivial in comparison with carditis or chorea, now became critical. A pivotal part of the reorientation was understanding that only tonsillitis caused by GABS bore a relationship to rheumatic fever, but once present, whether it produced any patient distress or not, it demanded prompt attention. Under the watchful eyes of doctors at the House of the Good Samaritan, such as T. Duckett Jones, patients who suffered relapses almost always demonstrated a confirmatory rise in antistreptolysin. From Jones's perspective, it was distressing that only about one-half of the children had complained of sore throats prior to relapse.[1] In other words, clinically "silent" throat infections also triggered rheumatic fever. Streptococcal infection, whether symptomatic or "silent," needed to be prevented or treated. After Coburn, the physician's first task thus was to stop GABS in its tracks, halting the march to Phases II and III. In a world beginning to teem with antibiotics,[2] a bacterial trigger emerged as an inviting target.

## Rheumatic "Activity"

Because the all-important sore throat could be so easily missed by both patient and physician, Phase II or Phase III unfortunately served as the frequent point where doctor and patient met, especially when another family member was already known to suffer from streptococcal infection. A rise in the antistreptolysin O titer or an elevation of the erythrocyte sedimentation rate indicated that the body was responding immunologically and that symptomatic rheumatic fever was likely to follow. So employed, these tests became diagnostic aids.

The erythrocyte sedimentation rate added a key dimension to clinical management. Coupled with the symptoms of Phase III—carditis, arthritis, chorea, nodules, erythema marginatum—and with the presence of fever and any abnormality on the electrocardiogram, the sedimentation rate became a measure of rheumatic "activity," a concept indicating that pathological processes, still not precisely understood, were under way. With its scaled measurement, the sedimentation rate served as the hallmark either of increasing severity of rheumatic fever or of therapeutic response.

Rheumatic "activity" was a peculiar concept: part bedside clinical assessment, part laboratory blood test. A physician's second task then was to monitor and, if possible, to modify and eliminate "activity."[3] Even though a murmur of newly acquired mitral stenosis disappeared, physicians learned to consider rheumatic fever "active" and in need of ongoing medical attention if the sedimentation rate remained elevated or if the electrocardiogram continued to show abnormalities. For example, children were kept in convalescent hospitals until all signs of "activity" had resolved.

### The Fading of Erythema Marginatum

Coburn's conception of "active" rheumatic fever and the disease's continuing biological evolution joined forces in a reassessment of the cardinal signs of rheumatic fever. In particular, erythema marginatum and chorea, now infrequent, came under scrutiny whether they should remain as central elements. Neither raised the sedimentation rate, leading some to conclude that rash and chorea were no longer principal components of "active" rheumatic fever. In 1938 Harry Keil, a biographer of William Charles Wells who also had a great interest in the evolution of rheumatic nodules, surveyed the prevalence of erythematous rashes and rheumatic fever at New York's Mount Sinai Hospital. Only a tenth of cases admitted to the hospital had evidence of any erythematous rash; of those, less than one-third sported classical erythema marginatum. To Keil, this rash was merely a cutaneous expression of streptococcal infection. In his experience, erythema marginatum seldom occurred in the absence of other manifestations of rheumatic fever. Keil concluded that the rash still belonged with the disease, but that it was now quite rare.[4]

### The Waning of Chorea

Chorea's fading sparked controversy. Its association with rheumatic fever, cemented for over a century, had from the start been variable. For example, in 1846 Dr. H. M. Hughes, in one of the earliest reports from Guy's Hospital, found that only about 8 percent of patients with chorea also suffered from rheumatism.[5] In contrast, five years later Germaine Sée at l'Hôpital des Enfants in Paris documented nearly seven times as many.[6] One controversy that remained lively in the twentieth century was the mechanical or pathological relationship between arthritis and carditis and brain disturbance. Put more bluntly, how did the diseased joints or heart convey illness to the brain? An early idea was that some inflamed part of a joint or heart valve broke off, or embolized, traveling through the bloodstream to the brain, where it then produced cerebral inflammation and chorea. The sepsis hypothesis, so popular before 1920, proposed a similar mechanism but with bacteria coursing through the blood and settling in the brain. Thwarting both notions was the observation, repeated over and again, that the brains of people dying from rheumatic fever with chorea appeared entirely normal. This contrasted sharply with the marked changes that rheumatic fever left in heart tissue.[7] Another difference, clearly separating chorea from other manifestations of rheumatic fever, was its conspicuous abnormal *behaviors,* very distinct from the physical signs of heart murmur, nodule, or rash. Chorea might begin as "sudden, irregular, purposeless, and incoordinate movements," but in the more serious cases chorea also included emotional lability, characterized by irritability, overactivity, uncontrolled outbursts, and silly laughter. So afflicted, most children could not concentrate and failed in their schoolwork. One estimate from Denver characterized 20 percent of victims of chorea as so psychologically scarred that they became delinquent or vagrant.[8] Standard treatment for other aspects of rheumatic fever, such as aspirin, seldom worked for chorea, prompting doctors to tailor remedies to the abnormal behaviors: sedatives in the nineteenth century, anticonvulsants, such as phenobarbital, in the twentieth. To many, chorea seemed not to belong with the other symptoms of rheumatic fever.

Freak insights, gained during treatment of a child who developed a severe allergy to phenobarbital, led physicians at Bellevue Hospital in New York to a new therapy for chorea. A child receiving phenobarbital developed classical signs of an allergic reaction: rash and a fever that exceeded 106 degrees. His doctors quickly stopped the drug, but the high fever persisted. In response to the extremely high fever, the patient's chorea subsided. It seemed plausible that high fever lessened chorea, suggesting a new avenue of treatment. Of course, only a few people were allergic to phenobarbital, but most reacted with very high fevers when given multiple injections of typhoid-paratyphoid vaccine, an immunization occasionally given in the 1920s to prevent typhoid fever. Seven daily doses of vaccine—and the high fever it caused—benefited most sufferers from chorea, cutting the average duration of the abnormal behaviors to one or two weeks from the usual period of several months.[9] Fever employed to treat one symptom of a disease, which, of course, had fever—though a far lower one—as another symptom, raised in some minds the question whether chorea should still be considered a cardinal part of rheumatic fever.

Working at the House of the Good Samaritan in 1935, T. Duckett Jones and Edward Bland were in a particularly good place to analyze chorea. "Good Sam," as the hospital was often called, opened its eighty beds to patients with rheumatic fever in 1921.[10] By 1935, Jones and Bland had access to carefully detailed histories from over twelve hundred patients. Jones and Bland drew stark contrasts to conclusions that William Osler had reached forty years earlier. Osler had stated: *"There is no known disease in which endocarditis is so constantly found, post-mortem, as chorea;* it is exceptional to find the heart healthy" (Osler's emphasis).[11] By 1935 chorea had changed markedly. Jones and Bland rarely encountered "violent chorea," the most severe form of the symptom. When present in its now milder form, chorea appeared to signal a blander course of rheumatic fever. Chorea seemed to protect from the most serious forms of heart disease; mortality from rheumatic fever with chorea as one of its manifestations was one-half that where chorea was entirely absent. Jones and Bland still thought chorea was a component of rheumatic fever, but clearly its relationship to the rest of the disease was changing.[12]

At Presbyterian Hospital in New York, Alvin Coburn reached a very different opinion. In his experience, children who started rheumatic fever with chorea alone seldom progressed to other manifestations and almost never to serious heart disease. In Coburn's view, chorea appeared in the 1930s to be emancipating itself from rheumatic fever. Equally striking was chorea's independence from prior throat infection with Group A beta-hemolytic streptococcus and from rheumatic "activity." In children with chorea alone, tonsils did not grow streptococci; the antistreptolysin titer did not rise; and the erythrocyte sedimentation rate remained normal. Coburn concluded: "The blood sedimentation rate is generally recognized as a highly sensitive index of rheumatic activity; yet in our experience and in that of a number of other observers uncomplicated chorea, even in patients known to be susceptible to rheumatic fever, is accompanied by normal sedimentation rates; this in our opinion is strong evidence against the rheumatic origin of chorea."[13]

Bellevue physicians were not prepared to go that far. A few of their patients with chorea, about 5 percent, still developed carditis, leading them to conclude that chorea remained a cardinal element of rheumatic fever, but they conceded that it was now almost a separate species. For them, chorea represented rheumatic fever without heart disease.[14]

Chorea's amelioration prompted O. F. Hedley, who had so carefully studied rheumatic fever in Philadelphia, to review all twenty-seven prior studies on chorea and rheumatic fever, published between 1887 and 1938. Hedley detailed its marked variability: chorea coincided with other manifestations of rheumatic fever in as few as 3 percent of cases or as many as 77 percent. He concurred with Jones, Bland, and Coburn that chorea was becoming far less likely to accompany more serious aspects of rheumatic fever. But as a statistician, Hedley had to point out that children with chorea still had a far greater chance of developing heart disease than children without chorea.[15] What went unquestioned by careful observers was that "chorea is a disorder which today steadily diminishes in frequency and severity."[16]

### Biological Change Prompts New Criteria for Diagnosis: T. Duckett Jones

In 1944, T. Duckett Jones struggled with the impact of rheumatic fever's changing biological nature on diagnosis. He was particularly concerned that many children and young adults—especially recruits in the military—were being too liberally diagnosed with rheumatic fever. Jones's experience at the House of the Good Samaritan was very different from Walter Cheadle's practice at the Hospital for Sick Children, Great Ormond Street, fifty years earlier. Then Cheadle had expected that nearly all children with rheumatic fever would suffer from most manifestations of rheumatic fever at some point during their initial bout or during a relapse. For Cheadle, rheumatic fever was a dramatic disease of signs and symptoms. For Jones, the issue was the scarcity of symptoms.

A precise diagnostic test for rheumatic fever eluded physicians. Although Jones agreed that a prior streptococcal throat infection was the necessary trigger, he concluded that a throat culture was not a diagnostic test. His new scheme, like Cheadle's, would remain one based on signs and symptoms, not laboratory tests. Using the same word that Cheadle had chosen, Jones divided symptoms and signs into "major manifestations" and "minor manifestations." The major manifestations were similar to those that Cheadle had listed in his "series." But each had undergone change to a milder form. Carditis, defined by cardiac enlargement, congestive heart failure, or an increase in the PR interval of the electrocardiogram, reflected the twentieth-century shift to myocarditis. Jones still included pericardial disease and endocardial disease as additional signs of heart involvement. Jones described joint disease as "arthralgia," or joint pain. Migrating polyarthritis—with swollen, red, and painful joints—was seldom present. Physicians had to rely on a patient's history of vague aches and pains of the joints that Jones realized accompanied both rheumatic fever and other infections. Chorea, if present, remained a diagnostic aid. Subcutaneous nodules, rare in the 1940s, were also helpful when present. A prior bout of rheumatic fever rounded out the "majors." Of note, Jones did not include erythema marginatum in his list of major manifestations. In Jones's scheme, diagnosis required two or more of these major manifestations.

Jones understood that even such loose criteria would exclude some children who might have rheumatic fever, so he created a list of lesser, or "minor," manifestations. These included fever, severe abdominal pain, chest pain, rashes (which might include erythema marginatum), nosebleeds, ill-defined lung findings, and abnormal laboratory tests, such as an elevated erythrocyte sedimentation rate or an elevated white blood count. Migratory polyarthritis was one of Jones's minor manifestations. In some respects, this was a peculiar list, almost certainly tailored to his experience. Nosebleeds, abdominal pain, pulmonary findings, and an increased white blood cell count, while occasionally mentioned by others, had never been so prominently displayed. In Jones's proposed scheme, a physician could also make a diagnosis of rheumatic fever with only one "major" manifestation *and* two or more "minor" manifestations. No combination of "minors" alone was sufficient.

Jones thought that his criteria met the challenge of the changing nature of rheumatic fever. But he realized that his diagnostic scheme remained imperfect. Specifically, he feared that too many would receive the diagnosis of rheumatic fever based on "arthralgia" plus fever and an elevated white blood cell count. In his view, such children did not have rheumatic fever, despite having one "major" and two "minor" manifestations.[17]

## Prevention of Rheumatic Fever: Tonsillectomy

Equally challenging were evolving ideas about prevention. Until the mid-1930s, tonsillectomy was the only widely employed means of preventing rheumatic fever. In most cases, physicians worried only about preventing relapses, although some public health officials encouraged the removal of diseased tonsils in all children whether or not they had suffered from rheumatic fever. Indeed, community hospitals filled operating rooms with youngsters who suffered repeated sore throats. In view of the popularity of the procedure, it was surprising that virtually all research studies maintained that tonsillectomy failed to prevent relapses,[18] reflecting the conclusion that Frederick Poynton had reached years earlier.[19] Unfortunately, no investigation approached the tonsillar question with the bacterial rigor that Coburn's theory demanded. Tonsillitis was a common symptom; the Group A beta-hemolytic streptococcus was only one of many causes of tonsillitis. Strikingly, no major study actually cultured throats to see whether surgical removal diminished infection with GABS. Leading the attack against tonsillectomy was May Wilson, who saw no benefit in the children she followed for years in New York.[20] Only at Johns Hopkins Hospital did physicians find that surgery slightly lessened the rate of relapse, but, once again, they obtained no bacterial cultures.[21] Despite the preponderance of opinion, many children with rheumatic fever, admitted for long stays in convalescent hospitals, underwent tonsillectomy. So concerned were their doctors about relapse that many grasped any straw.[22]

## Sulfonamide

For most physicians, a growing appreciation of the effectiveness of sulfonamide eliminated the need for a surgical approach to prevention. In addition, this early antibacterial drug initially held out the hope of cure. The introduction of sulfonamide came on the heels of Coburn's epidemiological proof of the streptococcal trigger.[23] Within months came thrilling reports that sulfonamide cured people with serious streptococcal illnesses, such as erysipelas, scarlet fever, and pelvic infections. These early successes prompted researchers to use the drug in cases of rheumatic fever.[24]

Among the first out of the blocks was Homer Swift. At Rockefeller Hospital, Swift treated eight patients suffering from clear symptoms of rheumatic fever, or Coburn's Phase III, with sulfanilamide, a closely related drug. Most immediately developed serious side effects from the drug, including fever, rash, gastrointestinal disturbances, lowered white blood cell count, and cyanosis. None of the patients experienced any improvement from their symptoms of rheumatic fever, leading to Swift's conclusion that sulfanilamide had no effect "once the condition is well established." In his view, the toxic effects of the drug outweighed negligible benefits.[25] Similar disappointing results occurred at the House of the Good Samaritan. Clearly symptomatic children received sulfanilamide; over one-half swiftly developed toxic reactions to the drug; none benefited; and most seemed worse from the experience. This ill-fated outcome prodded Benedict Massell and

Duckett Jones to conclude that "this drug is contraindicated in the presence of rheumatic fever."[26] In effect, both studies, authored by such prominent researchers, threw a weighty wet blanket on antibiotic enthusiasm. In hindsight, the drug in both studies was targeted at symptoms, not streptococci. It may be that neither group in the mid-1930s fully understood the role of the streptococcal catalyst in Coburn's scheme, which gave the germ no part to play after instigating the disease. What both studies demonstrated was that the use of sulfonamide carried grave risks. Sulfonamide was no cure for rheumatic fever.

Undaunted by earlier disappointments, Caroline Bedell Thomas at Johns Hopkins and Alvin Coburn at Pelham Home and Presbyterian Hospital in New York pressed on, but targeted sulfanilamide more closely at the streptococcus. Thomas, conceding that sulfanilamide was ineffective in treating the symptoms of rheumatic fever, set out to see whether the drug could prevent relapses by thwarting repeated streptococcal infections. Her patients were all victims of prior bouts of rheumatic fever, followed in a special clinic at Johns Hopkins. Her "controls" were patients who refused to take sulfanilamide on a daily basis. Thomas administered the drug during the fall and winter months, periods of greatest vulnerability to infection with streptococcus. As May Wilson later pointed out, Caroline Thomas, by selecting her control subjects in this nonrandom fashion, almost certainly biased her results.[27] Thomas measured success in preventing both infection with the streptococcus and relapses of rheumatic fever. From the onset of her investigation in 1936, Thomas's results startled. Virtually no patient receiving daily sulfanilamide became infected with the streptococcus, and none suffered a relapse of rheumatic fever. About 15 percent of control patients became infected with streptococcus; 10 percent of the control group relapsed.[28]

Alvin Coburn attacked the streptococcal catalyst in a slightly different fashion. He set out to treat convalescing patients at the Pelham Home with sulfanilamide at the first sign of throat pain. In other words, Coburn attempted to prevent Phase I from progressing to Phases II and III. He was foiled in this effort. He then turned to an approach similar to that of Caroline Thomas, giving prophylactic daily doses during the entire season of streptococcal infections. When he did so, his results were just as promising. Giving sulfanilamide year after year extended success. In addition, he experimented with lower doses of the drug, achieving comparable outcomes with fewer side effects. Of note, his patients were all in the hospital, so the issue of compliance was moot.[29]

Coburn addressed another objection raised by May Wilson. In her longitudinal study of New York children, Wilson demonstrated that children were less likely to relapse the older they became. She interpreted Coburn's success, which he construed as the consequence of sulfanilamide, as the natural course of rheumatic fever to ameliorate with time. To settle the issue, Coburn withdrew sulfanilamide from one hundred older patients who had been free of infection and relapse for several years. Thirty-two became infected with streptococcus; thirteen suffered relapses.[30]

Other sulfonamide forays were noticeably less successful. At Roosevelt Hospital in New York City, physicians had to halt use of sulfanilamide because half of their patients developed serious complications.[31]   Other research groups found that some patients, despite receiving sulfanilamide, relapsed, though less frequently than controls. Of note, these were studies of out-patients where the twice or thrice daily medicating was left to patients and families.[32]

Nevertheless, Caroline Thomas remained thoroughly convinced that sulfanilamide worked as a prophylactic drug. By 1942 none of her patients had relapsed, compared with over 10 percent of controls. She had lowered the dose of the drug and reduced the frequency from three times a day to two, without diminishing her success. In her hands, serious side effects were few. Thomas thought that her results were so persuasive that sulfanilamide should no longer be considered an experimental drug in rheumatic fever. All victims, once recovered from the initial bout of rheumatic fever, should receive daily sulfanilamide for at least five years.[33]

The American military in World War II heeded Thomas's advice and extended it to healthy recruits. Draftees, packed into barracks or ships, provided fodder for streptococcal infection. In 1942, one army camp reported that 10 percent of its 3,000 recruits contracted Group A beta-hemolytic streptococcal infection during a single epidemic.[34]   Alvin Coburn, who served in the navy, calculated the streptococcal burden for that branch of the military: 60,000 cases of scarlet fever, 21,000 cases of rheumatic fever, 1.3 million "man-days" lost.[35]   So concerned with streptococcal infection was the military that it set up a Commission on Hemolytic Streptococcal Infections.[36]   In the spring of 1943, the army air force began giving daily doses of sulfadiazine, a sulfonamide with fewer side effects, to 36,500 healthy soldiers. In the winter of 1943–44, the navy administered the drug to 600,000 healthy sailors. These were not carefully controlled research studies; rather, the goal was manpower productivity, free from disease. Nevertheless, all observers were struck with the markedly reduced numbers of streptococcal infections, reduced hospital stays, and greatly diminished cases of rheumatic fever.[37]

What no one anticipated was that giving sulfadiazine indiscriminately to all personnel almost immediately created strains of the streptococcus that were resistant to the antibiotic. Even more frightening, resistant strains moved quickly to other military installations where sulfadiazine had not been used, causing disease that could not be treated with the new drug. Coburn believed that the peculiar nature of crowded military life was partly responsible. Certainly, he observed, massive resistance had not occurred in civilian life. What escaped Coburn's analysis was one key difference between civilian and military studies. In civilian life, only people with a prior history of rheumatic fever received prophylactic sulfonamide. In the military, every recruit received the drug. What became clear was that everyone could not take sulfonamide all the time in order to prevent disease. The wonder drugs were capable of mutating bacteria.[38]

Aware of therapeutic successes in the military but not of the problem of resistance, civilian physicians pressed forward with sulfanilamide for prophylaxis. In 1944, for example, Caroline Thomas cited success in the military as further evidence supporting her claims.[39]   Further studies among civilians bolstered her position. By 1946 there were seventeen carefully performed clinical investigations, which, when tabulated, demonstrated clear advantage for patients with a prior history of rheumatic fever taking daily sulfonamide. Only about 2 percent of those receiving the drug relapsed, compared with almost 14 percent of controls.[40] In contrast to claims by Thomas and Coburn, most other researchers described troublesome side effects in up to a third of patients: rash, nausea, fever, or, in rare instances, a perilous drop in the white blood cell count.[41] Relying in part on experience in the military, some researchers favored sulfadiazine because of its fewer side effects.[42] So concerned were some physicians about May Wilson's assertion that "success" resulted from natural history and not from sulfonamide that they submitted her critique to Joseph Berkson, one of the nation's leading statisticians, for refereeing. Berkson disagreed with Wilson: he believed that the multiple sulfonamide studies had merit.[43]

By the end of the war, there was sufficient experience for researchers to suggest guidelines for general practice. All victims of a single bout of rheumatic fever who had carditis as a manifestation and all victims with two bouts in which heart disease was not a component should receive daily prophylaxis with one of the sulfonamide drugs. Still concerned that sulfonamide worsened the initial attack, researchers recommended that drug treatment begin two months after the initial "active" phase had ended. Patients were advised to use the drug for at least five years. Doubt existed whether patients who suffered from chorea alone, even in multiple bouts, benefited from sulfonamide.[44] For some, even five years of the drug was not enough; at Bellevue Hospital in New York City fully one-quarter relapsed once sulfonamide was stopped.[45]

In contrast to the large trials with sulfonamide, military physicians used penicillin in only a few small studies during the war. Once again Homer Swift, who worked in a Naval Research Unit at Rockefeller Hospital, was among the first to try the new antibiotic. Swift gave the drug to seven patients with symptoms of rheumatic fever, or Coburn's Phase III. Penicillin promptly eliminated streptococci from the throats but did nothing for heart disease, chorea, or arthritis.[46] Like the first experimenters with sulfonamide, others repeated the effort of targeting symptoms and not the streptococcal trigger, with similar disappointing results, leading one group to suggest that penicillin "is not only of no value but also may be harmful."[47] Despite these inauspicious efforts, military physicians at the end of the 1940s would pioneer in the more appropriate use of penicillin. Only at the House of the Good Samaritan did physicians glimpse the potential of penicillin. Giving injections of penicillin every two hours at the first sign of streptococcal sore throat immediately exterminated the bacteria, very different from sulfonamide, which merely suppressed streptococci. To doctors at "Good Sam," this superior effectiveness of penicillin might permit stopping the progression of rheumatic fever at Coburn's Phase I.[48]

## Treatment for Rheumatic Fever: The Convalescent Hospital

Sulfonamide prophylaxis solved a crucial clinical problem: the prevention of relapses. It was of no value in treatment or rehabilitation. "Active" rheumatic fever required care that could last for months or even years. Most physicians thought that the most appropriate site of treatment during the initial symptomatic portion of the illness was the children's hospital or children's ward of a general hospital. During this stage, concern focused on the heart and its potential decompensation. Once the heart disease appeared stable—but still "active" by cardiac examination, electrocardiogram, or sedimentation rate—a child entered the "convalescent" period, which often took place at another facility. The convalescent period extended until the cessation of all signs of clinical "activity." At Long Island College of Medicine, this averaged about two months;[49] at the Royal Hospital for Sick Children in Glasgow, the minimal stay was three months;[50] it was four months at the House of the Good Samaritan; six months at Children's Heart Hospital of Philadelphia; two years at Irvington House.[51] Always at issue was when to end treatment.[52]

Convalescent beds were always at a premium. In London, where many thought the English set an example, there were by one estimate about 1,200 places in hospitals for children convalescing from rheumatic fever in 1938.[53] Yet the London County Council estimated that about 23,000 children at any given time were under a doctor's care for "active" rheumatic fever.[54] O. F. Hedley reckoned that the United States in 1941 had fewer than 2,000 properly staffed and equipped convalescent beds. Leading his list were House of the Good Samaritan (80 beds); St. Francis Sanatorium for Cardiac Children, New York (50 beds); Irvington House, Irvington-on-Hudson, New York (150 beds); Pelham House, New York (30 beds); Children's Heart Hospital, Philadelphia (60 beds); Lymanhurst Cardiac Convalescent Home, Minneapolis (40 beds); and La Rabida Jackson Park Sanatorium, Chicago (100 beds).[55]

Pressing need demanded solutions. The Children's Mission of Boston estimated that 900 children needed convalescent care each year in that city alone. To help in meeting this requirement, Kenneth Blackfan, chairman of pediatrics at Harvard, suggested that physicians use some of the now empty beds at the tuberculosis sanatorium at Sharon. The children received care similar to that of those recovering from tuberculosis: "open-air" exposure, day and night, throughout the year. Parents were restricted to a short visit one afternoon each week. Even in such harsh physical and emotional environments most children fared well.[56]

The idea of employing underutilized sections of older tuberculosis sanitoria spread and in turn served as a stimulus for building sanitoria devoted entirely to the convalescent care of children with rheumatic fever. Among the first of this new type of institution was the St. Francis Sanatorium for Cardiac Children in Brooklyn, which Hedley included in his select list of centers. As its name suggests, it was run and financed by a religious order, the Franciscan Missionaries of Mary, with piggy-backed medical, teaching, and research programs. Medical care at St. Francis was similar to care received in nonreligious convalescent hospitals, but its founders claimed that its religious character attended better to the chronic nature of the disease.[57]

Physicians at the House of the Good Samaritan understood that their eighty beds met the needs of only a small proportion of Boston's children with rheumatic fever. To serve a greater number of patients, they pioneered in physician-supervised home or foster-home care. After an initial stay of about four weeks at either "Good Sam" or Massachusetts General Hospital, children were discharged home for strict bed rest. There were exacting selection criteria: no evidence of pericarditis or congestive heart failure. Physicians made monthly home visits, accompanied by a technician who drew blood samples for determination of the patient's sedimentation rate. Rheumatic "activity" lasted eight months on average. A group of patients who remained at the House of the Good Samaritan served as a control group, although it seems that those staying behind may well have been a good deal sicker. When Edward Bland evaluated the initial five years of the home care program, he concluded that home care yielded results that were the same or better than those of a convalescent hospital, and at about one-half the cost of care at "Good Sam.[58]

Some communities used special schools as sites for convalescent care. In doing so, they attended to both ailing hearts and ongoing educational needs. Syracuse, New York, was a model. A single physician, serving both public and parochial schools with a combined enrollment of 34,000 students, monitored the care of children convalescing from rheumatic fever. He determined the degree of restriction in physical activity, for example, whether a student should follow a limited schedule in a regular school or needed almost complete constraint in a school for handicapped children.[59]

Complete bed rest was the hallmark of convalescent care: no bathroom privileges, no feeding or washing oneself, no sitting up in bed. Children "must be taught to be passive, must be kept happy, warm [except, of course, for those assigned to Sharon Tuberculosis Sanitorium] and well fed, and must have physical, mental, and emotional rest" until all signs of rheumatic "activity" ceased.[60] The reason given for such draconian measures was the perceived fragility of the wounded heart. Only after signs of rheumatic "activity" had been gone for weeks was it considered safe for even modest physical exertion. In the home care program supervised by the House of the Good Samaritan, activity began with one hour out of bed *per week*.[61] Another rehabilitation program allowed a generous one-half hour daily in a chair at bedside.[62] As patients slowly emerged from the cocoon of bed rest, physicians monitored them closely for any sign of renewed rheumatic "activity." Most convalescent hospitals welcomed schoolteachers, who met individually with children at bedside.[63]

Military physicians challenged these rigid restrictions. Once-active men chafed when confined to bed. Enforced rest produced restlessness. Physical exertion such as sitting at the side of the bed, walking to the bathroom, shaving, and feeding led to no perceived additional cardiac stress. Some military physicians even advocated overnight passes (for married men).[64]

## Aspirin

Before 1950, most patients with rheumatic fever arrived at the doctor's office with symptoms, Coburn's Phase III. In particular, they had evidence of cardiac inflammation. Later, public health workers would educate physicians and patients to seek help at the first sign of a sore throat. Until midcentury, the only therapy for symptomatic rheumatic fever was aspirin. No one questioned its ability to break the fever or to end joint pain and swelling. The issue of whether aspirin healed heart disease remained unsettled. The emergence of myocarditis as the preeminent cardiac injury—with inflammation that smoldered for decades—added new difficulties in assessing the value of any drug. Nevertheless, it is clear that virtually all physicians recommended aspirin but remained divided in their opinion of its efficacy.[65]

Homer Swift suggested one line of reasoning that shed light on the clinical use of aspirin. Swift, it will be remembered, divided inflammation in rheumatic fever into two stages: an initial exudative period that was characterized by the accumulation of fluid, such as occurred in arthritis and pericarditis, and a later proliferative period, distinguished by the multiplication of cells, such as in myocarditis (the Aschoff body) and subcutaneous tendinous nodules. Endocarditis was difficult to place in just one camp. Swift thought that it had an early exudative phase and a later proliferative stage that resulted in deformed heart valves.[66] From his animal work, Swift thought that salicylate was effective in the exudative form of inflammation but not the proliferative stage. Swift's insight was reflected in clinical practice. Physicians could readily see the disappearance of fluid from the joints. Even though pericarditis, with its accumulation of fluid around the heart, was far less common in the twentieth century, it also responded somewhat to therapy with aspirin. In myocarditis, aspirin seemed of no value; in endocarditis opinions varied. For Swift, timing was a key element: to be effective aspirin needed to be given early.[67]

So effective was aspirin in treating fever and arthritis that some thought that it might serve as a preventive drug. In 1930 Clifton Leech at the Harriet Lane Home, the children's part of Johns Hopkins Hospital in Baltimore, gave children convalescing from rheumatic fever daily doses of aspirin long after their symptoms disappeared. So treated, these children seemed to suffer relapses less frequently.[68] A decade later, Alvin Coburn advocated giving children aspirin at the first sign of a sore throat in the hopes of averting a recurrence.[69]

The effect of aspirin on myocarditis proved difficult to appraise in clinical practice. One reliable sign of myocardial inflammation was the slowing of the conduction time between atria and ventricles, measured by the PR interval on the electrocardiogram. In the hands of many practitioners, aspirin, given at doses that suppressed fever and alleviated joint pain and swelling, failed to alter the abnormality on electrocardiogram.[70] Assessing the effect of aspirin on endocarditis was also difficult in practice. By the time a patient arrived at a doctor's office, the telltale evidence of endocarditis, the murmur of mitral or aortic valvular disease, was normally present. According to Swift's hypothesis, by the time a murmur was heard the period of aspirin's benefit to the endocardium was over.

## Coburn, "Activity," and Aspirin

The concept of rheumatic "activity," which combined clinical evaluation with laboratory confirmation, provided a novel way of assessing the value of aspirin. Helen Taussig, a pediatrician at Johns Hopkins who began her career studying rheumatic fever before shifting her interests to congenital heart disease as rheumatic fever waned, was among the first to suggest that aspirin speeded the return of the sedimentation rate to its normal value.[71] Alvin Coburn developed this idea.

Coburn argued that the treatment should be directed at "activity," not symptoms. In his view, physicians had erred in giving aspirin only as long as patients complained of fever, chest discomfort, or joint pain. Overt symptoms ended long before the cessation of "activity," measured by the sedimentation rate. Withdrawing aspirin too soon permitted ongoing cardiac damage. Coburn estimated that nearly 40 percent of patients relapsed when doctors and patients stopped aspirin at the point when fever and joint pain ended. Breaking new ground, Coburn proposed administering large doses of aspirin, up to ten grams a day, as soon as the diagnosis was made and continuing the drug until all signs of "activity" were extinguished for at least two weeks. This often meant that aspirin needed to be taken for months. To ensure that patients received sufficient aspirin, he advocated giving it intravenously—at least at the beginning of therapy—and measuring blood levels to make certain that the physician had not overshot or undershot his therapeutic mark.[72] When aspirin was used in this fashion, the patient experienced comfort from reduced fever and cessation of joint pain. In Coburn's hands, aspirin also dampened the effect of rheumatic carditis. None of his patients relapsed.

Coburn's advice to treat "activity" was heeded almost without question and continues to serve as one guidepost for therapy in rheumatic fever. His innovation provided a rationale for length and efficacy of therapy. And most doctors accepted that the best, and safest, way of monitoring aspirin was with guidance from the serum level. Some early reports supported Coburn's findings.[73] Not all were convinced, however, that his high-dose regimen of aspirin effectively treated heart disease. From Coburn's Presbyterian Hospital came reports that colleagues could not improve outcomes with Coburn's more aggressive approach.[74] Some encountered serious overdosing despite careful monitoring of the serum aspirin levels.[75] Others could not verify that aspirin hurried the return of the sedimentation rate to normal values.[76] Still others argued that high-dose aspirin benefited only pericarditis.[77]

What seems likely is that Coburn's more precise use of aspirin and "activity" collided with rheumatic fever's biological evolution. Always effective for fever, joint complaints, and pericardial fluid, salicylate, when first employed at the end of the nineteenth century, seemed more effective against heart disease simply because pericarditis was then more common. Aspirin was far less capable in treating the newer form of heart disease. Thus, as pericarditis waned, the perception waxed that aspirin was worthless in any form of heart injury. Nevertheless, when Coburn developed his aggressive high-dose aspirin treatment, rheumatic fever injured the heart far less seriously than it had when Thomas Maclagan first used salicin seventy-five years earlier. This lessening of impairment may well have left the impression of the benefits of Coburn's treatment.

## Radiation

A few physicians approached chronic myocardial inflammation with an entirely different therapeutic strategy. Beginning in the mid-1920s, Robert Levy, also at Presbyterian Hospital in New York, used radiation. His rationale was that x-ray killed inflammatory cells; in rheumatic fever Aschoff bodies were sites of inflammation. Over a period of many years, Levy selected a small number of patients with evidence of myocarditis and gave them four to twenty-five radiation treatments for a total dose of about 1500 rad, which in itself was capable of injuring the heart's muscle. Although Levy believed that his patients benefited from radiation, he was unable, of course, to obtain myocardial biopsies to verify his claims.[78] Never widely accepted, radiation nevertheless was assessed during World War II among naval personnel hospitalized with rheumatic fever. Giving much lower doses, naval physicians could detect no benefit.[79]

## Treatment for Congestive Heart Failure

Treating congestive heart failure with digitalis offered the hope of shortening the time a child spent in bed. Heart failure made the experience of rheumatic fever even more desperate for victims. Shortness of breath, swollen legs, and greatly enlarged livers worsened the quality of life. Some of the earliest trials of digitalis pushed the dose to the point where toxic effects were evident on the electrocardiogram. In this fashion, children's heart disease actually worsened.[80] The narrow range between effective dose and overdose in children proved a difficult one to achieve, but when it was attained, victims of rheumatic heart disease benefited.[81]

Physicians at the House of the Good Samaritan worked out the details. The first line of therapy for congestive heart failure was restricting fluid intake and lowering dietary salt. If the child remained symptomatic, doctors added a mercurial or xanthine diuretic, both drugs with side effects in the 1940s. When these efforts were not enough, they added digitalis, carefully monitoring for ill effects. In this manner, most children showed signs of improvement.[82]

## Conclusion

The concept of "activity," sulfonamide prophylaxis, and carefully monitored aspirin provided physicians with tools to combat rheumatic fever. Without question, they improved the lot of victims of the disease. One cannot leave this conclusion without a parting, sympathetic remembrance for all those children who spent months or years in convalescent homes, some exposed to cold and the elements, in enforced bed rest, with few visits from parents and family. Some endured rigor-producing fever for chorea; others serious side effects from early sulfonamide or digitalis; a few overdosage of radiation; most had tonsils removed. Their travail is part of the history of rheumatic fever.

CHAPTER 9

# Penicillin, Cortisone, and Heart Surgery, 1945–1965

⟊

$\mathcal{M}$idcentury was a heady time in rheumatic fever's history. Penicillin, not employed extensively for the treatment of streptococcal sore throat or in the prevention of recurrences of rheumatic fever before the late forties, largely replaced sulfonamide. Penicillin had several critical advantages over the older drugs. It killed streptococci instead of merely inhibiting bacterial replication. As such, penicillin proved strikingly more successful in treating the streptococcal infection (Coburn's Phase I) that immediately preceded the development of rheumatic fever (Coburn's Phase III), an obstacle that sulfonamide had failed to surmount. When compared with sulfonamide, penicillin had fewer unpleasant and life-threatening side effects. Penicillin was also effective in preventing relapses, and here too it demonstrated superiority over prior drugs. In the early fifties, pharmacologists reformulated penicillin into a long-acting injection of benzathine penicillin. Rather than pills several times each day, physicians and patients could now elect a single monthly shot. Always more popular with physicians, nurses, public health workers, and parents than with young children because of the considerable pain, monthly "bicillin" was almost foolproof in preventing relapses.

"Wonder" drugs were not limited to prevention. The early fifties ushered in two additional drugs—widely hailed as miraculous—for treating rheumatic fever, especially life-threatening myocarditis, a goal that had largely eluded aspirin. In untangling the hormonal web connecting the pituitary and adrenal glands, endocrinologists had identified a pituitary hormone, ACTH, that normally stimulated the adrenal glands to secrete cortisone. One property of cortisone was to reduce inflammation, the hallmark of symptoms in rheumatic fever. Physicians hoped to provide highly effective anti-inflammatory relief to patients either by administering ACTH, in doses that greatly exceeded the normal level of bodily hormone, or by giving large amounts of cortisone. The initial reception of these hormones was reminiscent of the introduction of salicylate seventy-five years earlier. First reports proclaimed dramatic deathbed rescues. Soon, concern over serious side effects and

*140*

the reappearance of symptoms after stopping hormones, or "rebound," dampened enthusiasm. Almost immediately, the American Heart Association and the British Medical Research Council collaborated to study the comparative benefits of hormones and aspirin. Here the epidemiological amelioration of rheumatic fever impeded determining whether hormones were superior to aspirin by limiting the number of critically ill children available for study. When the multinational collaborators completed the first phase of their investigation in 1955, they announced a stalemate which tempered some enthusiasm for cortisone but which paradoxically failed to convince many of those most closely involved in treating patients with rheumatic fever. When the therapeutic dust settled in the midsixties, there were so few children suffering from devastating carditis that most physicians selected therapy based on their experience rather than on rigorously vetted scientific proof. Many thought that the powerful drugs were no longer needed.

Aggressive heart surgery added to the excitement of the early fifties. Overcoming a decades-long reluctance to operate on heart valves, surgeons in the late forties began to repair and then to replace heart valves left permanently damaged despite all medical therapy. Most rheumatic injury to the heart evaded the surgeon; for example, there was no surgical treatment for myocarditis. Only the damaged endocardium was the surgeon's target. The most commonly injured valve, the mitral valve, fortunately was the least difficult for the surgeon to approach and mend. Even here, surgeons, with the aid of new professional colleagues—catheter-wielding cardiologists—had to select patients who were sick enough to justify the risks of surgery but who were not so ill that even a repaired heart valve would fail to alter a progressively fatal course. In tackling damaged heart valves, surgeons not only developed new surgical techniques and procedures but also encountered unpredictable consequences. Cutting through the tissues of the heart provoked a serious postoperative complication that surgeons later termed "post-pericardiotomy syndrome," initially provocative because it shared many characteristics with rheumatic fever, fueling concern that surgery was actually "reactivating" long-dormant rheumatic fever. Tissue removed from the left atrial appendage of the heart as a consequence of surgery provided pathologists with the first cardiac specimens from living patients in the history of the study of rheumatic fever. The finding that many had apparently fresh Aschoff bodies, long after the disease was thought "burned-out," prompted pathologists to rethink the natural history of the disease and the significance of the cardinal Aschoff body.

A clear mandate to remove the triggering streptococcus with penicillin seemed the unavoidable conclusion to laboratory research. Here the dramatic moderating of streptococcal diseases in general and rheumatic fever in particular hindered efforts. Office-based research pointed to obstacles. Much streptococcal infection was now asymptomatic. Some streptococcal disease mimicked the common cold. Only a fraction of streptococcal illnesses produced the "classical" symptoms of sore throat with accompanying signs of fever, swollen lymph nodes, and exudative pharyngitis. In most office practice, only 1 percent of streptococcal throat infections progressed to cause rheumatic fever. And these few cases were far milder by every measure than cases of a generation earlier. With the simple office throat culture, physicians had the means of diagnosing streptococcal disease quickly and accurately, but determining which patients required culturing was problematic. With every epidemiological study pointing toward the marked reduction in the incidence of rheumatic fever, some physicians in the fifties began to question whether close surveillance of the streptococcus in the office setting was even necessary. Even parents of the children at greatest risk, those with prior episodes of rheumatic fever, often neglected to take their offspring to the physician's office for monthly injections of penicillin. Most children did not suffer negative consequences.

The moderating nature of rheumatic fever and hormonal therapies that carried serious side effects prompted physicians to rethink Duckett Jones's criteria for diagnosis. Initially revised in 1955 and again in 1965, the new guidelines called for more objective evidence before reaching a diagnosis. Recommending a lifetime punctuated with painful monthly injections placed an increased burden of proof upon frontline physicians. At midcentury, the challenge for the physician was the diagnosis, prevention, and treatment of an increasingly rare disease.

## Penicillin

Penicillin altered rheumatic fever's clinical landscape. Although Alexander Fleming had observed the bacteria-killing nature of the penicillium mold in 1928, penicillin largely remained for the next decade an effective laboratory tool for sorting out bacteria on blood agar plates. In the late 1930s, Howard Florey and Ernest Chain at Oxford revitalized Fleming's idea and systematically explored it. The urgency of World War II brought an extraordinary cooperative transatlantic effort among university scientists, pharmaceutical industries, and the military which resulted in transforming penicillin from a promising laboratory mold into a most effective drug in sufficient quantities to meet the needs of infected soldiers.[1]

Victims of rheumatic fever were not among the first to receive penicillin. Sulfonamide—while imperfect—seemed adequate to meet the need of preventing relapses. But the mix of streptococcal infection and military life—both during and after the war—reversed the epidemiological downturn for rheumatic fever, prompting efforts to find more effective means of prevention. Much of the research of fundamental importance occurred in remote Cheyenne, Wyoming, at Fort Francis E. Warren Air Force Base and its Streptococcal Disease Laboratory. At first glance an unlikely setting, the Rocky Mountain states had enjoyed less of the downswing in incidence of rheumatic fever than other parts of the country. As such, this region emerged as an epidemiological "hot spot." The barrack life of recruits had always promoted more streptococcal illness and subsequent rheumatic fever than civilian life. While most of the nation welcomed the considerable lessening of rheumatic fever, the military continued to feel its crippling impact. A captive band of subjects, recruits provided considerable ease for careful study of the natural history of streptococcal illness and rheumatic fever, the bacteriological and immunological consequences they provoked, and the benefits of therapy. Into this fruitful concurrence of geography and military environment came a talented group of researchers who would dedicate much of their careers to this disease: Lewis

Wannamaker, Charles H. Rammelkamp, Jr., and Floyd W. Denny.[2] Of course, military life and its diseases were not perfect reflections of civilian life. For example, recruits were older by a decade than most civilians suffering an initial bout of rheumatic fever. Barrack life bred epidemics of streptococcal disease that proved more virulent than civilian "office practice," because, as the Fort Francis Warren group demonstrated, it selected out streptococci with more potent M proteins. Eventually, some would question whether insights gained in Wyoming were entirely applicable to Main Street.

Picking up a thread suggested by physicians at the House of the Good Samaritan,[3] the Fort Francis Warren group set out to see whether penicillin could abort the progression from streptococcal sore throat (Coburn's Phase I) to rheumatic fever (Coburn's Phase III), a crucial shortcoming of sulfonamide. These older drugs could prevent streptococci from multiplying but could not eliminate them from the pharynx. When physicians had stopped giving sulfonamide to patients, streptococci lingered in the throat to trigger rheumatic fever. In sharp contrast, penicillin promptly killed all streptococci. The question was one of timing: would penicillin overcome the necessary delay between the acquisition of bacteria on the tonsils and the start of antibiotic? Older studies had implied that streptococci needed some time to initiate the rheumatic havoc (Coburn's Phase II), but the span of the therapeutic window of opportunity was uncertain.

A close look at one of the initial investigations reveals the power of their method. They enrolled over *1,600* recruits who suffered from sore throats severe enough to produce exudates of pus on their tonsils. Researchers cultured all for streptococci and tested all serially for antistreptolysin-O. Randomly, they divided the recruits into a group that received penicillin and a control group that received no antibiotic, which was, of course, the prevailing approach in 1949 to the initial management of streptococcal tonsillitis. This random assignment eliminated a bias that had entered Caroline Bedell Thomas's earlier studies with sulfonamide when only those patients who were compliant received the drug. Only two men in the penicillin group subsequently developed rheumatic fever compared with seventeen in the control group. Penicillin was clearly more effective than no treatment. A crucial benefit to this study was the calculation that 2 percent of patients with untreated streptococcal sore throats ultimately went on to develop rheumatic fever, a prediction subsequently refined upward to 3 percent.[4]

Almost immediately, the treatment of streptococcal throat infections with penicillin became the recommendation of the American Heart Association. Because many physicians' offices did not have ready access to definitive culture techniques in the early 1950s, the AHA encouraged giving penicillin even in "suspected" cases.[5] With a similar study design, the Fort Francis Warren group determined that recruits benefited from penicillin even when the treatment began as long as nine days after the start of throat symptoms.[6] When long-acting benzathine penicillin became available, the Fort Francis Warren group demonstrated that a single injection eliminated streptococci from the throats of nearly 100 percent of sufferers. Once the streptococci were gone, the threat of rheumatic fever vanished.[7] So successful was long-acting penicillin that the navy began administering a single shot to all recruits in 1957.[8] Cementing the supremacy of penicillin over the more familiar sulfonamides, such as sulfadiazine, which doctors continued to use successfully in prophylaxis of recurrences, physicians at Fort Warren demonstrated once again that these drugs were unsuccessful in eliminating streptococci from throats and, as such, had no role in the treatment of the preceding streptococcal infection.[9]

### Long-Acting Injections of Penicillin (Bicillin) for the Prevention of Rheumatic Fever

The people with the most at stake were those recovering from rheumatic fever. Until now, the only measure of safety against relapse was the daily dosage of sulfonamide carried out for years. Would treatment with penicillin of subsequent streptococcal infections, instead of continuous prophylaxis, serve this population? At the House of the Good Samaritan, Benedict Massell too had a ready group of patients to study. Massell had taken over direction of much of the research at "Good Sam" after Duckett Jones became the medical director at the Helen Hay Whitney Foundation, which sponsored research in rheumatic fever. Massell was able to culture throats thrice weekly of patients convalescing from rheumatic fever. As soon as streptococci appeared (whether or not they produced symptoms in the child), he started penicillin. When he did so, only 6 percent of patients relapsed compared with nearly half of patients who served as controls. The lesson drawn was that penicillin used in this fashion was beneficial but not as effective as continuous prophylaxis with sulfadiazine, which, when followed, eliminated most relapses. In marked contrast to physicians at Fort Francis Warren, Massell studied only forty-six patients.[10]

A natural consequence of the Fort Francis Warren investigations was to see whether penicillin would also be effective in a scheme of continuous prophylaxis. Initially, penicillin was available only in injectable form and as such was considerably less attractive for daily use than oral sulfadiazine. In the early 1950s, penicillin became available in oral tablets. Dosage was five times the intramuscular route, and to be effective penicillin had to be given three or four times a day on an empty stomach, no mean task for parents to accomplish. Despite obstacles, penicillin proved highly efficacious. Its advantage over sulfadiazine was that physicians did not need to follow white blood counts looking for early signs of drug-induced toxicity.[11] The question arose whether patients and their families would be able to follow such a schedule for years. As a more palatable alternative, some doctors suggested, with initial clinical success, using oral penicillin intensively just one week each month.[12] For most physicians, the continuous daily prophylaxis with either sulfadiazine or penicillin was the safest recommendation for children who survived one bout of rheumatic fever.[13]

Long-acting penicillin, benzathine penicillin or "bicillin," changed the calculus of prophylaxis. Gene H. Stollerman, who began a career devoted to streptococcal illness and rheumatic fever at Irvington House, found in 1952 that a single monthly injection provided sufficient penicillin to prevent streptococcal infection. Its advantage, immediately appreciated by workers in the field, was that nurses, doctors, and parents could make certain that children received an adequate dose of the drug. Its disadvantage, also immediately appreciated by child recipients, was that the volume of penicillin required was sizable and its intramuscular injection painful.[14] Children balked so often that some physicians, including May Wilson, who was now working with a younger colleague, Wan Ngo Lim, at New York Hospital, offered oral penicillin coupled with frequent reminders from the office. Most doctors argued that monthly shots provided the most efficient means of prophylaxis.[15] In 1955 Stollerman formulated the general principles of prophylaxis: antibiotic for at least five years after the initial bout of rheumatic fever, preferably penicillin, in monthly injections because it eliminated the difficulties of multiple daily dosing.[16] The recommendation extended even to children who did not suffer carditis as a major manifestation of rheumatic fever, out of concern that a second or third bout might attack the heart.[17] Just how long to continue prophylaxis was a debated point. Clearly the risk of recurrence declined with time, especially after twenty years of age, but it never went away.[18] Despite this observation and the marked decline in rheumatic fever, the American Heart Association in 1965 recommended prophylaxis for life.[19]

Continuous penicillin posed theoretical problems. Would it lead to resistance of the group A beta-hemolytic streptococcus? Fortunately, that did not occur. Penicillin did result, however, in other resistant mouth flora, especially among non-hemolytic streptococci, that presented the worrisome possibility of untreatable bacterial endocarditis, always a concern for people with scarred heart valves.[20]

### Penicillin and Public Health Programs

Prophylactic penicillin offered communities a cheap alternative to long hospital stays for convalescent care. Newton, Massachusetts, was among the first to act. After consulting with Duckett Jones and Benedict Massell, public health officials set up a program to identify those children who needed prophylaxis. First, Jones and Massell joined community leaders in public forums to educate physicians regarding the need to provide penicillin. Next, Jones and Massell asked Newton's doctors to cull their files for cases. Then public health officials sent questionnaires home with all 14,000 of the community's schoolchildren asking parents whether their child had ever received the diagnosis of rheumatic fever. Responses revealed that 379 children had. The parents were directed to make an appointment with their physicians to confirm the memory and, if correct, to seek penicillin tablets for continuous prophylaxis. Newton's doctors substantiated the parents' recollections for 214 of the children. If parents could not afford the price of penicillin, the Newton Health Department supplied it without cost. The program enjoyed considerable success. The questionnaire revealed that only 16 percent of children who needed prophylaxis had received the antibiotic before the start of the project. The program raised this to 80 percent. Of note, despite intensive physician and parent education that reached into every home and the availability of free penicillin, one-fifth of those in need did not receive the drug.[21]

Officials in Youngstown, Ohio, went further; they set out to prevent even first attacks of rheumatic fever. Beginning in 1950, the same year that the Fort Francis Warren physicians reported the efficacy of treating the preceding bout of streptococcal sore throat, Youngstown public health officials went to work. A close look at their program illustrates the immensity of the project. It began with an intensive educational campaign—public lectures, Parent-Teacher Association programs, radio shows, and newspaper articles—that targeted, separately, physicians and nurses, schoolteachers and principals, and parents and children. The following year, officials put their program into gear. Any child with a sore throat was directed to report to the school nurse, who obtained a throat culture. The parent of an absent child received a phone call to determine whether the absence was due to tonsillitis. If so, the parent was urged to obtain a throat culture either at school or at a physician's office. Through both routes, nearly nine hundred cultures were obtained in 1951. Six percent of the cultures grew hemolytic streptococci. Both the parent and the child's physician received telephone notification of a positive culture with instruction for the child to seek medical attention. The following day, the school nurse once again called the parent to ask what action had been taken. Foolproof? Not at all. Despite these efforts, only half of the children received any penicillin; less than a third received a full course of the drug.[22]

Community and state programs proliferated. In 1950 two states offered free antibiotics to needy patients; in 1958 the number grew to twenty-nine. These antibiotic programs joined the Crippled Children's Program public sector efforts—which had grown to include all but one state in aiding "cardiac cripples."[23]

### Inadequacy of Public Health Programs: The Biological Evolution of Rheumatic Fever and Physician Error

Despite identification and treatment programs, children with rheumatic fever still found their way to doctors' offices. Leaders in the field analyzed the reasons for these "preventable" cases. After talking with parents and children, physicians at Irvington House discovered that over 40 percent of bouts of rheumatic fever were preceded by totally asymptomatic streptococcal illnesses, which had been detected only through rising antistreptolysin-O titer in the blood.[24] Two-thirds of patients arriving with rheumatic fever at the House of the Good Samaritan had not consulted a doctor for the preceding illness, largely due to the mild nature of the symptoms. The third who had attended a doctor received either an incorrect diagnosis or inadequate therapy.[25] A different, but no less distressing, story came from doctors at La Rabida Sanitarium in Chicago. Only one-third of patients with sore throats received a throat culture. Even more disturbing, only one-third of blood agar plates had been interpreted correctly by the physician as demonstrating the presence of hemolytic streptococci.[26] With these problems in mind, Benedict Massell advised parents and physicians: mothers should take a sick child's temperature four times a day. If the fever ever reached 101 degrees, she should consult a physician. Unless the cause of the fever was clearly identified, a physician should obtain a throat culture. The appearance of any beta-hemolytic colonies on the bacterial plate should dictate penicillin. Even these stringent guide-lines, of course, did not detect totally asymptomatic cases or prevent physician error.[27]

Programs for prophylaxis of recurrences fared no better. Two-thirds of children discharged from Herrick House, a convalescent hospital thirty miles west of Chicago, were no longer taking penicillin at a follow-up visit. About half of the parents gave as a reason that they had stopped bringing their children to a doctor. The prescription had simply run out. As woeful, the other half selected doctors who did not understand the need for continuous prophylaxis. Some of these physicians stopped the penicillin because there was no evidence of heart disease, a sign, of course, of the measure's success and the need for its continuance.[28] A survey conducted by the U.S. Public Health Service and the American College Health Association of over 500,000 first-year students entering 137 colleges during a five-year period in the late 1950s revealed the immensity of the problem. Only half of the adolescents in need of prophylaxis had ever been enrolled in a program; merely 12 percent arrived at college taking penicillin.[29] A similar poll of military recruits in 1960 revealed that only 7 percent of those in need received antibiotics.[30] One interpretation of this neglect was that rheumatic fever had disappeared from the public mind as a health menace.

### ACTH and Cortisone

"A new era in the study and treatment of rheumatic diseases began on April 13, 1949," Benedict Massell precisely proclaimed, when Philip Hench and colleagues at the Mayo Clinic first gave patients cortisone and ACTH.[31] Cortisone and ACTH hormones, known to physiologists for over a decade as "compound E" and "compound F," had not been available in sufficient amounts for human trials until 1948. The first patients to receive the hormones were victims of Addison's Disease, who lacked normal levels of cortisone. Hench, who had edited annual critical surveys of literature dealing with rheumatological diseases since 1935, turned his attention to the potent anti-inflammatory characteristics of these compounds. Hench proposed their use, at much higher doses, in degenerative arthritis in adults and rheumatic fever in children. His supposition was that both drugs should lower fever, lessen the pain and swelling of arthritis, and reverse the carditis—all signs of inflammation—in rheumatic fever. Hench understood that giving pituitary ACTH resulted in patients' secreting higher than normal amounts of adrenal cortisone. In essence, giving either preparation resulted in increasing the level of cortisone available to lessen inflammation. At first, Hench treated just seven patients. He was impressed with the prompt response in abating symptoms and urged further study.[32]

Massell and physicians at the House of the Good Samaritan immediately accepted the task of exploring the effects of hormones, and later in 1949 they administered ACTH to ten of their sickest patients. Like many physicians who regularly treated those seriously ill with rheumatic fever, Massell understood that aspirin had serious limitations, especially in healing carditis. His initial experience with hormones rendered him an ardent convert. He had good reason for his passion: even in these precariously ill patients fever vanished in a day, joint pain in one to three days, joint swelling in two to three days, pericarditis and congestive heart failure in less than two weeks. The sedimentation rate returned to normal in less than one month; nodules melted in less than two months. Large doses of ACTH had side effects: acne, stretch marks, headaches, and in a few cases psychiatric disturbances. More immediately, ACTH promoted fluid retention that initially worsened congestive heart failure. To Massell, the benefits of hormone were "striking" and far outweighed the complications, hitting a chord that was struck again and again throughout the medical profession.[33]

What followed was a cascade of reports from many hospitals that treated children with rheumatic fever. For the most part they described experiences with a small number of patients, often just during the period when the drug was administered. In part, the small numbers were dictated by the epidemiological downswing of the disease: no hospital had enough patients, especially with life-threatening carditis, to conduct a study that would achieve statistical significance. There were other problems. What was the appropriate dose, for how long should treatment last, what signs should the clinician follow, how many side effects could be tolerated? Treatment with cortisone was often followed by a new phenomenon: a distressing "flare" or "rebound" of symptoms once medication was stopped. What did these new symptoms mean for the prognosis of the patient? Despite shortcomings, these early reports were uniformly enthusiastic, especially in the treatment of the sickest patients—those with pericarditis (fortunately now rare) and myocarditis complicated by congestive heart failure.[34]

A second wave of hormonal clinical trials suggested chinks in the armor. At Bellevue Hospital in New York City, physicians confirmed that hormones were strikingly effective in treating fever and arthritis and in improving the general "well being" of the patient, for example, improving appetite. At issue, did hormone benefit the heart? In a discussion that bore striking resemblance to the debate on the value of salicylate seventy-five years earlier, the Bellevue doctors thought cortisone helped with pericarditis, perhaps aided myocarditis, but almost certainly did not prevent damage to heart valves.[35] Several groups concluded—again from the perspective of their small numbers of patients—that hormone produced no benefit to the heart but ladened the patient with serious side effects.[36]

A third wave, still relying on small numbers but profiting now from the experiences of others, attempted to sort things out. May Wilson believed that timing predicted success with hormones. Patients in her care uniformly did well when treated with hormone during the initial five days of the symptoms.[37] Some physicians believed that children required still higher doses, despite concerns over serious side effects.[38] Benedict Massell entered this round of the debate with only slightly tempered enthusiasm. Reviewing his experience at the House of the Good Samaritan and the now extensive literature, he reached a conclusion virtually identical with that of May Wilson: prompt use of cortisone, before the development of permanent heart damage, was clearly beneficial to children.[39]

## Sorting out Therapy: The British Medical Research Council and the American Heart Association

The paucity of patients and the flush of excitement accompanying the dramatic first usage of cortisone were just two of the impediments to assessing the true worth of steroid hormones. The very nature of rheumatic fever, with manifestations so variable that it required Duckett Jones's algorithm just to make a diagnosis, confounded clear-headed study.[40] After the first enthusiasm for hormone waned, the need plainly emerged to establish its worth compared with aspirin, the flawed but nonetheless accepted treatment. Complicating matters still further was the question whether it made a therapeutic difference which hormone was used, ACTH or cortisone. Early studies comparing hormones and aspirin could establish no obvious superiority, but these investigations, carried out in single hospitals, also suffered from lack of sufficient numbers of patients.[41] Even Benedict Massell, hormonal advocate, conceded in 1953 that the relative merit of competing drugs was an unresolved issue.[42]

In the hope of settling these therapeutic perplexities, the Medical Research Council of Great Britain and the American Heart Association collaborated in a carefully constructed, twelve-hospital study. Its coordinators included many of the major leaders and institutions most closely involved with rheumatic fever.[43] Each of the over five hundred patients had to meet Jones's criteria for diagnosis, modified only to make it more rigorous by requiring observable swelling and limitation of motion of joints, or arthritis, in place of Jones's original inclusion of simple joint pain, or arthralgia. All patients received penicillin treatment for current streptococcal infection and were placed on penicillin prophylaxis. All endured the rigors of enforced bed rest. The patients were randomly assigned to one of three drug regimens: aspirin (at a dose somewhat lower than Coburn's suggested schedule), cortisone, or ACTH. The duration of all three drugs was six weeks. Patients were kept in the hospital under observation during this period and for three weeks after stopping the drugs. Patients returned for clinic appointments monthly for six months and then every other month. The protocol thus seemed nearly perfect: the best investigators and institutions, rigorous diagnostic criteria, uniform administration of drugs, in-hospital observation, close follow-up, and conclusions subjected to demanding statistical tests. "Nearly" perfect in that detractors pointed out that there was not a group receiving no drug at all.

The conclusions astonished many, including some of the participating physicians. Despite a few minor differences, no drug showed superiority. Equally powerful was the conclusion that no drug cured rheumatic fever. All worked well with fever and joint symptoms. None was particularly effective with chorea and erythema multiforme. No clear advantages emerged in treating the all-important heart disease, although there were only a few patients in the "seriously ill" category, despite the large number enrolled in the study.[44]

The study also clarified the nature and seriousness of the "rebound" phenomenon that occurred when hormone was stopped. Nearly half of patients developed new fever; more than half had marked change in the erythrocyte sedimentation rate; some suffered from new arthritis; fewer from distressing new cardiac symptoms.[45] While not insurmountable problems, they needed to be factored into any decision about therapy.

Benedict Massell disagreed with the findings of the "cooperative report" even though the conclusions were based in part on his patients and his evaluations of the drugs they received. He insisted that hormones given early in the course of rheumatic fever performed better than aspirin.[46] Physicians from Sheffield promptly modified the findings to suggest that aspirin and cortisone, used together, performed better than either alone, a conclusion based on only six patients.[47]

Some took substantive aim at the "cooperative report." Believing that the six-week duration was too short, six American hospitals (Bellevue, Babies, Mount Sinai, and Montefiore Hospitals in New York City, House of the Good Samaritan in Boston, and Babies' Hospital in Cleveland) joined forces in the late 1950s to see whether twelve weeks of hormone, now in the form of prednisone, demonstrated an advantage over aspirin. Enrolling only fifty-seven patients among them, these researchers—the Combined Rheumatic Fever Study Group—again could demonstrate no clear advantage.[48] This conclusion was reinforced by a five-year follow-up analysis of patients initially enrolled in the British/American Cooperative Study, which continued to demonstrate no advantage for either drug in the long-term prognosis of patients.[49]

The conviction that steroid was superior to aspirin died hard. The Combined Rheumatic Fever Study Group tested May Wilson's assertion of a decade earlier that a short course of high-dose (in fact, three times the accepted maximum dose) prednisone early in the disease improved a child's odds. It did not. These researchers remarked that further studies were unlikely "in view of the declining severity of rheumatic fever." Since aspirin and prednisone yielded similar results, aspirin's fewer side effects tipped the balance in its favor.[50] In 1965, a ten-year follow-up analysis of the British/American Cooperative Study maintained its judgment that both drugs, while flawed, worked equally well.[51]

Despite the thrust of these multi-centered studies, belief in the superior value of steroids persisted. The discrepancy caught the eye of medical editorial writers, who explained the aberrancy to readers: most physicians who had considerable experience with rheumatic fever became convinced early on that hormones were superior to aspirin in helping the sickest patients, now very few in number. These seriously ill patients were not enrolled randomly in the large studies; instead all received cortisone. Large studies had not actually answered the questions put to them; and epidemiological realities rendered additional studies unnecessary.[52]

### Mitral Valve Surgery

At midcentury, surgeons, who had played virtually no role in the history of rheumatic fever except in performing tonsillectomies, grabbed a portion of center stage with operations which successfully repaired damaged heart valves. The early history of surgery to correct mitral stenosis has captured the fascination of both surgeons and historians, focusing in particular on the lag between early suggestions for surgical repair in the first years of the century and initial surgical success and (mostly) failures in the 1920s, and on a second delay until the late 1940s when surgeons in the United States (Boston[53]—Dwight E. Harkin, Laurence B. Ellis, Paul F. Ware, and Leona R. Norman; Philadelphia[54]—Robert Glover, Charles Bailey, and Thomas J. E. O'Neill; and Baltimore—Alfred Blalock) and England[55] (Charles Baker, R. C. Brock, and Maurice Campbell) took up their scalpels with considerable success.[56]

Much epidemiological history separated initial suggestions, surgical attempts of the 1920s, and surgical success of the 1940s. In all three periods, the surgical target was the damaged mitral valve. Yet the nature of rheumatic heart disease had changed considerably in fifty years. In 1900 rheumatic fever frequently injured all tissues of the heart, especially mitral and aortic heart valves and myocardium. Isolated mitral valve injury was rare, and many thought that it did not exist. Affected heart valves were often severely calcified. In most cases, a greatly weakened heart muscle accompanied the damaged heart valves. Rheumatic carditis was thus a multi-tissue disease. Even if one were bold enough to attempt to fix the mitral valve, a surgeon faced a major reconstructive task almost certainly beyond surgical remedy in 1900. Despite some operative success with chest diseases, surgeons understood that just entering the thoracic cavity carried grave risk. By the late 1940s, rheumatic heart disease was a very different illness. The myocardial component, while the most common cardiac injury, was less debilitating. Even so, surgeons still worried that any operation on the mitral valve might not succeed because of the weakened heart muscle. Equally important, rheumatic endocarditis was far less likely to leave terribly scarred valves. In other words, between 1900 and 1950, both rheumatic myocarditis and valvular disease moderated significantly.

Moderating biology, however, was only part of the story. Surgeons, who in the 1920s had selected desperately ill cases, in the 1940s refined their targets for surgical attack. Although the surgical goal in the 1940s was reopening the scarred heart valve, surgeons such as Dwight Harkin properly realized that rheumatic fever had also injured the myocardium. In many patients, myocarditis smoldered decades after the initial bout of rheumatic fever. At issue was assessing how great an impediment myocardial injury presented. Here surgeons made use of the clinical concept of "rheumatic activity." Any surgeon needed to make certain that all signs of "active" myocarditis, such as arrhythmia or congestive heart failure, were long past. For these assurances, the surgeon relied on the patient's history—long free from relapse—and on a normal electrocardiogram and sedimentation rate. Even so, there were concerns that a weakened myocardium might not withstand the surgical assault. In selecting appropriate cases for surgery, Harkin and others wanted patients who had evidence of isolated mitral stenosis and not the commonly accompanying injuries of mitral regurgitation or aortic valve disease. In other words, surgeons selected highly specific candidates for operation.

Harkin was also aware of the earlier surgical scorecard, with only two patients surviving in the 1920s in ten attempts. In fact, he had consulted frequently with Elliott Cutler and Claude Beck, learning from their pioneering experiences.[57]

In 1954 Claude Beck stated that the changing nature of rheumatic mitral valve disease had helped to usher in the successful surgery of the forties. In the 1920s, the mitral valves he and Cutler had operated upon were severely scarred and calcified, greatly hindering surgery. In the 1940s, injured valves were less likely to be calcified and much more amenable to repair. Beck commented:

> I have been asked this question: "why did [Elliott C.] Cutler stop the operation for mitral stenosis?" There were several reasons. The valves we examined were calcified and rigid, and it looked as though a piece of valve should be cut away in order to relieve stenosis. It is probable that the pathology of the mitral valve has been changed by the use of sulfonamides and antibiotics, for we did not then see soft, pliable valves that could be opened by finger dilatation.[58]

Beck's bestowal of credit to antibiotics was both generous and almost certainly wrong. When Harkin and others began operating on injured heart valves, only a few of their patients had received penicillin. These patients had suffered their initial bouts with rheumatic fever decades earlier, even before the first use of sulfonamide. Evolving biology, not drugs, set the surgical stage.[59] Harkin was also familiar with the considerable animal experimentation of the 1930s and 1940s.[60] Indeed, his own laboratory work had developed a surgical technique for the repair of the mitral valve that relieved the obstruction without creating an incompetent valve.[61] Harkin was also emboldened by successes in repairing cardiac injuries in World War II and by early achievements in the surgical treatment of tetralogy of Fallot, a complex congenital heart malformation. In developing operations for heart wounds and "blue babies," surgeons had done much in improving techniques for thoracic surgery.[62] In sum, the reasons for the timing of surgery's entry in the history of rheumatic fever were dictated by evolving biology, laboratory research, and advances in surgical technique.

Early surgery on the mitral valve was nothing if not dramatic. After entering the chest and cutting through the pericardium, the surgeon identified the left atrium. Animal experiments had demonstrated that this was the safest and most direct route to the mitral valve. The surgeon then made an incision into the left atrial appendage, large enough to admit his index finger. The heart was beating, the operative field was blood-filled, and the surgeon's only direct assessment of the mitral valve was with his fingertip. Surgeons diverged in approaches at this point. Harkin, after evaluating the injured state of the mitral valve, used his finger to split the fused leaflets, an operation he called "finger valvuloplasty." Charles Bailey and others employed a small knife attached to the index finger to cut the narrowed valve, a procedure termed "commissurotomy." In either approach, the goal was increased forward flow of blood without creating catastrophic mitral regurgitation.[63] Bailey and colleagues had operated on over two hundred patients by 1951,[64] four hundred by 1952.[65] As one colleague stated, surgery on the mitral valve had quickly "passed through its pioneer phase."[66]

## Surgical Selection of Patients

Part of the initial success was the shrewd selection of patients. Surgeons classified the degree of impairment that the damaged mitral valve caused, eliminating those patients who were thought beyond surgical hope. By the early 1950s, characteristics of the "ideal" patient emerged: only mitral valve disease without evidence of calcification, injury severe enough to cause symptoms such as shortness of breath on exertion but not yet causing pulmonary hypertension or right-sided heart failure, no clinical evidence of active myocarditis, and young adults under fifty years of age. By the end of the 1950s, surgeons developed techniques to repair the aortic valve as well and demonstrated that adolescents also benefited from surgery if all signs of "active" myocarditis were long vanished.[67] In the view of many surgeons, valvular repair joined penicillin as a preventive measure in that successful surgery averted further strain on both valve and heart muscle.[68]

Surgeons investigated their concern about the weakened myocardium and in doing so provided insight into the evolution of rheumatic fever. As part of surgical repair of the mitral valve, the surgeon often needed to remove a small piece of the left atrial appendage. In essence, these were the first "biopsies" of living hearts that pathologists had ever received for study. At issue was whether these specimens showed evidence of active myocarditis. Nearly one-half contained lesions that most pathologists identified as Aschoff bodies, many of which appeared newly formed. This indicated that mitral valve disease was frequently associated with myocarditis, even active myocarditis—long a worry of both surgeons and physicians—but that the inflammation was now so mild that it did not undermine surgical results.[69]

## Surgical Outcomes

Surgical therapy opened opportunities for patients but was not without risk. An analysis of outcome at Columbia-Presbyterian Hospital in New York showed that half of the patients operated on in the 1950s enjoyed objective relief of symptoms. A fifth received no benefit from surgery; a tenth were made worse; and one quarter had died either as a result of surgery or in spite of surgery.[70] The postoperative experience for patients was often quite rocky. An unanticipated complication was the provocation of symptoms—fever, chest pain, accumulation of pericardial fluid, congestive heart failure, and arthritis—that mimicked a recurrence of rheumatic fever. To some these distressing symptoms, coupled with the finding of Aschoff bodies in the atrial appendages, indicated that surgery had "reactivated" dormant rheumatic fever. Careful sorting out of cases and the realization that these symptoms could occur after any operation that involved cutting the pericardium permitted surgeons to understand that this was a general problem of heart surgery and not a peculiar complication of rheumatic heart disease.[71]

Physicians in practice had to decide which of their patients were the most likely candidates for successful surgery. One physician stated the task: "The realization that rheumatic heart disease represents a pancarditis and surgery per se affects only one facet of the illness, namely the mechanical block to the forward flow of blood, should allow the development of a philosophy concerning the surgical approach."[72] Despite this catholic philosophy, the availability of surgery for some patients nevertheless focused considerable attention on the mitral valve. In particular, newer diagnostic techniques, such as the phonocardiogram, heart catheterization to measure pressures, and cineangiography to assess valvular function, aided physicians, high-technology cardiologists, and surgeons in selecting candidates.[73] In spite of shortcomings, surgery provided a new lease on active life for a sizable number of carefully selected patients.

## Therapy and Moderating Biology Alter Diagnosis

Penicillin (either as preventive or life-long prophylaxis), the availability of controversial and highly toxic hormones, and surgical repair of scarred heart valves collectively heightened the need for more precise diagnosis. Therapy raised the stakes for physicians and patients by inserting both risk and immediacy into decision making.[74] There were concerns of both "under-call" and "over-call." Parents insufficiently aware of the jeopardy that an untreated streptococcal sore throat caused their children often failed to seek a doctor's attention. Physicians, long schooled to downplay a simple "cold," had to reorganize their approach to often-minor complaints. Over-diagnosis was of equal concern: a lifetime of monthly bicillin injections demanded diagnostic accuracy. Some physicians made a casual decision about the presence or absence of streptococci without the benefit of either throat culture or antistreptolysin-O titer, its "method . . . too complicated and time-consuming to make it a feasible test for the average physician's office laboratory."[75]

Many communities addressed the problem of inaccurate diagnosis with consultative clinics, often staffed by cardiologists, that offered to confirm or modify the diagnosis reached previously by a child's primary care doctor.[76] Rheumatic fever's changing nature lay at the heart of diagnostic difficulties: it simply was not the highly dramatic illness it once had been. One physician from Levittown, New York, who served as a consultant for many generalists, explained: "Major and minor [Jones] criteria, when present, are of utmost diagnostic importance, but these are absent in the great majority of cases seen in the [referral] clinic; the 'typical' case, in our experience, has no explosive attack and few or none of the orthodox classical manifestations."[77]

A frequent source for referral occurred when a doctor, in the course of evaluating a child for a febrile illness, heard a heart murmur not appreciated during prior examinations. Children with fevers often complained of aches and pains; some acted a bit peculiarly. Were these symptoms the start of carditis, arthritis, and chorea? Should the child be on penicillin, aspirin, or cortisone; should the child be hospitalized; did the heart need the attention of specialized diagnostic technologies; did a surgeon need to be called? At most referral appointments, which occurred sometime after the acute illness, the child was entirely well; the fever gone; aches, pains, and unusual behaviors departed; and heart murmur, when still present, thought to be "functional," an odd term that meant "not completely normal but certainly not pathologic." Most referral centers agreed with the diagnosis of rheumatic fever in about one case in four.[78] These were largely mild cases. Incidentally, this worry over the meaning of heart murmurs left its mark on patients and parents long after rheumatic fever receded from view. Even decades later, the detection of any additional heart noise often engendered needless fear.

### Revised Jones Criteria

Therapies and the ever-moderating symptoms forced an "official" second edition of the Jones criteria in 1955. Researchers taking part in the Cooperative Study on cortisone, ACTH, and aspirin had called for the modifications so that all participants were in agreement on which children should be entered in the study. Duckett Jones took part in the revision just before his death. The same division of "major" and "minor" criteria remained, with two "majors" or one "major" and two "minors" needed to make a diagnosis. In several ways, the criteria were made more objective. For example, great lengths were taken to make as certain as possible that cardiac signs represented structural injury to the heart. Arthritis, with clear signs of redness, swelling, and limitation of movement of two or more joints, replaced mere joint pain, or arthralgia. Chorea needed to be demonstrable to the observer and of "moderate" severity. Minor manifestations were also tightened. Arthralgia, booted from the "majors," became a "minor," joining fever; a prolonged PR interval on the electrocardiogram; an elevated erythrocyte sedimentation rate, increased white blood cell count, or positive C-reactive protein; evidence of preceding Group A beta-hemolytic streptococcal infection; and a previous history of rheumatic fever.[79]

Stricter standards for diagnosis did not eliminate all errors, but at some referral centers the rate of over-diagnosis fell considerably.[80] Diagnostic criteria were made more objective still with a second revision in 1965. For the first time, diagnosis required evidence of the preceding streptococcal infection in addition to the same requisites of majors and minors.[81]

C-reactive protein served for some physicians as a surer sign of rheumatic "activity" than the erythrocyte sedimentation rate. A nonspecific but very sensitive indicator of inflammation, C-reactive protein, unlike the sedimentation rate, did not appear in the blood unless inflammation was present and disappeared once activity ceased. As such, it proved to be a more sensitive indicator for length of therapy, especially with cortisone, or beginning of relapse. Unfortunately, its measurement required complicated laboratory procedures, limiting its use in the 1950s and 1960s to larger hospitals.[82]

### Changing Clinical Management

Moderating severity of rheumatic fever accelerated the trend away from strict bed rest. At Herrick House, physicians in the 1950s began to worry about the psychological strain of prolonged inactivity. Children now felt better earlier in the course of their illnesses, emboldening doctors to encourage bathroom privileges, eating at tables, walking, fishing, hiking, and swimming.[83] In Sheffield, England, physicians also questioned the wisdom of protracted bed rest, but they conceded that it was no longer possible to perform a controlled clinical study because there were so few children hospitalized with serious rheumatic fever.[84]

In earlier years, the recommendation for reduced activity extended even to care after leaving the convalescent hospital. These restrictions often encouraged children and their families, friends, and teachers to believe that the victims of rheumatic fever were handicapped far in excess of their actual impairment. Physicians at Irvington House documented that many severely restricted children changed career goals or refrained from marriage and child-bearing. The military needlessly rejected many from service, merely on the strength of the history of having had the disease.[85] These practices died slowly. In one survey of physician practices in the late 1950s, nearly all doctors routinely limited physical activities, although less severely than a decade earlier.[86] For other physicians, bed rest remained the keystone of treatment into the 1960s.[87]

Interest in the psychological consequences of bed rest raised concerns about the emotional experience of the children and their families with rheumatic fever. Many children felt responsible for contracting the illness by wearing light clothes during winter, playing in the rain, and getting chilled.[88] One child explained, "I stayed out playing in the rain after the baby-sitter told me to come in." Another described the experience in the hospital: "I felt I was never going to get out of the hospital. [The nurses] break your toys and bother you a lot; they make you do all sorts of things and get in your way; they keep you in bed longer if they don't like you or what you do; I got out of bed once when I wasn't supposed to, and the next day they said I was worse and put me in a room by myself; That's when I really got sick."[89] Coming home from the hospital was often as difficult as leaving. Siblings resented the special attention that a sick child received and in some cases exploited. One child exclaimed, "They won't spank me; they wouldn't dare; I've been sick. I make my father do what I want him to; When he won't, I just grab my chest; he knows that I might die anytime."[90] Parents admitted being overly protective: "I don't dare let Joe ride a bicycle, [he might] drop dead." Another parent told her daughter, "Don't jump rope, Margaret, or you'll drop dead." Yet another overlooked truancy: "John has been sick and we can't expect much from him."[91] Both parents and children feared visits to the follow-up clinic. One child lamented, "It's so awful to have it hanging over you. Maybe some day you'll have it again. It's so terrible."[92]

Children who experienced chorea were particular targets for psychological study because of the apparent injury to the brain and nervous system.[93] Here the experts divided, some believing that chorea resulted in long-standing emotional difficulties;[94] others asserting that chorea healed without residual effect.[95] Despite varying opinions, all understood that the issue was moot: chorea was vanishing.

At the end of the 1950s, Currier McEwen, a physician at Bellevue Hospital, summarized the turbulent ten years of therapy. Prevention of the first attack and antibiotic prophylaxis until adulthood or beyond against relapse remained the cornerstone. Bed rest was no longer "strict," although a child could still expect a considerable period of severely limited activity. McEwen made a distinction between aspirin and cortisone even though all studies had failed to support any significant differences. He used aspirin alone if there was no evidence of carditis. When a child had definite signs of heart disease, he used prednisone for ten days followed by aspirin until all signs of rheumatic activity were extinguished. Children who failed to respond to aspirin and prednisone could expect a date with the surgeon.[96]

# The Waning of Rheumatic Fever: Molecular Biology, Epidemiology, and History, 1945–1965

$\mathcal{A}$t the end of World War II, J. Alison Glover, who had documented the steady decline of rheumatic fever throughout the twentieth century, offered an explanation for the downfall. While acknowledging the benefits of improvements in diet, housing, and standard of living, Glover suggested a more fundamental biological reason: "It seems probable that the main cause of the decline is of a more subtle kind, a change in the relationship between man and the *streptococcus pyogenes.*"[1] Glover offered several possibilities: Were humans more immune? Were humans "less likely to exhibit the rheumatic reaction"? Or was the streptococcus less virulent? Provocative questions when posed in 1946; by 1965 observations from molecular biology provided insights for epidemiologists and historians.

After the war, many laboratory researchers turned the tools of biochemistry and immunology more closely on the streptococcus to probe what it was about this germ's nature that provoked human destruction. These scientists took the streptococcus apart—structurally and biochemically—and analyzed whether and how each component provoked human chemical systems and tissues. Group A beta-hemolytic streptococcus became one of the most meticulously examined of all bacteria. Not all of these efforts pertained directly to rheumatic fever, but many significantly altered how scientists and physicians thought about germ and illness. Of vital relevance to historians of disease, ideas from molecular biology cast light on the movement of rheumatic fever through history. Molecular biology thus arose as a critical historical tool.

At first glance, these highly technical bench-laboratory studies might appear to be of interest only to that small group of scientists who were intrigued by the streptococcus. But these analyses explored interstices where germs abutted human populations. It was here that biology emerged as an essential historical aid. The discourse was that of highly specialized medical science; the import illuminated how one disease traveled through history. One scientific insight was that streptococcal proteins could serve as biologically active catalysts of *human* chemical reactions. For example, streptokinase was found to activate the human chemical reaction that dissolved blood clots. Another finding was that "M" proteins, which composed part of the bacterial cell wall, were responsible for virulence, epidemiological movement through populations, and ultimately human immunity. A third revelation was that these same M proteins, as well as other bacterial components, cross-reacted with human tissues, such as myocardium. Human antibodies produced to destroy an M protein—and consequently the streptococcus—served as well to attack the human myocardium. Rheumatic fever thus became a peculiar example of autoimmune disease. Initially performed in laboratory animals, these studies were confirmed in human heart tissue removed during heart surgery to repair damaged heart valves. Taken together, these studies indicated that streptococcus and humans were locked in an intimate ecological relationship. The streptococcus derailed the workings of the human body; changes in bacterial makeup provoked rheumatic fever. In other words, disease, epidemiology, molecular biology, and history merged.

### Epidemiological Demise of Rheumatic Fever

Glover's conclusion about the epidemiological demise of rheumatic fever received confirmation from virtually all quarters. A physician in Birmingham, England, explained, "Rheumatic fever seems to be a dying disease; the wards of children's hospitals are no longer full of rheumatic children, and rheumatic schools are not now hard pressed to accommodate patients seeking admission."[2] Even though rheumatic fever remained the major cause of heart disease in children, many predicted that even this special status would soon change, overtaken by congenital heart malformations.[3]

Physicians at the House of the Good Samaritan were in a particularly good place to document the changing nature of rheumatic fever. "Good Sam's" longitudinal experience with 3,500 children by 1950 was the most comprehensive in the United States. In every aspect, rheumatic fever was a milder disease in 1950 than in 1921 (table 10.1). Of particular note was the conspicuous difference in "marked cardiac enlargement," signaling a vast reduction in children who suffered congestive heart failure, clear evidence that rheumatic heart disease was moderating.[4] The mortality rate fell to about 1 percent at the House of the Good Samaritan in 1960.[5] Physicians at "Good Sam" credited a combination of factors: improved standard of living for the poorest urban dwellers in Boston, the medical focus on streptococcal disease with prompt treatment and prophylaxis, and the obvious mutation of rheumatic fever into a blander disease. Doctors at the Hospital for Sick Children in Toronto, evaluating a smaller number of children, recorded a similarly remarkable drop in severity and deaths.[6]

Public health officials from many cities contributed evidence of rheumatic fever's decline. In New York City, school health doctors identified fewer than one-half as many children with residual rheumatic heart disease attending school in

TABLE 10.1    *Declining severity of rheumatic heart disease,*
*House of the Good Samaritan, 1921–1951*

|  | Percentage with valvular disease | "Marked" cardiac enlargement | No cardiac enlargement | Deaths after five years |
|---|---|---|---|---|
| 1921–22 | 75% | 30% | 20% | 24% |
| 1930–31 | 65 | 23 | 20 | 20 |
| 1940–41 | 58 | 14 | 38 | 8 |
| 1950–51 | 60 | 14 | 45 | 3 |

SOURCE: Edward F. Bland, "Declining Severity of Rheumatic Fever, A Comparative Study of the Past Four Decades," *New England Journal of Medicine* (1960), 262: 597–599.

1953 as they had three decades previously.[7] Deaths from rheumatic heart disease fell in New York City by over 80 percent in the forties alone. In 1940, rheumatic fever was the second leading cause of death among children five to nine years old; first among those ten to fourteen; and second among those fifteen to nineteen. In 1950, rheumatic fever was not even in the top five causes of death for children five to nine years old, and had fallen to third place in the two older age groups.[8] Similar declines were recorded in New Haven, Connecticut,[9] Rochester, New York,[10] San Francisco,[11] Shreveport, Louisiana,[12] and Cardiff, Wales.[13] The military in both Britain[14] and the United States[15] rejected recruits far less frequently for reasons of crippling rheumatic heart disease in the years that followed World War II. Only in the Rocky Mountain states did rheumatic fever persist at its prior intensity, a finding that paralleled military experience at Fort Francis Warren in Wyoming.[16] American vital statistics painted the composite picture: deaths from rheumatic fever declined 70 percent between 1919 and 1945, a trend that actually accelerated during the late forties. Of note, these American statistics demonstrated that the remarkable decline was not shared equally along racial lines. Nonwhite children experienced a drop of only twenty-five percent.[17]

The Framingham Study described the state of rheumatic heart disease in 1956 among adults in one small city just west of Boston. Although primarily designed for following hypertension and arteriosclerotic heart disease, the Framingham Study shed light on rheumatic fever because it permitted physicians to examine the hearts of all adults in that city. What doctors discovered was that nearly 3 percent of citizens between thirty and sixty years of age still had signs of old rheumatic heart disease, mostly the murmurs of mitral stenosis. So mild had rheumatic heart disease become that fully five out of six experienced no limitation of life-style: individuals discovered their prior heart insult only as a result of enrolling in the larger study.[18] A survey of college students revealed a similar prevalence of rheumatic heart disease. About 2 percent of entering freshmen at over one hundred colleges reported having had a bout of rheumatic fever, with physicians confirming mild residual heart damage in about one-third of these.[19]

One measure of diminishing virulence was the downturn in the likelihood for rheumatic fever to relapse. May Wilson called attention to this aspect drawn from her close study of nearly eight hundred children at New York Hospital. Wilson recorded that over 20 percent of her patients had relapsed in 1936 compared with only 7 percent in 1951, the year when she started to prescribe antibiotics to prevent relapse.[20] A similar, but less profound, decline in recurrences was recorded among children in Cardiff.[21]

Rheumatic nodules were slowly disappearing. Physicians at Bellevue Hospital noted that 11 percent of patients between 1928 and 1942 had nodules. As Thomas Barlow and Walter Cheadle had noted sixty years earlier, the presence of nodules carried a graver risk of mortality. At Bellevue, 22 percent of children with nodules died, many times greater than children without nodules. From 1943 to 1958, the incidence of nodules fell to 9 percent, and mortality declined to 9 percent. In the twentieth century, nodules, when present, continued as an ominous prognostic sign.[22] Chorea, too, was disappearing. A review of nearly three hundred patients with chorea admitted to Babies' Hospital in New York between 1929 and 1941 revealed far less dramatic neurological involvement, with "movements . . . so subtle as to escape recognition," unless brought into relief with a detailed examination.[23]

Rheumatic fever had become a fundamentally different disease. As an editorial writer in the *Journal of the American Medical Association* noted in 1962, the incidence of the disease was much less, each symptom was milder, and, taken as a whole, rheumatic fever was far less severe than it had been a generation earlier.[24] So mild were the residual effects that women could aspire to become pregnant and bear children with little or no consequences.[25] Gene Stollerman captured rheumatic fever's vanishing nature:

> In many cities in the United States, convalescent hospitals and homes for children with rheumatic fever have closed their doors or changed their admission policies to include patients with related diseases . . . it is becoming more difficult to find cases of Sydenham's chorea and subcutaneous nodules to demonstrate to medical students, and fulminating, fatal rheumatic pancarditis has become relatively rare.[26]

### Moderating Biology: Military Setting

Stollerman firmly tied the alteration of rheumatic fever to shifting streptococcal epidemiology and to the fluid nature of the molecular biology of the streptococcus. One pillar of Stollerman's understanding was built solidly upon research at Fort Francis Warren in the early 1950s. In this military setting, severe epidemics of streptococcal disease swept through barracks housing new recruits from around the country. What separated these infections from the streptococcal sore throats encountered in private practice was the severity of illness, sheer numbers of victims, and geographical clustering of cases. This unique military setting allowed researchers to gather hundreds of cases in short periods of time. By contrast, in civilian practice it was unusual for everyone in a family, classroom, or church congregation to fall ill to serious streptococcal illness all at once. Streptococcal infection in the military setting also produced more rheumatic fever—around 3 percent of cases—than in civilian practice. Physicians at the Wyoming military installation suspected that its location in the Rocky Mountain area, with its greater prevalence of streptococcal illness, was one reason for so many cases of rheumatic fever, but comparisons with other military facilities, for example, those in North Carolina, revealed a similar vulnerability.[27]

Fort Warren physicians sought answers for the severity of streptococcal illness in the biochemical constituents of the streptococci they were isolating. What set these infections apart was the inclusion of specific M proteins—there were more than forty described by the 1950s—in the bacterial cell wall that made fighting off infection difficult. Investigators speculated that these streptococci, armed with potent M proteins, were responsible for the epidemic nature of the outbreaks and the seriousness of cases. They suspected, but could not prove, that these same M proteins were "rheumatogenic" in their ability to provoke rheumatic fever. Confounding their research was the growing awareness that, even in this special setting, nearly one-half of streptococcal infections were now so mild that they produced no symptoms.[28]

## Moderating Biology: Main Street Practice

Stollerman was not certain that military lessons were entirely relevant to the civilian office setting. In particular, he was well aware of the milder nature of streptococcal illness and the waning of rheumatic fever. Stollerman questioned whether the ground swell for the prompt and liberal use of penicillin in practice was actually necessary.[29] He called attention to careful epidemiological studies carried out by Milton Saslaw, a pediatrician in Miami, Florida, which showed that streptococcal infection remained common, but mild. Up to 40 percent of children in Miami had throat culture–proven streptococcal infections each winter. Many were entirely asymptomatic, detected only as a consequence of the study. Yet rheumatic fever was rare: only 1 percent of streptococcal infections in Miami triggered rheumatic fever.[30] Stollerman conducted a similar study in Chicago with children who came to his clinic with complaints of sore throat. His findings demonstrated the new complexities of rheumatic fever: throat swabs from 2,545 children with sore throat revealed that about 40 percent, or 1,051, had GABS. Of the latter group, one-half received penicillin, and none developed rheumatic fever. Of the remaining one-half who did not receive antibiotics, two developed rheumatic fever, or 1 percent, confirming the results from Miami.[31] What Stollerman took from studies at Fort Warren, Miami, and Chicago was that epidemic streptococcal disease in military settings produced much sicker patients and was far likelier to result in rheumatic fever than counterparts in office settings. He explained the disparity: in civilian practice the presence of virulent M proteins was a rarity. Epidemics did occur in office practice, but were uncommon. For example, Oxford, England, experienced such an epidemic in 1960;[32] the Rocky Mountain states would encounter another in the 1980s.

These insights produced a quandary for practitioners. Doctors and patients were confronted by a mild—often asymptomatic—triggering illness. Left untreated, only 1 percent of infections provoked rheumatic fever. Even this undesired consequence was a faint shadow of its crippling past. In many practices, streptococcal infection mimicked the common cold. Depending on circumstances, children could expect five to ten colds each year. Perhaps only one-fourth of these were due to streptococcal illness.[33] The policy of one practice in rural Colorado, an area with considerable streptococcal infection, illustrated the considerable work required to prevent rheumatic fever. This group of physicians cultured the throat of every child who came to the office with symptoms of a cold. When a culture grew beta-hemolytic streptococci, the physicians requested that every member of the family come to the office for a throat culture. After treatment of all documented cases, everyone was asked to return for additional cultures to document successful eradication. It worked, but at enormous effort.[34]

## Molecular Biology of the Streptococcus

The molecular biology of the streptococcus offered new paths of thinking about rheumatic fever. Maclyn McCarty, who worked down the hall from Rebecca Lancefield and Homer Swift at the Rockefeller Hospital, provided many of the insights.[35] "The interactions between host and parasite, or its products," McCarty concluded in 1952, "which result in the typical lesions of [rheumatic fever] are thought to involve antigen-antibody mechanisms." The streptococcus contained so many "biologically active products" that it seemed likely to McCarty that one or more jolted the human body into a disease state mediated through the production of destructive antibodies.[36] One early example had been the discovery of streptolysin—a streptococcal substance that destroyed red blood cells—which provided the basis for the much-used diagnostic tests, either with the throat culture blood agar plate or serum antistreptolysin-O titer. For another illustration, Rebecca Lancefield and others had described over forty-five different M proteins. These constituents of the bacterial cell wall accounted for virulence by interfering with phagocytosis, one of the human defenses against bacterial invasion. M proteins were also responsible for human immunity to streptococcal disease by stimulating the production of antibodies—directed against the specific M protein—which in turn protected against future infections of the same type.[37] Yet another example of streptococcal/human interaction came from blood coagulation. Long known to inhibit blood clots, streptokinase was found to be a nonhuman "activator" of inactive human plasminogen into biologically active plasmin, the normal way the body dissolves its own blood clots.[38]

McCarty saw a pattern in these streptococcal chemicals. Each directly interacted with human biology—red cell lysis, inhibition of phagocytosis, and dissolving clots. Each streptococcal protein provoked the production of human antibodies. It seemed likely to McCarty that either a streptococcal component or a human antibody produced in reaction to a streptococcal component was the agent responsible for rheumatic fever. In the early 1950s, he was quick to concede that these evocative examples did not constitute proof.[39] A kidney disease, acute glomerulonephritis, provided McCarty with instruction. Acute glomerulonephritis also followed streptococcal illness, with resulting antigens and antibodies responsible for renal injury.[40]

Finding the specific destructive links in what many came to term "the poststreptococcic state" proved elusive.[41] Decades earlier, Homer Swift had proposed that hypersensitivity to the streptococcus supplied one key to rheumatic fever. Despite creative laboratory efforts, Swift had never been able to re-create all aspects of rheumatic fever in animals, a fate shared by other researchers who employed newer immunological approaches, such as serum sickness and the arthus reaction.[42] And no one had succeeded in showing that the immune system of patients with rheumatic fever was actually in "overdrive," producing disease-causing antibodies in excess.[43]

The experimental questions changed in the late 1950s: Could a human-produced antibody that was targeted at the vulnerable tissues, such as the myocardium, be detected in patients with rheumatic fever? If so, could it be shown that the stimulus responsible for provoking the antibody was streptococcal in origin? Finally, could such an antibody actually cause disease?[44]

In some ways these questions were refinements of one experimental inquiry that had spanned over half a century: could experimental streptococcal infection succeed in producing the cardinal Aschoff body? The immunological techniques of antibody production and detection of the 1950s and 1960s certainly differentiated newer attempts from the old, and their conclusions called into question whether the Aschoff body should have been the "gold standard" for research all along.

In his last contribution to the study of rheumatic fever before his death in 1953, Homer Swift teamed up with his colleague George Murphy in one final attempt to produce experimental Aschoff bodies. They infected the skin of rabbits with successive inoculations of whole streptococci over a period that ranged from three to twenty months. They achieved the closest cellular approximation yet to human Aschoff bodies, but in their final analysis, Swift and Murphy concluded that they had fallen short of exact reproduction.[45]

## Cross-Reactivity between the Streptococcus and Humans

Melvin Kaplan, a physician at Western Reserve School of Medicine working in collaboration with staff at the House of the Good Samaritan, provided the insights that led to a new conception of rheumatic fever. In the early 1960s, Kaplan detected antibodies attached to atrial appendages removed by surgeons when reconstructing mitral heart valves. Not all atrial appendages, to be sure. In fact he initially found antibodies in less than one-third. This finding suggested to Kaplan that these antibodies were the agents of ongoing inflammation. It was perplexing to him that these antibodies were attached to heart tissue at spots distinct from the location of active Aschoff bodies.[46] Next, Kaplan obtained sera (and thus antibodies) from patients with newly diagnosed rheumatic fever and found that these antibodies attached to heart tissue from patients with old rheumatic fever which had also been removed at the time of valvular surgery. When mixed together, the antibodies attached to heart antigens, again in spots separate from Aschoff bodies. These observations raised a number of issues. First, were the hearts of humans who had suffered from rheumatic fever different from normal human hearts in that they possessed targets for antibody attachment? Second, were hearts, years after recovery from rheumatic fever, similar to hearts at the time of initial attack, or had the disease altered the chemical structure of the heart? Third, did antibody attachment actually damage the heart? Fourth, what provoked antibody formation in the first place?[47]

The obvious provocateur of antibody was the Group A beta-hemolytic streptococcus. Kaplan isolated streptococcal cell walls, injected them into rabbits and produced antistreptococcal cell wall antibodies. He next mixed these antibodies with surgically removed heart tissue. The streptococcal antibodies attached to human heart tissue from rheumatic fever patients. In other words, Kaplan found that an element of streptococcal cell wall was immunologically cross-reactive with human heart tissue. The site of antibody attachment was the heart's sarcolemma and myocyte, not Aschoff bodies. Kaplan believed that M protein was the likely element in the streptococcal cell wall that stimulated antibody production.[48] Up to this point, Kaplan's human heart tissue had been obtained at surgery. Since these patients had actually suffered from rheumatic fever decades earlier, this begged the question whether a similar streptococcal antibody/human heart attachment could be demonstrated at the point of initial illness. With so few children dying from fulminant rheumatic fever in the mid-1960s, this demonstration was a tall order. Nevertheless, Kaplan repeated the experiment with autopsy specimens from five children. Streptococcal antibodies in great numbers attached to the same areas of sarcolemma and myocyte.[49] To Kaplan, such prolific attack strongly suggested that these antibodies were the cause of the children's death.

Other laboratories quickly repeated Kaplan's work and were generally supportive.[50] Maclyn McCarty used these insights as one focus of his T. Duckett Jones Memorial Lecture in 1964, entitled "Missing Links in the Streptococcal Chain Leading to Rheumatic Fever." McCarty reviewed the many streptococcal components, such as streptolysin, streptokinase, M proteins (which now numbered over fifty), that interacted with human tissues. He was intrigued with Kaplan's demonstration of cross-reactivity of streptococcal antigens with human myocardium. In 1965—when this history ends—McCarty cautioned that proof of pathological destruction lay in the future.[51]

It is worth noting differences between Kaplan's work and the half-century of attempts that preceded him. In part, his use of immunological techniques of antibody creation and detection separated his work from that of others. His use of human heart tissue was clearly different and could not have been done before cardiac surgery supplied the needed specimens. Prior researchers had always been stymied by the fact that rheumatic fever seemed limited to humans.

One issue was the meaning of Kaplan's work for the persistent belief that

Aschoff bodies represented the cardinal injury in rheumatic fever. Kaplan's antibodies did not attach to Aschoff bodies, an observation noted but strangely drawing only limited comment in the 1960s. His studies indicated that the Aschoff body was unique, or pathognomonic, to rheumatic fever but not pathologic.[52] In other words, Kaplan's work challenged the validity of one goal of scientific inquiry since the time of Frederick Poynton and Alexander Paine, suggesting that the pursuit of the Aschoff body had been a misdirected passion. In other respects, Kaplan's disease-producing antibodies blended nicely with earlier theories. For example, the cross-reacting streptococcal/human antibodies fleshed out the immunologic havoc that Alvin Coburn had predicted in the mid-1930s with Phase II.

## Molecular Biology and History

Physicians continue to think about rheumatic fever in terms of cross-reactivity between human tissues and the streptococcus.[53] This idea from molecular biology joined forces with the historical record of patient case histories and hospital reports to clarify details about rheumatic fever over the past two centuries. In the years between 1965 and the present, scientists have expanded the scope of Kaplan's initial observations, discovering similar immunological connections with brain, skin, endocardium, and joint tissue. These insights from molecular biology offer an explanation for the epidemiological comings and goings of rheumatic fever over the past two centuries. Before the end of the eighteenth century the streptococcus only contained components that cross-reacted with human joints. Arthritis was thus the only complaint that patients brought to doctors. In the nineteenth century, the streptococcus possessed elements that cross-reacted with pericardium, endocardium, myocardium, brain, skin, and connective tissue, leading initially to heart symptoms of the type that caused patients, such as Miss A. L. and Mr. T. M., to seek relief, and later to the chorea that so distressed Francis Hill. Over the course of the twentieth century, the streptococcus lost these provocative components. Streptococcal infections continued to occur commonly, but they did not trigger rheumatic fever. Cross-reactivity also helped in understanding the variability of rheumatic fever in different patients. For example, it explained why one patient suffered from chorea and another from pericarditis: the provoking streptococcus contained the necessary elements.

In the 1980s, small epidemics of rheumatic fever descended on several communities in the Midwest and the Rocky Mountains. To be sure, the cases were milder than the ones Walter Cheadle had faced a century earlier. But with arthritis and heart disease, these children easily caught the eye of practitioners, reminiscent of the way in which the complaints of Miss A. L. and Mr. T. M. had captured the attention of William Charles Wells nearly two centuries earlier.[54] Cross-reactivity also helped to explain this encore of rheumatic fever: for a short period streptococci once again contained the antigens that were targeted at human tissues. When Gene Stollerman analyzed the M proteins from the triggering streptococci, he found types not present in recent decades.[55]

These epidemics underscored the likelihood that rheumatic fever will return in the future at understandable, but unpredictable, moments. Alvin Coburn, silent for more than a decade about rheumatic fever, observed in 1961, "One may reasonably anticipate that cyclical fluctuations in the incidence and severity of rheumatic fever are to be expected in the future; moreover, the fundamental problem— why only a small percentage of humankind is susceptible to rheumatic fever—has barely been recognized."[56]

Cross-reactivity did not immediately help in solving the puzzle of why some people responded to the ubiquitous and ever-changing streptococcus while most did not. Even in the most deleterious setting, such as a military barrack, only 3 percent of streptococcal sufferers developed rheumatic fever. Virtually every worker in the field accepted May Wilson's contention that victims of rheumatic fever were genetically different. Most, however, did not accept her assertion that susceptibility was passed through simple Mendelian autosomal recessive means,[57] an idea that she continued to assert into the 1950s[58] and which received some support from family studies in New Haven[59] and among kibbutz children in Israel.[60] Others attempted, with limited success, to link susceptibility to rheumatic fever with inheritance of ABO blood groups.[61] In 1965, cross-reactivity anticipated the discovery that only vulnerable people possessed the capacity of producing destructive antibodies. In the 1980s, with the aid of previously unavailable tissue-typing techniques, researchers discovered some of these foundations of genetic susceptibility in rheumatic fever.[62]

The changing molecular biology of the streptococcus only partly explained the decline of rheumatic fever. The streptococcus did not mutate overnight. Epidemiological studies by Arthur Newsholme and Alison Glover indicated that bacterial change began toward the end of the nineteenth century. Alterations of living patterns that lessened the passage of streptococci, such as those decreasing living density, certainly helped to prevent streptococcal disease and rheumatic fever. After sulfonamide became widely available in the 1940s, it diminished relapses. Penicillin provided even more effective intervention. Public health programs that committed both parents and physicians to streptococcal vigilance managed to prevent the streptococcus from triggering rheumatic fever. Additionally, the widespread use of antibiotics for other infections, such as otitis media, pneumonia, and sinusitis, has succeeded in ridding children of asymptomatic resident streptococci. Still, the containment of rheumatic fever owed much to its biological mutability.

In 1965, rheumatic fever had nearly vanished from the medical landscape. Each symptom and sign that had made rheumatic fever so visible to patients and doctors, had disappeared. There was only the occasional new victim; those few who died had been afflicted long before. Accidents, suicide, homicide, and AIDS replaced rheumatic fever as leading causes of death among children. School health nurses neither peered at suspicious tonsils nor swabbed them; surgeons no longer removed them. Convalescent hospitals closed and specialized classrooms for "cardiac cripples" ceased to concern local school boards. Agonizing monthly clinic visits for injections of bicillin dwindled, and many doctors forgot Jones's criteria for diagnosis. Their students never learned them. To be fair, doctors still ferreted out streptococcal infections, but some physicians doubted the need to treat them. Parents persisted in worrying more about a diagnosis of streptococcal tonsillitis than—let's say—a diagnosis of "viral" sore throat. The detection of a heart murmur still conjured up parental fear more properly relegated to another era. Rheumatic fever was gone, but it had left its mark on medicine's memory.

# Epilogue

$\twoheadrightarrow$

*T*he history of rheumatic fever has much to say to historians and physicians. One insight that emerges is that rheumatic fever changed biologically over the course of the last two centuries, gathering symptoms and severity over the nineteenth century only to moderate just as spectacularly during the twentieth century. Rheumatic fever was not unique in this regard. Diseases come and go, worsen and ameliorate, targeting different populations along the way. Most diseases do not mutate as quickly or as dramatically as rheumatic fever, but most travel a dynamic historical course. That diseases change markedly over time will not come as a surprise to physicians. Health problems that faced them as medical students are almost always quite different from diseases that confront them at retirement. This observation does not necessarily imply progress, only difference. Those who have lived through the twentieth century's plagues, such as cancer, heart disease, and the pandemic of human immunodeficiency virus, know that health conditions are as likely to worsen as to improve. Historians need to appreciate fully disease mutability. Commonly historians study diseases over periods that span many more years than those encompassing a single physician's career. They should anticipate that any disease under historical scrutiny will undergo fundamental biological changes. Historians of disease need to root their studies deeply in biology.

A corollary is that microbes change with time. The streptococcus provides vivid proof, but mutability can be seen with other common germs, such as influenza virus and *corynebacterium diphtheriae*. Similarly, the effectiveness of therapy changes with mutations in either disease or germ. For example, salicylate was more effective in treating rheumatic heart disease at the end of the nineteenth century because pericarditis was then the predominant heart injury. When myocarditis came into prominence in the twentieth century, aspirin was less effective. Contemporary medical practice offers other examples. When I entered medical school, virtually all middle ear infections were treatable with antibiotics. As I write these words, I have under my care several children with ear infections caused by bacteria that no antibiotic will touch. By the end of my medical career, I suspect that I will approach all infections with the understanding that resistance to antibiotics is the rule and not the exception. This has bearing on rheumatic fever. The streptococcus is likely to persist in mutating. No therapy has ever successfully treated all aspects of rheumatic fever. At some future point, existing antibiotics may cease to prevent streptococcal infection and thus rheumatic fever.

A second insight that emerges from the history of rheumatic fever is that the relationship of humans and germs is a complex one. Here the physician, molecular biologist, and historian must work closely together. The streptococcus in rheumatic fever illustrates just how intricate the relationship can be. Streptococcal infections are tied to geographical, climatic, and social environments. Historians have an important role in illustrating this intricacy. Understandings about germs and the diseases they cause never emerge whole cloth. Here rheumatic fever does not disappoint. At the end of the nineteenth century, germ theory offered a plausible explanation for rheumatic fever. Yet the knowledge of bacteria and the laboratory techniques available to Frederick J. Poynton and Alexander Paine in 1900 fell far short of answering the questions put to them. The ideas which they and others pursued were firmly rooted in the medical bacteriology of the day. "Sepsis" theory made good common sense and good scientific sense. Before bacteriology could provide insights into rheumatic fever, streptococci needed to be sorted out by groups and types and then taken apart molecularly. During this interval, epidemiologists provided physicians with useful insights with their study of rheumatic fever in homes, schools, barracks, and tropics. Eventually a congruence emerged of streptococcal bacteriology, immunology, and epidemiology. The concepts of bacterial "trigger" and "cross-reactivity" were entirely innovative ideas that emerged from the interplay of several biomedical disciplines. Complex disease ecology is not unique to rheumatic fever, an observation that historians must take to heart. It is not fully creditable to write about diseases caused by influenza virus, plague's *Yersinia pestis,* or poliovirus without understanding how each microbe afflicts human populations. To historians falls the task of assembling the pieces of the ecological puzzle.

This is not to imply at all that the currents of medicine's history have been entirely determined by biology. Patients and physicians struggling with rheumatic fever provide an excellent example of the nature of the physician/patient relationship in the nineteenth and twentieth centuries. It was not a story solely of clinical triumphs. Signs and symptoms often did not point directly to diagnosis, confirmatory laboratory tests were lacking, and ready cures evaded. At each point of rheumatic fever's history, physicians offered—and patients accepted—therapies that extended the soundest hope of relief from symptoms. Nevertheless, patients and physicians often directed their attention to different aspects of the disease. Distressing joint pain, fever, and chorea worried patients more than doctors. Heart disease, often imperceptible to the patients, concerned physicians. Aspirin and steroids helped but did not cure. Antibiotics forced both patients and physicians to reorient thinking about the seriousness of once-trivial sore throats. It will not come as a surprise either to patients or to physicians on medicine's front lines to learn that vagaries and frustrations characterize confrontations with disease: the child who fails to grow and develop; hypertension or cancer that responds to no drug;

delusions that persist for years; addictions that nag; obesity that defies any diet; the couple who cannot conceive. Patients, doctors, *and* historians seek cures, but the usual content of medicine is fundamentally of a different nature. Patients bring complaints and physicians respond. This interaction may include information, experience, diagnostic technologies, medicines, advice, comfort, encouragement, or hope. Occasionally cures ensue. More often, the patient endures the disease. I do not wish to leave the impression that children in offices, hospitals, or convalescent homes received nothing of benefit from the doctors in charge of their care for rheumatic fever. Carefully administered aspirin and steroids alleviated some of the suffering. Antibiotics, when taken, treated streptococcal sore throats and prevented relapses. Surgery helped selected patients. Physicians never found a cure for rheumatic fever, but this failure need not detract from their efforts.

Rheumatic fever's dramatic rise and fall should not camouflage the efforts of those who sought to confront it. Although it is possible to glimpse rheumatic fever's biological fluidity at the end of the eighteenth century, medical innovations in the nineteenth and twentieth centuries brought the evolving disease into ever-sharpening focus. Care of patients within hospitals, the stethoscope and electrocardiogram, bacterial culturing, and Walter Cheadle's and Duckett Jones's innovative diagnostic schemes "collaborated" with mutating biology to bring rheumatic fever into finely honed relief. The decline of rheumatic fever provides another clear picture of this collaboration. Ameliorating biology was the driving force, but the transformation from deadly disease to bland infection took almost a century. During this period knowledge of the role of the streptococcal trigger permitted the identification of worrisome crowded environments, such as military barracks. When antibiotics became available, physicians exploited them initially to prevent relapses among rheumatic fever victims and ultimately to prevent even first attacks. Antibiotics were particularly crucial when streptococcal infections were more likely to provoke rheumatic fever.

In 1986 Floyd Denny observed, "We have raised an entire generation of young physicians who have never seen a case of acute rheumatic fever." This happy state of affairs stemmed both from biological changes and from efforts that Denny and many others had expended over the past two centuries. To be sure, medical students will not find rheumatic fever in the clinic. They must travel instead to the medical history library.

# NOTES

## Preface

1. Richard F. Gillum, "Trends in Acute Rheumatic Fever and Chronic Rheumatic Heart Disease: A National Perspective," *American Heart Journal* (1986), 111: 430–432; and U.S. Department of Health, Education, and Welfare, Public Health Service, *Vital Statistics of the United States 1970* (Washington, D.C.: Government Printing Office, 1975), vol. II–Mortality, part A, sect. 1: 1–121.
2. Personal communication Thomas Eliot Frothingham; see also Edward F. Bland, "Rheumatic Fever: The Way It Was," *Circulation* (1987), 76: 1190–1195.
3. Lowell A. Rantz, "Hemolytic Streptococcal Infections," in *Preventive Medicine in World War II, Communicable Diseases: Transmitted Chiefly through Respiratory and Alimentary Tracts*, ed. John Boyd Coates, Jr. (Washington D.C.: Office of the Surgeon General, 1958), vol. IV, 229–257; and Rantz, "Rheumatic Fever," in *Internal Medicine in World War II: Infectious Diseases*, ed. John Boyd Coates, Jr. (Washington, D.C.: Office of the Surgeon General, 1963), vol. II, 225–238.
4. Alvin F. Coburn and Donald C. Young, *The Epidemiology of Hemolytic Streptococcus during World War II in the United States Navy* (Baltimore: Williams and Wilkins Co., 1949).
5. W. Paul Holbrook, "The Army Air Forces Rheumatic Fever Control Program," *Journal of the American Medical Association* (1944), 126: 84–87; Floyd W. Denny, Lewis W. Wannamaker, William R. Brink, Charles H. Rammelkamp, Jr., and Edward A. Custer, "Prevention of Rheumatic Fever, Treatment of the Preceding Streptococcic Infection," *Journal of the American Medical Association* (1950), 143: 151–153; and Lewis W. Wannamaker, Charles H. Rammelkamp, Jr., Floyd W. Denny, William R. Brink, Harold B. Houser, Edward O. Hahn, and John H. Dingle, "Prophylaxis of Acute Rheumatic Fever: By Treatment of the Preceding Streptococcal Infection with Various Amounts of Depot Penicillin," *American Journal of Medicine* (1951), 10: 673–695.
6. T. Duckett Jones, "The Diagnosis of Rheumatic Fever," *Journal of the American Medical Association* (1944), 126: 481–484; David D. Rutstein, Walter Bauer, Albert Dorfman, Robert E. Gross, John A. Lichty, Helen B. Taussig, and Ruth Whittemore, Committee on Standards and Criteria for Programs of Care (American Heart Association), "Jones Criteria (Modified) for Guidance in the Diagnosis of Rheumatic

Fever," *Modern Concepts of Cardiovascular Disease* (1955), 24: 291–293; and Gene H. Stollerman, Milton Markowitz, Angelo Taranta, Lewis W. Wannamaker, and Ruth Whittemore, "Jones Criteria (Revised) for Guidance in the Diagnosis of Rheumatic Fever," *Circulation* (1965), 32: 664–668.

7. Richard L. Varco and Ivan D. Baronofsky, "The Surgical Problem in Rheumatic Valvular Heart Disease," in *Rheumatic Fever: A Symposium*, ed. Lewis Thomas (Minneapolis: University of Minnesota Press, 1952), 249–264.

8. Arthur Newsholme, "The Milroy Lectures on the Natural History and Affinities of Rheumatic Fever: A Study in Epidemiology," *Lancet* (1895), 1: 589–596, 657–665.

9. Homer F. Swift, "The Chronicity of Rheumatic Fever," *New England Journal of Medicine* (1934), 211: 197–203.

10. Irvine Loudon, "Maternal Mortality: 1880–1950. Some Regional and International Comparisons," *Social History of Medicine* (1988), 1: 183–228.

11. Gene H. Stollerman, "Changing Streptococci and Prospects for the Global Eradication of Rheumatic Fever," *Perspectives in Biology and Medicine* (1997), 40: 165–189.

12. I refer to these researchers throughout this book. Some—but certainly not all—of the most insightful historical accounts include: Stollerman, "Changing Streptococci"; Gene H. Stollerman, "Rheumatic Fever," *Lancet* (1997), 349: 935–942; Stollerman, "Rheumatic Carditis," *Lancet* (1995), 346: 390–392; Stollerman, "The Nature of Rheumatogenic Streptococci," *Mount Sinai Journal of Medicine* (1996), 63: 144–158; Stollerman, "Factors That Predispose to Rheumatic Fever," *Medical Clinics of North America* (1960), 44: 17–28; Stollerman, "History," *Rheumatic Fever and Streptococcal Infection* (New York: Grune and Statton, 1975), 1–19; Benedict F. Massell, *Rheumatic Fever and Streptococcal Infection: Unraveling the Mysteries of a Dread Disease* (Boston: Francis A. Countway Library of Medicine, distributed by the Harvard University Press, 1997); Walter Butler Cheadle, *The Various Manifestations of the Rheumatic State as Exemplified in Childhood and Early Life, Lectures Delivered before the Harveian Society of London* (London: Smith, Elder, and Co., 1889); Thomas John Maclagan, *Rheumatism, Its Nature, Its Pathology, and Its Successful Treatment,* 2nd ed. (London: Adam & Charles Black, 1896); Alfred Mantle, "A History of the Present-Day Accepted Aetiology of Acute Rheumatism," *Practitioner* (1912), 88: 185–192; F. J. Poynton and Alexander Paine, *Researches on Rheumatism* (London: J. & A. Churchill, 1913); Carey Franklin Coombs, *Rheumatic Heart Disease* (Bristol: John Wright and Sons, Ltd., 1924); Homer F. Swift, "The Pathogenesis of Rheumatic Fever," *Journal of Experimental Medicine* (1924), 39: 497–508; Swift, "Rheumatic Fever," *American Journal of the Medical Sciences* (1925), 170: 631–647; Swift, "Rheumatic Fever," *Journal of the American Medical Association* (1929), 92: 2071–2083; Swift, "The Chronicity of Rheumatic Fever," *New England Journal of Medicine* (1934), 211: 197–203; Swift, "Rheumatic Heart Disease: Pathogenesis and Etiology in Their Relation to Therapy and Prophylaxis," *Medicine* (1940), 19: 417–440; and Swift, "The Etiology of Rheumatic Fever," *Annals of Internal Medicine* (1949), 31: 715–738; Harry Keil, "Dr. William Charles Wells and His Contribution to the Study of Rheumatic Fever," *Bulletin of the Institute of the History of Medicine* (1936), 4: 789–816; Keil, "The Rheumatic Subcutaneous Nodules and Simulating Lesions," *Medicine* (1938), 17: 261–380; Keil, "The Rheumatic Erythemas: A Critical Survey," *Annals of Internal Medicine* (1938), 11: 2223–2272; Keil, "A Note on Edward Jenner's Lost Manuscript on 'Rheumatism of the Heart,'" *Bulletin of the History of Medicine* (1939), 7: 409–411; May Georgiana Wilson, *Rheumatic Fever: Studies in the Epidemiology, Manifestations, Diagnosis, and Treatment of the Disease during the First Three Decades* (New York: Commonwealth

Fund, 1940); John R. Paul, *The Epidemiology of Rheumatic Fever: A Preliminary Report with Special Reference to Environmental Factors in Rheumatic Heart Disease and Recommendations for Future Investigations* (New York: Metropolitan Life Insurance Company, 1930); Paul, *The Epidemiology of Rheumatic Fever and Some of Its Public Health Aspects*, 2nd ed. (New York: Metropolitan Life Insurance Company, 1943); J. Alison Glover, "Milroy Lectures on the Incidence of Rheumatic Diseases," *Lancet* (1930), 1: 499–505; George E. Murphy, "On Muscle Cells, Aschoff Bodies, and Cardiac Failure in Rheumatic Heart Disease," *Bulletin of the New York Academy of Medicine* (1959), 35: 619–651; George Murphy, "The Evolution of Our Knowledge of Rheumatic Fever, an Historical Emphasis on Rheumatic Heart Disease," *Bulletin of the History of Medicine* (1943), 14: 123–47; Alvin Frederick Coburn, *The Factor of Infection in the Rheumatic State* (Baltimore: Williams and Wilkins, 1931); Maclyn McCarty, "Lewis Wannamaker in the Campaign against Rheumatic Fever," *Zentralblatt für Bakteriologie, Mikrobiologie, und Hygiene-Series A* (1985), 260: 151–164; McCarty, "Maxwell Finland Lecture: An Adventure in the Pathogenic Maze of Rheumatic Fever," *Journal of Infectious Diseases* (1981), 143: 375–385; McCarty, "Present State of Knowledge Concerning Pathogenesis and Treatment of Rheumatic Fever," *Bulletin of the New York Academy of Medicine* (1952), 28: 307–320; McCarty, "Missing Links in the Streptococcal Chain Leading to Rheumatic Fever: The T. Duckett Jones Memorial Lecture," *Circulation* (1964), 29: 488–493; Edward F. Bland, "Declining Severity of Rheumatic Fever: A Comparative Study of the Past Four Decades," *New England Journal of Medicine* (1960), 262: 597–599; Bland and T. Duckett Jones, "Rheumatic Fever and Rheumatic Heart Disease: A Twenty Year Report on 1000 Patients Followed since Childhood," *Circulation* (1951), 4: 836–843; Bland, "Rheumatic Fever: The Way It Was"; Charles H. Rammelkamp, Jr., Lewis W. Wannamaker, and Floyd W. Denny, "The Epidemiology and Prevention of Rheumatic Fever," *Bulletin of the New York Academy of Medicine* (1952), 28: 321–334; Floyd W. Denny, "T. Duckett Jones and Rheumatic Fever in 1986," *Circulation* (1987), 76: 963–970; Denny, "A 45–Year Perspective on the Streptococcus and Rheumatic Fever: The Edward H. Kass Lecture in Infectious Disease History," *Clinical Infectious Diseases* (1994), 19: 1110–1122; Rebecca C. Lancefield, "Cellular Constituents of Group A Streptococci Concerned in Antigenicity and Virulence," *Streptococcal Infections*, ed. Maclyn McCarty (New York: Columbia University Press, 1954), 3–18; and Lewis W. Wannamaker and John M. Matsen, *Streptococci and Streptococcal Diseases: Recognition, Understanding, and Management* (New York: Academic Press, 1972).

13. Philip S. Hench, Walter Bauer, Almon A. Fletcher, David Ghrist, Francis Hall, and Preston White, "The Present Status of the Problem of 'Rheumatism,' A Review of Recent American and English Literature on 'Rheumatism' and Arthritis," beginning in 1935 in the *Annals of Internal Medicine*. (Title varies slightly from year to year, as do the collaborators.) These reviews cited between 400 and 1,100 articles and books each year, proving a rich source on research for this period. *Annals of Internal Medicine* (1935), 8: 1315–1374; (1936), 9: 883–982; (1936), 10: 754–909; (1938), 11: 1089–1247; (1939), 12: 1005–1104; (1940), 13: 1655–1739, 1837–1990; (1941), 14: 1383–1448; (1941), 15: 1002–1108.

14. Arthur L. Bloomfield, *A Bibliography of Internal Medicine: Communicable Diseases*. (Chicago: University of Chicago Press, 1958), 133–163.

15. Massell, *Rheumatic Fever and Streptococcal Infection*, 287–377.

16. Exceptions are Peter C. English, "Emergence of Rheumatic Fever in the Nineteenth Century," *Milbank Quarterly* (1989), 67: (suppl. 1), 33–49; English, "Emergence of

Rheumatic Fever in the Nineteenth Century," *Framing Disease: Studies in Cultural History* (New Brunswick, N.J.: Rutgers University Press, 1992), 20–32; and Thomas G. Benedek, "Rheumatic Fever and Rheumatic Heart Disease," *Cambridge World History of Human Disease*, ed. Kenneth Kiple (Cambridge: Cambridge University Press, 1993), 970–977.

17. Charles E. Rosenberg and Janet Golden, eds., *Framing Disease: Studies in Cultural History* (New Brunswick, N.J.: Rutgers University Press, 1992).


## Prologue

1. John Swan, *The Entire Works of Dr. Thomas Sydenham, Newly Made English from the Originals: Wherein the History of Acute and Chronic Diseases, and the Safest and Most Effectual Methods of Treating Them, Are Faithfully, Clearly, and Accurately Delivered* (London: Edward Cave at St. John's Gate, 1749); William Cullen, *First Lines of the Practice of Physic, for the Use of Students in the University of Edinburgh*, 2nd ed. (Philadelphia: Steiner and Cist, 1781); and Baron Van Swieten, *Commentaries upon Boerhaave's Aphorisms Concerning the Knowledge and Cure of Diseases* (Edinburgh: Charles Elliot, 1776),.

2. William Charles Wells, "On Rheumatism of the Heart," *Transactions of a Society for the Improvement of Medical and Chirurgical Knowledge* (1812), 3: 373–424.

3. W. S. Church, "An Examination of Nearly Seven Hundred Cases of Acute Rheumatism, Chiefly with a View to Determining the Frequency of Cardiac Affections, and Especially Pericarditis, at the Present Time," *St. Bartholomew's Hospital Reports* (1887), 23: 269–287.

4. G. W. Bury, "A Statistical Account of Four Hundred Cases of Acute Rheumatism Admitted into the Wards of the Middlesex Hospital during the Years 1853–59," *British and Foreign Medico-Chirurgical Review* (1861), 28: 194–198.

5. P. H. Pye-Smith, "Analysis of the Cases of Rheumatism, and Other Diseases of the Joints, Which Have Occurred in the Hospital during Three Consecutive Years: With Remarks on the Pathological Alliances of Rheumatic Fever," *Guy's Hospital Reports* (1874), 19: 311–356.

6. Audrey B. Davis, *Medicine and Its Technology: An Introduction to the History of Medical Instrumentation* (Westport, Conn.: Greenwood Press, 1981); Dale C. Smith, "Austin Flint and Auscultation in America," *Journal of the History of Medicine and Allied Sciences* (1978), 33: 129–149; and Malcolm Nicolson, "The Introduction of Percussion and Stethoscopy to Early Nineteenth-Century Edinburgh," in *Medicine and the Five Senses*, ed. W. F. Bynum and Roy Porter (London: Cambridge University Press, 1993), 134–153.

7. Jean-Baptiste Bouillaud, *New Researches on Acute Articular Rheumatism in General; and Especially on the Law of Coincidence of Pericarditis and Endocarditis with This Disease, as Well as on the Efficacy of the Method of Treating It by Repeated Blood-Letting at Short Intervals,* trans. James Kitchen (Philadelphia: Haswell, Barrington, and Haswell, 1837).

8. Dr. Yonge, "Case of Cerebral Disturbance: Dependent upon Disease of the Pericardium," *Guy's Hospital Reports* (1840), 5: 276–281 (reported by Dr. Bright).

9. Alvin F. Coburn, *The Factor of Infection in the Rheumatic State* (Baltimore: Williams and Wilkins, 1931); and Coburn, "Observations on the Mechanism of Rheumatic Fever," *Lancet* (1936), 2: 1025–1030.

10. John Rodman Paul, *The Epidemiology of Rheumatic Fever: A Preliminary Report with*

*Special Reference to Environmental Factors in Rheumatic Heart Disease and Recommendations for Future Investigation* (New York: Metropolitan Life Insurance Co., 1930), 30.

11. Philip S. Hench, "Recent Studies on Arthritis and Rheumatism in the United States," *Annals of Rheumatic Diseases* (1941), 2: 172–192.

12. For two examples, see Carey F. Coombs, "The Diagnosis and Treatment of Rheumatic Heart Disease in Its Early Stages," *British Medical Journal* (1930), 1: 227–230; and Thomas T. Mackie, "Rheumatic Fever: An Analytical Study of Three Hundred and Ninety-Three Cases of Rheumatic Fever and Eighty-Nine Cases of Chorea," *American Journal of the Medical Sciences* (1926), 172: 199–221.

13. One example from Syracuse, New York: J. G. Fred Hiss, "A Plan for Rehabilitation for Rheumatic Subjects," *Journal of Pediatrics* (1945), 26: 230–236.

14. L. Aschoff, "Zur Myocarditisfrage," *Verhandlungen der deutschen pathologischen Gesellschaft* (1904), 8: 46–53.

15. Leon Gordis, "The Virtual Disappearance of Rheumatic Fever in the United States: Lessons in the Rise and Fall of Disease," *Circulation* (1985), 72: 1155–1162.

16. Milton Markowitz, "The Decline of Rheumatic Fever: Role of Medical Intervention," *Journal of Pediatrics* (1985), 106: 545–550.

17. T. Maclagan, "The Treatment of Acute Rheumatism by Salicin," *Lancet* (1876), 1: 342–343, 2: 601–604.

18. George E. Murphy, "Salicylate and Rheumatic Activity: An Objective Clinical-Histologic Study of the Effect of Salicylate on Rheumatic Lesions, Those of Joints and Tendon Sheaths in Particular," *Bulletin of the Johns Hopkins Hospital* (1945), 77: 1–42.

19. Homer F. Swift, Johannes K. Moen, and George K. Hirst, "The Action of Sulfanilamide in Rheumatic Fever," *Journal of the American Medical Association* (1938), 110: 426–434.

20. Alvin F. Coburn and Lucile V. Moore, "The Prophylactic Use of Sulfanilamide in Streptococcal Respiratory Infections, with Especial Reference to Rheumatic Fever," *Journal of Clinical Investigation* (1939), 18: 147–155.

21. Caroline Bedell Thomas and Richard France, "A Preliminary Report of the Prophylactic Use of Sulfanilamide in Patients Susceptible to Rheumatic Fever," *Bulletin of the Johns Hopkins Hospital* (1939), 64: 67–77.

22. Alvin Frederick Coburn and Donald Cook Young, *The Epidemiology of Hemolytic Streptococcus during World War II in the United States Navy* (Baltimore: Williams and Wilkins, 1949).

23. Arlie R. Barnes, Harry L. Smith, Charles Slocum, Howard F. Polley, and Philip S. Hench, "Acute Rheumatic Fever Treated with Cortisone and Corticotropin," *Rheumatic Fever: A Symposium*, ed. Lewis Thomas (Minneapolis: University of Minnesota Press, 1952), 274–290.

24. Floyd W. Denny, "T. Duckett Jones and Rheumatic Fever in 1986," *Circulation* (1987), 76: 963–970.

25. Melvin H. Kaplan and Mary Meyeserian, "An Immunological Cross-Reaction between Group-A Streptococcal Cells and Human Heart Tissue," *Lancet* (1962), 1: 706–710. See also Elia M. Ayoub, "Cross-Reacting Antibodies in the Pathogenesis of Rheumatic Myocardial and Valvular Disease," 451–464, Gene H. Stollerman, "Hypersensitivity and Antibody Responses in Streptococcal Disease," 501–513, and Maclyn McCarty, "Theories of Pathogenesis of Streptococcal Complications," 517–530, in Lewis W. Wannamaker and John M. Matsen, eds., *Streptococci and Streptococcal*

*Diseases: Recognition, Understanding, and Management* (New York: Academic Press, 1972).

26. Maclyn McCarty, "An Adventure in the Pathogenic Maze of Rheumatic Fever," *Journal of Infectious Diseases* (1981), 143: 375–385.

27. Patricia Ferrieri, "Acute Rheumatic Fever: The Come-Back of a Disappearing Disease," *American Journal of Diseases in Children* (1987), 141: 725–727; Don M. Hosier, Josepha M. Craenen, Douglas W. Teske, John J. Wheller, "Resurgence of Acute Rheumatic Fever," *American Journal of Diseases in Children* (1987), 141: 730–733; Milton Markowitz and Michael A. Gerber, "Rheumatic Fever: Recent Outbreaks of an Old Disease," *Connecticut Medicine* (1987), 51: 229–233; L. George Veasy, Susan E. Wiedmeier, Garth S. Orsmond, Herbert D. Ruttenberg, Mark M. Boucek, Stephen J. Roth, Vera F. Tait, Joel A. Thompson, Judy A. Daly, Edward L. Kaplan, and Harry R. Hill, "Resurgence of Acute Rheumatic Fever in the Intermountain Area of the United States," *New England Journal of Medicine* (1987), 316: 421–427; Ellen R. Wald, Barry Dashefsky, Cindy Feidt, Darleen Chiponis, and Carol Byers, "Acute Rheumatic Fever in Western Pennsylvania and the TriState Area," *Pediatrics* (1987), 80: 371–374; and Blaise Congeni, Christopher Rizzo, Joseph Congeni, and V. V. Sreenivasan, "Outbreak of Acute Rheumatic Fever in Northeast Ohio," *Journal of Pediatrics* (1987), 111: 176–179.

28. Gene H. Stollerman, "The Nature of Rheumatogenic Streptococci," *Mount Sinai Journal of Medicine* (1996), 63: 144–158; for a similar hypothesis, see Floyd W. Denny, Jr., "A 45–Year Perspective on the Streptococcus and Rheumatic Fever: The Edward H. Kass Lecture in Infectious Disease History," *Clinical Infectious Diseases* (1994), 19: 1110–1122; and Gene H. Stollerman, "Rheumatogenic Group A Streptococci and the Return of Rheumatic Fever," *Advances in Internal Medicine* (1990), 35: 1–25.

### Chapter 1   *The New Face of Rheumatism*

1. William Charles Wells, "On Rheumatism of the Heart," *Transactions of a Society for the Improvement of Medical and Chirurgical Knowledge* (1812), 3: 373–424.

2. John Swan, *The Entire Works of Dr. Thomas Sydenham, Newly Made English from the Originals: Wherein the History of Acute and Chronic Diseases, and the Safest and Most Effectual Methods of Treating Them, Are Faithfully, Clearly, and Accurately Delivered* (London: Edward Cave at St. John's Gate, 1749), "Of the Rheumatism," 245–246. See Andrew Cunningham, "Thomas Sydenham: Epidemics, Experiment, and the 'Good Old Cause,'" *The Medical Revolution of the Seventeenth Century*, ed. Roger French and Andrew Wear (Cambridge: Cambridge University Press, 1989), 164–190; Kenneth Dewhurst, "An Oxford Medical Quartet: Sydenham, Willis, Locke, and Lower," *Oxford Medicine: Essays on the Evolution of the Oxford Clinical School to Commemorate the Bicentenary of the Radcliffe Infirmary, 1770–1970,* ed. Kenneth Dewhurst (Oxford: Sanford Publications, 1970), 23–31; Dewhurst, *Dr. Thomas Sydenham (1624–1689): His Life and Original Writings* (London: Wellcome Historical Medical Library, 1966); Geoffrey Guy Meynell, *Materials for a Biography of Dr. Thomas Sydenham (1624–1689): A New Survey of Public and Private Archives* (Folkestone: Winterdown Books, 1988); and Meynell, *A Bibliography of Dr. Thomas Sydenham (1624–1689)* (Folkestone: Winterdown Books, 1990).

3. Guenter B. Risse, "Cullen as Clinician: Organization and Strategies of an Eighteenth-Century Medical Practice," *William Cullen and the Eighteenth-Century Medical World*, ed. Reginald Passmore, Andrew Doig, Joan Ferguson, and Iain Milne (Edinburgh:

Edinburgh University Press, 1993), 133–151; Risse, *Hospital Life in Enlightenment Scotland: Care and Teaching at the Royal Infirmary of Edinburgh* (Cambridge: Cambridge University Press, 1986), 150–152; A. L. Donovan, *Philosophical Chemistry in the Scottish Enlightenment: The Doctrines and Discoveries of William Cullen and Joseph Black* (Edinburgh: Edinburgh University Press, 1975); Christopher Lawrence, "Cullen, Brown, and the Poverty of Essentialism," in *Brunonianism in Britain and Europe*, ed. W. F. Bynum and Roy Porter (London: Wellcome Institute for the History of Medicine, 1988), suppl. no. 8 *Medical History*, 1–21; W. F. Bynum, "Cullen and the Study of Fevers in Britain, 1760–1820," in *Theories of Fever from Antiquity to the Enlightenment*, ed. W. F. Bynum and Vivian Nutton (London: Wellcome Institute for the History of Medicine, 1981), suppl. no. 1 *Medical History*, 135–147; and Inci Altug Bowman, "William Cullen (1710–90) and the Primacy of the Nervous System," Ph.D. diss., Indiana University, 1975, 178–198.

4. William Cullen, *First Lines of the Practice of Physic, for the Use of Students, in the University of Edinburgh,* 2nd ed. (Philadelphia: Steiner and Cist, 1781), 156.

5. Ibid., 157.

6. Baron van Swieten, *Commentaries upon Boerhaave's Aphorisms Concerning the Knowledge and Cure of Diseases* (Edinburgh: Charles Elliot, 1776), vol. 13, 88.

7. Ibid., 6.

8. William Balfour, "Observations on the Pathology and Cure of Rheumatism," *Edinburgh Medical and Surgical Journal* (1815), 11: 168–187.

9. Cullen, *First Lines*, 158.

10. William Shearman, "On the Distinction between Rheumatism and Inflammation," *London Medical Repository* (1826), 26: 340–344.

11. L. A. Dugas, "Remarks on the Pathology and Treatment of Rheumatism," *Southern Medical and Surgical Journal* (1836–37), 1: 15–22. See also Thomas H. Webb's Fiske Fund Prize Dissertation of the Rhode Island Medical Society, "What Are the Causes and Nature of Rheumatism, and the Best Mode of Treatment to Be Employed Therein," *Boston Medical and Surgical Journal* (1837), 16: 117–122, 133–139, 149–152, and 187–191.

12. Edward J. Seymour, "On the Most Effectual Treatment of Acute Rheumatism in Hospital Practice in the Last Eight Years," *Medico-Chirurgical Review and Journal of Practical Medicine* (1838), 29: 657–660.

13. Samuel Fish, "Large Doses of Opium in Rheumatism," *Boston Medical and Surgical Journal* (1837), 17: 44–47.

14. William Charles Wells, "On Rheumatism of the Heart," *Transactions of a Society for the Improvement of Medical and Chirurgical Knowledge* (1812), 3: 373–424. For a discussion of Wells's contribution, see Harry Keil, "Dr. William Charles Wells and His Contribution to the Study of Rheumatic Fever," *Bulletin of the History of Medicine* (1936), 4: 789–816; and Keil, "A Note on Edward Jenner's Lost Manuscript on 'Rheumatism of the Heart,'" *Bulletin of the History of Medicine* (1939), 7: 409–411.

15. Van Swieten, *Commentaries upon Boerhaave's Aphorisms,* vol. 13, p. 32.

16. Cullen, *First Lines*, 156.

17. John Haygarth, *A Clinical History of Diseases. [1], A Clinical History of the Acute Rheumatism. 2. A Clinical History of the Nodosity of the Joints, 1805,* reprinted with an introduction by Lawrence A. May (Oceanside, N.Y.: Dabor Science Publications, 1977).

18. Matthew Baillie, *The Morbid Anatomy of Some of the Most Important Parts of the Human Body*, 2nd ed. (London: J. Johnson and G. Nicol, 1797), 44–46.

19. David Dundas, "An Account of a Peculiar Disease of the Heart," *Medico-Chirurgical Transactions* (1809), 1: 37–46.
20. James Russell, "Case of Rheumatism of the Heart, Successfully Treated," *Edinburgh Medical and Surgical Journal* (1814), 10: 18–21.
21. R.T.H. Laennec, *A Treatise on the Diseases of the Chest: In Which They Are Described According to Their Anatomical Characters, and Their Diagnosis Established on a New Principle by Means of Acoustick Instruments* (London: T. & G. Underwood, 1821), 266.
22. W. P. Dewees, "A Case of Rheumatism with Metastasis, Producing Carditis, Pericarditis, Peripneumonia, and Pleuritis," *American Journal of the Medical Sciences* (1828), 2: 473–475.
23. Joseph-Irénée Itard, "Considérations sur le rhumatisme du coeur," thèse présentée et soutenue à la faculté de médecine de Paris, le 13 juillet 1824, pour obtenir le grade de docteur en médecine.
24. Dewees, "A Case of Rheumatism with Metastasis."
25. Wells, "On Rheumatism of the Heart."
26. David Dundas, "An Account of a Peculiar Disease of the Heart," *Medico-Chirurgical Transactions* (1809), 1: 37–46.
27. W. S. Church, "An Examination of Nearly Seven Hundred Cases of Acute Rheumatism: Chiefly with a View to Determining the Frequency of Cardiac Affections, and Especially Pericarditis, at the Present Time," *St. Bartholomew's Hospital Reports* (1887), 23: 269–287.
28. G. W. Bury, "A Statistical Account of Four Hundred Cases of Acute Rheumatism Admitted into the Wards of the Middlesex Hospital during the Years 1853–59," *British and Foreign Medico-Chirurgical Review* (1861), 28: 194–198.
29. P. H. Pye-Smith, "Analysis of the Cases of Rheumatism, and Other Diseases of Joints, Which Have Occurred in the Hospital during Three Consecutive Years: With Remarks on the Pathological Alliances of Rheumatic Fever," *Guy's Hospital Reports* (1874), 19: 311–356.
30. Audrey B. Davis, *Medicine and Its Technology: An Introduction to the History of Medical Instrumentation* (Westport, Conn.: Greenwood Press, 1981); Dale C. Smith, "Austin Flint and Auscultation in America," *Journal of the History of Medicine and Allied Sciences* (1978), 33: 129–149; Malcolm Nicolson, "The Introduction of Percussion and Stethoscopy to Early Nineteenth-Century Edinburgh," in *Medicine and the Five Senses*, ed. W. F. Bynum and Roy Porter (London: Cambridge University Press, 1993), 134–153; John Harley Warner, *Against the Spirit of the System: The French Impulse in Nineteenth-Century American Medicine* (Princeton, N.J.: Princeton University Press, 1998); and Jacalyn Duffin, *To See with a Better Eye: A Life of R.T.H Laennec* (Princeton, N.J.: Princeton University Press, 1998).
31. James B. Herrick, "Jean-Baptiste Bouillaud and His Contributions to Cardiology," *Bulletin of the Society of Medical History of Chicago* (1940), 5: 230–246; and Erwin Heinz Ackerknecht, *Medicine at the Paris Hospital, 1794–1848* (Baltimore, Johns Hopkins Press, 1967), 108–109. See also Alain Contrepois, "Towards a History of Infective Endocarditis," *Medical History* (1996), 40: 25–54.
32. Jean-Baptiste Bouillaud, *New Researches on Acute Articular Rheumatism in General; and Especially on the Law of Coincidence of Pericarditis and Endocarditis with This Disease, as Well as on the Efficacy of the Methods of Treating It by Repeated Blood-Lettings at Short Intervals*, trans. James Kitchen (Philadelphia: Haswell, Barrington, and Haswell, 1837), iii.
33. Ibid., 20–21.

34. Ibid., 2.

35. Ackerknecht, *Medicine at the Paris Hospital;* Toby Gelfand, *Professionalizing Modern Medicine: Paris Surgeons and Medical Science and Institutions in the 18th Century* (Westport, Conn.: Greenwood Press, 1980); *The Parisian Education of an American Surgeon. Letters of Jonathan Mason Warren (1832–1835),* with notes and introduction by Russell M. Jones (Philadelphia: American Philosophical Society, 1978); and Dora B. Weiner, *The Citizen-Patient in Revolutionary and Imperial Paris* (Baltimore: Johns Hopkins University Press), 1993.

36. Alfred Stillé, "Case of Rheumatism, Endo-pericarditis, Pleurisy, and Double Pneumonia, with Autopsy," *Medical Examiner* (1840), 3: 21–25; for other examples, see also Dr. Grisolle, "Rhumatisme articulaire aigu, péricardite; endocardite épanchement pleurétique droit, traitement par les saignées a haute dose, mort," *Journal hebdomadaire des progrès des sciences et institutions médicales* (1836), 2: 244–254; V. Cazeneuve, "Observations sur la coïncidence du rhumatisme articulaire avec la péricardite et l'endocardite suives de quelques réflexions sur les adhérences du péricarde, et sur la nature du rhumatisme articulaire," *Recueil de mémoires de médecine, de chirurgie et de pharmacie militaires* (1838), 45: 183–254; Lucien Corvisart, "Rhumatisme articulaire, et endo-péricardite aigue," *Bulletin de la société anatomique de Paris* (1848), 23: 306–310, 332–342; Q. J. Henry Tenneson, "Considérations sur le rhumatisme du coeur, thèse pont le doctorat en médecine," Paris, 1864; and Jean-Numa Dutrénit, "Considérations sur l'endocardite rhumatismale," thèse Montpellier, 1866.

37. Saul Jarcho, "Pericarditis Supervening on Rheumatism (Roots, 1836)," *American Journal of Cardiology* (1966), 18: 594–598.

38. Thomas Sydenham, *The Works of Thomas Sydenham*, trans. from the Latin edition of Dr. Greenhill (London: Sydenham Society, 1848), vol. II, 257–258.

39. Pamela Bright, *Dr. Richard Bright (1789–1858)* (London: Bodley Head, 1983); and Diana Freeman Berry and Campbell Mackenzie, *Richard Bright (1789–1858): Physician in an Age of Revolution and Reform* (London: Royal Society of Medicine, 1992).

40. Richard Bright, "Cases of Spasmodic Disease Accompanying Affections of the Pericardium," *Medico-Chirurgical Transactions* (1839), 22: 1–19.

41. Specifically, Bright cited *Syllabus or Outlines on the Practice of Medicine* (Guy's Hospital, 1802) and a case report, J. Copland, *London Medical Repository* (1821), vol. 15.

42. Dr. Yonge, "Case of Cerebral Disturbance: Dependent upon Disease of the Pericardium," *Guy's Hospital Reports* (1840), 5: 276–281 (reported by Dr. Bright).

43. Dr. Hughes, "Dr. Hughes's Digest of One Hundred Cases of Chorea," *Guy's Hospital Reports* (1846), 4: 360–395 (377, 379).

44. James Richard Smyth, "Rheumatic Fever: With Rheumatic Pericarditis and Pleuritis; Bleeding in Structural Disease of the Heart; Remedial Employment of Mercury," *Lancet* (1839–40), 1: 721–725.

45. Dr. Burrow, "Rheumatic Fever for the Ninth Time, Associated with Pericarditis and Chorea, Fatal Result," *Lancet* (1859), 1: 288–289.

46. Dr. Hodges, "Rapidly Fatal Case of Acute Rheumatism, With Very Slight Pericarditis, and Little or No Abnormal Effusion," *Boston Medical and Surgical Journal* (1855), 53: 188.

47. Lionel S. Beale, "Clinical Lecture on the Treatment of Rheumatic Fever; and of the Use of Alcohol in Serious Cases of This Disease," *British Medical Journal* (1862), 1: 81–83, 111–112.

48. J. Knight, "An Address Delivered before the Oneida County Medical Society in January (1847), on the Treatment of Rheumatism," *New York Journal of Medicine* (1847), 8: 180–184.

49. Charles Clay, "Sulphur in Rheumatic Affections," *Lancet* (1839–40), 2: 783–784; Clay, "Additional Observations on Sulphur Lotum, in Rheumatic Affections: and the Operation for Varicose Veins in the Legs," *Lancet* (1840–41), 1: 417; and Dr. Aran, "Researches upon the Treatment of Acute Articular Rheumatism by the Local Application of Anesthetic Agents," *Edinburgh Medical and Surgical Journal* (1852), 77: 112–120.

50. J. J. De Roches, "Two Cases of Acute Rheumatism, Treated with Opium: And Some Observations on the Comparative Merits of That Method, and of the Treatment Which Is Founded on the Principle of Depletion," *Edinburgh Medical and Surgical Journal* (1805), 1: 154–159.

51. Samuel Fish, "Corroborative Testimony in Favor of Large Doses of Opium in Rheumatism," *Boston Medical and Surgical Journal* (1837), 16: 330–332; and J. Mauran, "Opium in Rheumatism," *Boston Medical and Surgical Journal* (1837), 16: 169–172.

52. John T. Banks, "Acute Rheumatism: Endocarditis Followed by Pericarditis and Pleuropneumonia," *Dublin Hospital Gazette* (1854–55), n.s. 1: 53–55.

53. Quotation began his case report. D. J. Corrigan, "Observations on the Treatment of Acute Rheumatism by Opium," *Dublin Journal of the Medical Science* (1840), 16: 256–277.

54. Ibid., 262–264.

55. Haygarth, *A Clinical History of Diseases*, 1–146; Dr. Duncan, "Treatment of Acute Rheumatism by the Sulphate of Quinine, " *Lancet* (1830), 2: 201–202; and David D. Davis, "On the History of the Employment of Cinchona Bark in the Treatment of Acute Rheumatism," *Lancet* (1840–41), 1: 718–722.

56. Bouillaud, *New Researches*, 22.

57. Dr. Taylor, "Clinical Lecture: Delivered at University College Hospital," *Lancet* (1841–42), 1: 345–349.

58. Dr. O'Connor, "Cases of Acute Rheumatism Successfully Treated with Bicarbonate of Potash," *Lancet* (1856), 2: 487–488; and O'Connor, "Clinical Remarks on a Case of Consecutive Attacks of Acute Rheumatism, Followed by Pericarditis, Endocarditis, and Pleuritis: Recovery," *Lancet* (1862), 2: 10–12.

59. James Alexander, *Rheumatism: Its Nature, Causes and Cure. Gout: Its Nature, Causes, Cure, and Prevention* (London: John Churchill, 1858), viii.

60. John Roberton, "Rheumatic Fever: Its Dangers and Its Treatment," *British Medical Journal* (1864), 1: 659–660.

CHAPTER 2    *Acute Rheumatism and Hospitals*

1. Dorothy Porter and Roy Porter, *Patient's Progress: Doctors and Doctoring in Eighteenth-Century England* (Oxford: Polity Press, 1989).

2. See, for example, H. M. Hughes, "Digest of One Hundred Cases of Chorea Treated in the Hospital," *Guy's Hospital Reports* (1846), 2nd series, 4: 360–395; Alfred Baring Garrod, "On a Successful Method of Treating Acute Rheumatism by Large and Frequent Doses of Bicarbonate of Potash," *Medico-Chirurgical Transactions* (1855), 38: 111–156; F. Sibson, "Table of Cases of Acute Rheumatism Treated by Large Doses of Opium," *British Medical Journal* (1857), 2: 1000–1004; and W. H. Dickinson, "Tables Illustrating the Effects of Remedies upon Uncomplicated Acute Rheumatism," *Lancet* (1869), 1: 116–118, 153–155, 183–185, and 252–255.

3. Lindsay Patricia Granshaw, "The Rise of the Modern Hospital in Britain," in *Medicine in Society: Historical Essays*, ed. Andrew Wear (Cambridge: Cambridge University Press, 1992), 197–218; Granshaw, "'Fame and Fortune by Means of Bricks and Mortar': The Medical Profession and Specialized Hospitals in Britain, 1800–1948," in *The Hospital in History,* ed. Granshaw and Roy Porter, (London: Routledge, 1989), 199–220; Granshaw, "The Hospital," in *Companion Encyclopedia of the History of Medicine*, ed. W. F. Bynum and Roy Porter (London: Routledge, 1993), vol. 2, 1180–1203.

4. See, for example, W. Brockbank, *Portrait of a Hospital, 1752–1948: To Commemorate the Bi-Centenary of the Royal Infirmary, Manchester* (London: William Heineman, 1952), 72–95; Lindsay Patricia Granshaw, "St. Thomas's Hospital, London, 1850–1900," Ph.D. diss., Department of History and Philosophy of Science, Bryn Mawr College, 1981, 119; and John Langdon-Davies, *Westminster Hospital: Two Centuries of Voluntary Service* (London: John Murray, 1952), 208–209.

5. Some historians have used rheumatism to illustrate a view that hospitals admitted only patients who were mildly ill with "chronic" or "lingering" illnesses; this view fails to take into account that many patients with acute rheumatism in the nineteenth century were severely, but not fatally, ill with chorea or heart disease. See, for example, Charles E. Rosenberg, *The Care of Strangers: The Rise of America's Hospital System* (New York: Basic Books, 1987).

6. Roy Porter, "Hospitals and Surgery," in *Cambridge Illustrated History of Medicine*, ed. Roy Porter (Cambridge: Cambridge University Press, 1996), 202–245.

7. Roy Porter, "Cleaning Up the Great Wen: Public Health in Eighteenth-Century London," in *Living and Dying in London*, ed. W. F. Bynum and Roy Porter (London: Wellcome Institute for the History of Medicine, 1991), 61–75; and Roy Porter, ed., *Patients and Practitioners: Lay Perceptions of Medicine in Pre-Industrial Society* (Cambridge: Cambridge University Press, 1985).

8. J. G. Humble, "Westminster Hospital: First 250 Years," *British Medical Journal* (1966), 1: 156–162.

9. H. C. Cameron, *Mr. Guy's Hospital, 1726–1948* (London: Longmans, Green, and Co., 1954); William B. Ober, ed., *Great Men of Guy's* (Metuchen, N.J.: Scarecrow Reprint Corp., 1973),.

10. Hilary Aidan St. George Saunders, *The Middlesex Hospital, 1745–1948* (London: Max Parrish, 1949). See also Guenter Risse, "Medicine in the Age of the Enlightenment," in *Medicine in Society: Historical Essays*, ed. Andrew Wear (Cambridge: Cambridge University Press, 1992), 149–195.

11. Charles J. MacAllister, *The Origin and History of the Liverpool Royal Southern Hospital, with Personal Reminiscences* (Liverpool: W. B. Jones, and Co., 1936).

12. Edward Mansfield Brockbank, *Sketches of the Lives and Work of the Honorary Medical Staff of the Manchester Infirmary, from its Foundation in 1752 to 1830 When It Became the Royal Infirmary* (Manchester: Manchester University Press, 1904).

13. Guenter B. Risse, *Hospital Life in Enlightenment Scotland, Care and Teaching at the Royal Infirmary of Edinburgh* (Cambridge: Cambridge University Press, 1986), 150–152; Granshaw, "St. Thomas's Hospital," 76; and Samuel West, "The Form and Frequency of Cardiac Complications in Rheumatic Fever," *Practitioner* (1888), 41: 104–113. Chorea, much of it related to acute rheumatism, was also a common admitting diagnosis at Hospital for Sick Children, Great Ormond Street; see Elizabeth M. R. Lomax, *Small and Special: The Development of Hospitals for Children in Victorian Britain* (*Medical History*, suppl. 16) (London: Wellcome Institute for the History of Medicine, 1996), 184.

14. J. Rosser Matthews, *Quantification and the Quest for Medical Certainty* (Princeton: Princeton University Press, 1995), 14–38.

15. Obit., "The Late Dr. Edmund Lyon of Manchester," *British Medical Journal* (1863), 1: 224; Brockbank, *Sketches*, 253–256; and W. Brockbank, *Portrait of a Hospital.*

16. Edmund Lyon, "Statistics of Rheumatism," *Transactions of the Provincial Medical and Surgical Association, London* (1840–41), 9: 338–344.

17. P. H. Pye-Smith, "Analysis of the Cases of Rheumatism, and Other Disease of Joints, Which Have Occurred in the Hospital during Three Consecutive Years: With Remarks on the Pathological Alliances of Rheumatic Fever," *Guy's Hospital Reports* (1874), 3rd series, 19: 311–356.

18. George William Fleetwood Bury, "A Statistical Account of Four Hundred Cases of Acute Rheumatism Admitted into the Wards of the Middlesex Hospital during the Years 1853–59," *British and Foreign Medico-Chirurgical Review* (1861), 28: 194–198.

19. Samuel Wilks and G. T. Bettany, *A Biographical History of Guy's Hospital* (London: Warwick House, 1892), 242–245.

20. H. M. Hughes, "Digest of One Hundred Cases of Chorea Treated in the Hospital," *Guy's Hospital Reports* (1846), 2nd series, 4: 360–395.

21. Obit., *Lancet* (1914), 1: 1578–1579; Obit., *British Medical Journal* (1914), 1: 1215–1216; and Obit., *Guy's Hospital Reports* (1921), 71: 137–142. See P. H. Pye-Smith, ed., *The Principles and Practice of Medicine* (edited and completed from the manuscript of the late Charles Hilton Fagge), 2nd ed. (London: J. and A. Churchill, 1888), vol. 2, 810–834 (section on acute rheumatism).

22. Pye-Smith, "Analysis of the Cases of Rheumatism." See also Germaine Sée, "De la chorée: rapports du rhumatisme et des maladies du coeur avec les affections nerveuses et convulsives," *Mémoires de l'académie de médecine* (1850), 15: 414–420; Morris J. Lewis, "A Partial Study of the Seasonal Relations of Chorea and Rheumatism," *Journal of Nervous and Mental Disease* (1886), n.s., 13: 761–766; H. Walter Syers, "Chorea and Rheumatism," *Lancet* (1889), 2: 1271; and Stephen MacKenzie, "On the Relationship of Chorea to Rheumatism, with Special Reference to the Heart Murmur Which So Frequently Attends Chorea," *Transactions of the International Medical Congress* (London, 1881), 4: 97–105.

23. Bury, "A Statistical Account."

24. Pye-Smith, "Analysis of the Cases of Rheumatism."

25. W. S. Church, "An Examination of Nearly Seven Hundred Cases of Acute Rheumatism, Chiefly with a View to Determining the Frequency of Cardiac Affections, and Especially Pericarditis, at the Present Time," *St. Bartholomew's Hospital Reports* (1887), 23: 269–287.

26. Ian H. Porter, "The Nineteenth-Century Physician and Cardiologist Thomas Bevill Peacock (1812–82)," *Medical History* (1962), 6: 240–254; Thomas B. Peacock, *On Malformations, etc, of the Human Heart: With Original Cases* (London: John Churchill, 1858); Peacock, *On Some of the Causes and Effects of Valvular Disease of the Heart* (London: John Churchill, 1865); and Peacock, *On the Prognosis in Cases of Valvular Disease of the Heart* (London: J. and A. Churchill, 1877). See also F. G. Parsons, *The History of St. Thomas's Hospital* (London: Methuen and Co., 1936), vol. 3, 242.

27. Thomas B. Peacock, "On Rheumatic Carditis," *St. Thomas's Hospital Reports* (1875), n.s., 6: 1–20; and Peacock, "Statistical Report on Cases of Rheumatic Fever Treated

during the Years 1872–1876, Inclusive," *St. Thomas's Hospital Reports* (1879, 1880), n.s. 10: 1–20.

28. Church, "An Examination." For another analysis of heart disease and acute rheumatism at St. Bartholomew's Hospital, see Samuel West, "The Form and Frequency of Cardiac Complications in Rheumatic Fever," *Practitioner* (1888), 41: 104–113; and Samuel West, *How to Examine the Chest: A Practical Guide for the Use of Students*, 2nd ed (London: J. & A. Churchill, 1890).

29. MacAlister, *Origin and History*, 38, 40–46; Obit., *Lancet* (1913), 1: 424; and Obit., *British Medical Journal* (1913), 1: 367–368.

30. William Carter, "Ten Years' Hospital Experience of Acute and Sub-Acute Rheumatism," *Liverpool Medico-Chirurgical Journal* (1881), 1: 88–101.

31. Obit., *Lancet* (1906), 2: 1181–1182; and Obit., *British Medical Journal* (1906), 2: 1158.

32. H. Walter Syers, "An Analysis of Five Hundred Consecutive Cases of Acute Rheumatism," *Lancet* (1888), 1: 1292.

33. W. H. Dickinson, "Tables Illustrating the Effects of Remedies upon Uncomplicated Acute Rheumatism," *Lancet* (1869), 1: 116–118, 153–155, 183–185, and 252–255.

34. E. L. Fox, "Clinical Observations on the Temperature of Disease: I. Acute Rheumatism," *Medical Times and Gazette* (1870), 1:15; and Thomas Stevenson, "On the Urine in Acute Rheumatism," *Guy's Hospital Reports* (1866), 3rd series, 12: 431–443.

35. George K. Behlmer, "Ernest Hart and the Social Thrust of Victorian Medicine," *British Medical Journal* (1990), 301: 711–713.

36. William M. Ord, ed., *Collected Works of Francis Sibson*, 4 vols. (London: Macmillan and Co., 1881), biography xix–xliii.

37. E. A. Hart, "Acute Rheumatism Treated by Large Doses of Opium," *British Medical Journal* (1857), 2: 963–964; and Sibson, "Table of Cases."

38. Archibald E. Garrod, *A Treatise on Rheumatism and Rheumatoid Arthritis* (London: Charles Griffin and Co., 1890), 21.

39. W. H. Brock, "The Life and Work of William Prout," *Medical History* (1965), 9: 101–126; and Brock, *From Protyle to Proton: William Prout and the Nature of Matter, 1785–1985* (Bristol: Adam Hilger, 1985).

40. William Prout, *An Inquiry into the Nature and Treatment of Gravel, Calculus, and Other Diseases Connected with a Deranged Operation of the Urinary Organs* (London: Baldwin, Cradock, and Joy, 1821), 127–139, 176.

41. Alfred Baring Garrod, *The Nature and Treatment of Gout and Rheumatic Gout*, 2nd ed. (London: Walton and Maberly, 1863), 523–572; Garrod, *The Essentials of Materia Medica and Therapeutics,* 3rd ed. (London: Longmans, Green, and Co., 1870), 119–120; Obit., *British Medical Journal* (1908), 1: 58–59; and Obit., *Lancet* (1908), 1: 65–67.

42. Archibald E. Garrod, *A Treatise on Rheumatism and Rheumatoid Arthritis* (London: Charles Griffin and Co., 1890), 21–23; Charles Hilton Fagge and Philip Henry Pye-Smith, *A Textbook of Medicine,* 4th ed., 2 vols. (London: J. and A. Churchill, 1901), 486–498.

43. James Alexander, *Rheumatism: Its Nature, Causes, and Cure. Gout: Its Nature, Causes, Cure, and Prevention* (London: John Churchill, 1858), viii–ix.

44. William F. Channing, "The Alkaline Treatment of Rheumatism," *Boston Medical and Surgical Journal* (1855), 52: 335–336.

45. J. H. Salisbury, "Remarks on the Structure, Functions, and Classification of the Parent

Gland Cells, with Microscopic Investigations Relative to the Causes of the Several Varieties of Rheumatism, and Directions for Their Treatment," *American Journal of the Medical Sciences* (1867), 54: 359–377.

46. John Langdon-Davies, *Westminster Hospital, Two Centuries of Voluntary Service* (London: John Murray, 1952), 262.

47. P. W. Latham, "Some Points in the Pathology of Rheumatism, Gout, and Diabetes," *Lancet* (1886), 1: 626–629, 673–677, 723–726, 771–774, and 817–820.

48. See Balthazar W. Foster, "The Synthesis of Acute Rheumatism," *British Medical Journal* (1871), 2: 720–722; and Samuel Gee, "Rheumatic Fever without Arthritis, *St. Bartholomew's Hospital Reports* (1888), 24: 21–23.

49. J. M. DaCosta, "Acute Articular Rheumatism," *Medical Record* (1874), 9: 481–482. For other detractors, see Austin Flint, "Heart Complication in Acute Articular Rheumatism," *Boston Medical and Surgical Journal* (1883), 109: 409–410; and T. J. Maclagan, "The Pathology and Treatment of Rheumatic Endocarditis," *Lancet* (1883), 1: 517–518.

50. J. B. Chapin, "Treatment of Rheumatism, with Statistical Results of 25 Cases Treated in the New York Hospital," *New York Medical Times* (1854), 3: 385–388. For alkaline therapy at the Massachusetts General Hospital, see Dr. Perry, "Cases of Rheumatism Treated by Carbonate of Soda," *Boston Medical and Surgical Journal* (1855), 52: 481–482.

51. Alfred Baring Garrod, "On A Successful Method of Treating Acute Rheumatism by Large and Frequent Doses of Bicarbonate of Potash," *Medico-Chirurgical Transactions* (1855), 38: 111–156.

52. Jules Kosky, *Mutual Friends: Charles Dickens and Great Ormond Street Children's Hospital* (London: Weidenfeld and Nicolson, 1989), 206; Obit., *Lancet* (1913), 1: 203–204; Obit., *British Medical Journal* (1913), 1: 141–143; and W. Howship Dickinson, *Occasional Papers on Medical Subjects, 1855–1896* (London: Longmans, Green and Co., 1896). See also Elizabeth M. R. Lomax, *Small and Special: The Development of Hospitals for Children in Victorian Britain* (*Medical History*, suppl. 16) (London: Wellcome Institute for the History of Medicine, 1996).

53. W. H. Dickinson, "On the Treatment of Acute Rheumatism, Considered with Regard to the Liability at Affects of the Heart under Different Remedies," *Medico-Chirurgical Transactions* (1861–62), 45: 343–354; for an expanded version, see Dickinson, "Tables Illustrating the Effects of Remedies upon Uncomplicated Acute Rheumatism," *Lancet* (1869), 1: 116–118, 153–155, 183–185, and 252–255.

54. Thomas K. Chambers, "Treatment of Rheumatic Fever," *British Medical Journal* (1866), 1: 187–188; Chambers, "Clinical Lecture on the Treatment of Acute Rheumatism," *Lancet* (1862), 2: 199–201; Chambers, *Lectures, Chiefly Clinical,* 4th ed. (London: John Churchill and Sons, 1865), 126–148.

55. Dale C. Smith, "Austin Flint and Auscultation in America," *Journal of the History of Medicine and Allied Sciences* (1978), 33: 129–149; see also Austin Flint, *Collected Essays and Articles on Physiology and Medicine,* 2 vols. (New York: D. Appleton and Co., 1903).

56. Austin Flint, "A Contribution toward the Natural History of Articular Rheumatism: Consisting of a Report of Thirteen Cases Treated Solely with Palliative Measures," *American Journal of the Medical Sciences* (1863), n.s., 46: 17–36.

57. Review, Henry W. Fuller, *On Rheumatism, Rheumatic Gout, and Sciatica: Their Symptoms, Pathology, and Treatment,* 2nd ed. (London: Churchill, 1856), in *British Medical Journal* (1857), 1: 257–258.

58. Noel G. Coley, "George Owen Rees, M.D., FRS (1813–1889): Pioneer of Medical Chemistry," *Medical History* (1986), 30: 173–190

59. G. Owen Rees, "On the Treatment of Rheumatism by Lemon Juice," *Lancet* (1850), 2: 651; Rees, "Cases of Rheumatic Fever Treated by Citric Acid," *Lancet* (1851), 1: 571–572; Rees, "On the Remedial Effects of Lemon-Juice in Rheumatism and on Sources of Fallacy Connected with Its Use," *Lancet* (1853), 1: 534–535; Rees, "Four Cases of Rheumatic Fever, Treated with Mint-Water Only," *Guy's Hospital Reports* (1865), 3rd series, 11: 429–434; Rees, "Cases of Acute Rheumatism Treated by Lemon Juice, with Remarks," *Guy's Hospital Reports* (1866), 3rd series, 12: 479–494; and William Pepper, "Lemon Juice as a Remedy in Rheumatism," *Transactions of the College of Physicians of Philadelphia* (1850–53), n.s., 1: 124–142. See Samuel Wilks and G. T. Bettany, *A Biographical History of Guy's Hospital* (London: Warwick House, 1892), 251–261.

60. Samuel Wilks and G. T. Bettany, *A Biographical History of Guy's Hospital* (London: Warwick House, 1892), 261–274; Theodore Dyke Acland (ed.), *A Collection of the Published Writings of William Withey Gull: vol. 1, Medical Papers* (London: New Sydenham Society, 1894).

61. Obit., *Lancet* (1891), 1: 1408–1410.

62. William Gull and Henry Sutton, "Remarks on the Natural History of Rheumatic Fever," *Medico-Chirurgical Transactions* (1869), 52: 43–84 (67); Henry G. Sutton, "Cases of Rheumatic Fever Treated for the Most Part By Mint Water," *Guy's Hospital Reports* (1865), 3rd series, 11: 392–428; Sutton, "A Second Report of Cases of Acute Rheumatism Treated in the Wards of Guy's Hospital: With Remarks on the Natural History of the Disease," *Guy's Hospital Reports* (1866), 3rd series, 12: 509–539; and Gull and Sutton, "Remarks on the Natural History of Rheumatic Fever," *British Medical Journal* (1869), 1: 57–58, 130–131.

63. For other therapeutic suggestions, see J. Russell Reynolds, "Remarks on the Treatment of Acute Rheumatism by Tincture of Pure Perchloride of Iron," *British Medical Journal* (1869), 2: 649; R. Randle Buck, "The Treatment of Acute Rheumatism by Tincture of Perchloride of Iron," *British Medical Journal* (1870), 1: 260. J. M. DaCosta, "A Contribution to the Therapeutics of Acute Rheumatism, Based on a Series of Cases Treated with Bromide of Ammonium," *Pennsylvania Hospital Reports* (1869), 2: 53–82; A. W. Barclay, "On the Employment of Quinine in the Treatment of Rheumatic Fever," *St. George's Hospital Reports* (1873), 6: 101–116; and James Andrew, "On the Treatment of Rheumatic Fever by a Non-Nitrogenous Diet," *St. Bartholomew's Hospital Reports* (1874), 10: 359–368.

64. "Treatment of Acute Rheumatism," *British Medical Journal* (1869), 1: 8–9. See also Henry Kennedy, "Remarks on the Treatment of Acute Rheumatic Fever," *British Medical Journal* (1869), 1: 397–398; Charles H. Robinson, "Cases of Acute Rheumatism Treated Principally by the Alkaline Method," *Lancet* (1869), 1: 812–813; and "Debate of the Treatment of Rheumatic Fever (at the Royal Medical and Chirurgical Society)," *Lancet* (1869), 1: 160–162.

65. "Treatment of Acute Rheumatism," *Medical Record* (1873), 8: 131 (Bellevue Hospital), 503 (Roosevelt Hospital).

66. R. Clement Lucas, "On the Treatment of Acute Rheumatism with Acids," *Lancet* (1874), 1: 296–297.

67. John M. Riddle, *Dioscorides on Pharmacy and Medicine* (Austin: University of Texas Press, 1985), 44.

68. C. E. Buss, "Über die Anwendung der Salicylsäure als Antipyreticum," *Deutsches Archiv für klinische Medicin* (1875),15: 457–501.

69. Thomas Maclagan, "The Treatment of Acute Rheumatism by Salicin," *Lancet* (1876), 1: 342–343, 2: 601–604. See also Joseph L. Miller, "The Specific Action of Salicylates in Acute Articular Rheumatism," *Journal of the American Medical Association* (1914), 63: 1107–1110; and P. J. Hanzlik, "Actions and Uses of the Salicylates and Cinchophen in Medicine," *Medicine* (1926), 5: 197–373. For biographical information about Maclagan, see Obit., *Lancet* (1903), 1: 1000; and Obit., *British Medical Journal* (1903), 1: 766.

70. T. J. Maclagan, *Rheumatism: Its Nature, Its Pathology, and Its Successful Treatment,* 2nd ed. (London: Adam and Charles Black, 1896).

71. Dr. Stricker, "Über die Resultate der Behandlung der Polyarthritis Rheumatica mit Salicylsäure," *Berliner Klinische Wochenschrift* (1876), 13: 1–2; and L. Riess, "Nachtrag zur innerlichen Anwendung der Salicylsäure, insbesondere bie dem acuten Gelenkrheumatismus," *Berliner Klinische Wochenschrift* (1876), 13: 86–89.

72. For example, see Edward Headlam Greenhow, *The Treatment of Rheumatic Fever with Salicin and Salicylate of Soda* (London: Spottiswoode, 1880).

73. M. E. Broadbent [daughter], ed., *Life of Sir William Broadbent* (London: John Murray, 1909).

74. W. H. Broadbent, "Treatment of Rheumatic Fever by Salicylic Acid," *Lancet* (1876), 1: 530–531; Thomas Maclagan, letter to editor, *Lancet* (1876), 1: 585; and W. H. Broadbent, letter to editor, *Lancet* (1876), 1: 619.

75. S. L. Abbott (reported by M. Hutchinson), "Acute Rheumatism, with Valvular Lesions, Remarkable Character of Pulse, Salicylic Acid Treatment," *Boston Medical and Surgical Journal* (1876), 95: 117–119.

76. Berthier, "La salicylate et le rheumatism; La grande vogue du jour vielle question de thérapeutique général à ce propos," *Revue médicale française et étrangère* (1877), 2: 481–487.

77. William Osler, "Acute Rheumatism Treated with Salicylate of Soda: Delirium Apparently Caused by the Remedy," *Canada Medical and Surgical Journal* (1879), 7: 493–495; anon., "Delirium in Acute Rheumatism after Salicylate of Soda," *British Medical Journal* (1881), 1: 159–161; and T. D. Acland, "Delirium Following the Treatment of Acute Rheumatism by Salicylic Acid," *British Medical Journal* (1881), 1: 337.

78. Albert Wood, "Case of Rheumatism Following Mild Scarlet Fever in Which Salicylic Acid Was Used," *Boston Medical and Surgical Journal* (1876), 95: 45–46; Henry Clarke, "Three Cases of Polyarthritis Treated by Salicylic Acid," *Boston Medical and Surgical Journal* (1876), 95: 42–46; D. W. Hodgkins, "Salicylic Acid in Acute Rheumatism," *Boston Medical and Surgical Journal* (1876), 94: 595–596; Ralph C. Huse, "Salicylic Acid in Acute Rheumatism," *Boston Medical and Surgical Journal* (1876), 94: 595; Dr. Russell, "Eight Cases of Acute Rheumatism Treated by Salicylic Acid; Notice of a Case of Rheumatic Hyperpyrexia Treated by the Same Medicine," *British Medical Journal* (1877), 1: 454–455; F. W. Brigham, "Five Cases of Rheumatism Treated with Salicylic Acid," *Boston Medical and Surgical Journal* (1876), 95: 46; Dr. Remmington, "Three Cases of Acute Articular Rheumatism," *Boston Medical and Surgical Journal* (1876), 95: 44–45; S. K. Towle, "Salicylic Acid in Acute Rheumatism," *Boston Medical and Surgical Journal* (1876), 94: 593–595; A. Clarke, "Salicylate of Soda in Rheumatism," *Medical Record* (1876), 11: 663–665; George M. Edebohls, "An Interesting Case of Acute Articular Rheumatism—Unusual Number and Severity of Complications," *Medical Record* (1877), 12: 776–777; and T. J.

Maclagan, "The Treatment of Acute Rheumatism by Salicin and Salicylic Acid," *Lancet* (1879), 1: 875–877.

79. Anon., "The Treatment of Acute Rheumatism in the Hospitals of Chicago," *Medical Record* (1887), 12: 758–759; and V. Y. Bowditch, "Massachusetts General Hospital: Cases of Acute Rheumatism in 1878–1879," *Boston Medical and Surgical Journal* (1879), 101: 134–139

80. W. Howship Dickinson, *Occasional Papers on Medical Subjects, 1855–1896* (London: Longmans, Green, and Co., 1896).

81. Germain Sée, "Étude sur l'acide salicylique et les salicylate," *France médicale* (1877), 24: 449–466.

82. Anon., "Acute and Subacute Rheumatism in the Years 1877–78," *St. George's Hospital Reports* (1877–79), 9: 216–233; and Isambard Owen, "The Salicylate Treatment of Acute and Subacute Rheumatism," *Lancet* (1881), 2: 1081.

83. Reginald Southey, "On the Treatment of Acute Rheumatism by Salicylate of Soda," *St. Bartholomew's Hospital Reports* (1879), 15: 7–14.

84. David W. Finley and R. H. Lucas, "Note on the Salicylate and Alkaline Treatment of Acute Rheumatism, with an Analysis of 150 Cases," *Lancet* (1879), 2: 420–421.

85. Francis Warner, "Analysis of Statistics Illustrating the Action of Salicin Compounds in the Treatment of Acute and Subacute Rheumatism," *Lancet* (1881), 2: 1080.

86. De Havilland Hall, "The Salicylate Treatment of Acute Rheumatism," *Lancet* (1881), 2: 1081–1082.

87. C. Hilton Fagge, "Remarks on the Use of the Salicylates in Acute Rheumatism," *Lancet* (1881), 2: 1030–1033; and Donald W. C. Hood, "Statistics in Connexion with Treatment of Acute Rheumatism by the Salicylate. Being an Analysis of 1200 Cases at Guy's Hospital," *Lancet* (1881), 2: 1119.

88. James Russell, "Salicylic Acid Treatment Contrasted with Other Remedies in the Treatment of Acute Rheumatism," *British Medical Journal* (1882), 1: 459.

89. William Osler, "Acute Rheumatism Treated with Salicylate of Soda: Delirium Apparently Caused by the Remedy," *Canada Medical and Surgical Journal* (1879), 7: 493–495; anon., "Delirium in Acute Rheumatism after Salicylate of Soda," 159–160; and Acland, "Delirium Following the Treatment of Acute Rheumatism by Salicylic Acid."

90. William R. D. Blackwood, "The Treatment of Acute Articular Rheumatism," *Medical Record* (1879), 15: 213; and T. J. Maclagan, "Note on the Danger Attending the Use of Salicylic Acid on Acute Rheumatism," *Lancet* (1880), 1: 327.

91. Robert Sinclair, "The Alkaline, Salicin, and Salicylate of Soda Treatment of Acute Rheumatism," *Lancet* (1880), 1: 281–282.

92. Ibid.

93. Alfred Stillé, "The Treatment of Acute Rheumatism," *Medical Gazette* (1881), 8: 276.

94. W. S. Cheesman, "Heart-Lesions in Rheumatic Fever," *Medical Record* (1882), 21: 202–203.

95. T. Gilbart-Smith, "Cardiac Complications in Acute Rheumatism: Prior to and Subsequent to the Introduction of the Salicyl Compounds," *Lancet* (1882), 1: 135–137.

96. T. J. Maclagan, "Rheumatic Endocarditis," *British Medical Journal* (1883), 1: 713–714.

97. Charles H. May, "Statistics of Four Hundred Cases of Rheumatism, With Special Reference to Treatment," *Medical Record* (1884), 25: 57–62, 87–92, 116–121, and 173–178.

98. Anon., "Treatment of Rheumatism in the Philadelphia Hospitals," *Medical News* (1886), 49: 627–629; see also anon., "The Treatment of Rheumatism in the New York Hospitals," *Medical News* (1886), 49: 655–657.

99. John M. Eyler, *Sir Arthur Newsholme and State Medicine, 1885–1935* (Cambridge: Cambridge University Press, 1997).

100. Arthur Newsholme, "The Natural History and Affinities of Rheumatic Fever: A Study in Epidemiology," *Lancet* (1895), 1: 589–596.

CHAPTER 3    *Cheadle and the "Typical Case"*

1. W. B. Cheadle, "Harveian Lectures on the Various Manifestations of the Rheumatic State: As Exemplified in Childhood and Early Life," *Lancet* (1889), 1: 821–827, 871–877, and 921–927. See also Cheadle, "A Clinical Illustration of Certain Phases of the Rheumatic Diathesis," *Lancet* (1886), 1: 483–484.

2. J. Knight, "An Address Delivered Before the Oneida County Medical Society in January (1847) on the Treatment of Rheumatism," *New York Journal of Medicine* (1847), 8: 180–184.

3. Alexander Murray, "Observations on a Form of Scarlet Fever Succeeded by Rheumatic Affections, in Illustration of the West India Epidemic," *Edinburgh Medical and Surgical Journal* (1830), 33: 294–303. See also A. Siebert, "Rheumarthritis und Scarlatina," *Deutsche Klinik* (1851), 3: 275–277.

4. Nathaniel J. Haydon, "On the Connexion of Rheumatism with Scarlatina," *Lancet* (1854), 1: 301–302.

5. Hughes Willshire, "On Some Points in the Pathology of Rheumatism in Children," *Lancet* (1854), 1: 138–139.

6. Dr. O'Connor, "Scarlatina Complicated with Acute Rheumatism, Bronchitis and Pericarditis Supervening: Recovery," *Lancet* (1861), 2: 473–474.

7. Dr. Bolles, "Scarlet Fever, Acute Rheumatism, Peri and Endocarditis, and Acute Nephritis: Partial Recovery, Relapse, and Death," *Boston Medical and Surgical Journal* (1876), 94: 426–428.

8. T. F. Raven, "Note on the Association of Rheumatism with Scarlatina," *British Medical Journal* (1886), 1: 440.

9. Sir James K. Fowler (Obit.), *British Medical Journal* (1934), 2: 91–92.

10. J. Kingston Fowler, "On the Association of Affections of the Throat with Acute Rheumatism," *Lancet* (1880), 2: 933–934.

11. Alfred Mantle, "The Etiology of Rheumatism Considered from a Bacterial Point of View," *British Medical Journal* (1887), 1: 1381–1384.

12. B. Mayston Bond, "Scarlatinal Rheumatism," *Lancet* (1890), 1: 52. See also E. Bloch, "Zur Aetiologie des Rheumatismus," *Münchener Medicinische Wochenschrift* (1898), 45: 445–448.

13. Henry Ashby, "On the Nature of the So-Called Scarlatinal Rheumatism," *British Medical Journal* (1883), 2: 514–515.

14. William Osler, *The Principles and Practice of Medicine: Designed for the Use of Practitioners and Students of Medicine* (New York: D. Appleton and Co., 1892), p. 332. For a discussion of the role of tonsils in health, see William Henry Thayer, "Observations on Rheumatism Especially as Involving the Tonsils," *New York Medical Journal* (1890), 52: 90–93.

15. William Charles Wells, "On Rheumatism of the Heart," *Transactions of a Society for the Improvement of Medical and Chirurgical Knowledge* (1812), 3: 373–424. The most

thorough history of rheumatic nodules is Harry Keil, "The Rheumatic Subcutaneous Nodules and Simulating Lesions," *Medicine* (1938), 17: 261–380.

16. Thomas Barlow, "On Subcutaneous Nodules Connected with Fibrous Structures, Occurring in Children, the Subjects of Rheumatism and Chorea," *Transactions of the International Medical Congress* (1881), 4: 116–128. See also Samuel West, "Clinical Notes and Observations: Rheumatic Fever—Numerous Nodules—Pericarditis and Endocarditis," *St. Bartholomew's Hospital Reports* (1886), 22: 213–215; J. A. Coutts, "Subcutaneous Rheumatic Nodules," *Illustrated Medical News* (1889), 3: 267–271; and M. E. Troisier, "Les nodosités rhumastismales sous-cutanées," *Bulletins et mémoires de la société médicale des hôpitaux de Paris* (1883, 1884), 20 (pt. 2), 45–67.

17. Archibald E. Garrod, "On the Relation of Erythema Multiforme and Erythema Nodosum to Rheumatism," *St. Bartholomew's Hospital Reports* (1888), 24: 43–54. See also A. Sevester, "Érythème marginé: Rapports de cette affection avec le rhumatisme," *Progrès (le) médical* (1873), 1: 318; and E.E.A. Ferrand, "Les exanthème du rhumatisme," *Bulletins de la société médicale d'émulation de Paris* (1867), n.s., 1: 419–423.

18. P. H. Pye-Smith, "Analysis of the Cases of Rheumatism, and Other Diseases of Joints, Which have Occurred in the Hospital during Three Consecutive Years: With Remarks on the Pathological Alliances of Rheumatic Fever," *Guy's Hospital Reports* (1874), 3rd series, 19: 311–356.

19. James F. Goodhart, "On the Rheumatic Diathesis in Childhood," *Guy's Hospital Reports* (1880), 3rd series, 25: 103–138.

20. Archibald E. Garrod and E. Hunt Cooke, "An Attempt to Determine the Frequency of Rheumatic Family Histories Amongst Non-Rheumatic Patients," *Lancet* (1888), 2: 110.

21. August Hirsch, *Handbook of Geographical and Historical Pathology*, trans. Charles Creighton (London: New Sydenham Society, 1886), 3: 745–765. For an extensive survey in Great Britain, see Thomas Whipham, "Reports of the Collective Investigation Committee of the British Medical Association. Report on Inquiry no. III. Acute Rheumatism," *British Medical Journal* (1888), 1: 387–404.

22. Arthur Newsholme, "The Milroy Lectures on the Natural History and Affinities of Rheumatic Fever: A Study in Epidemiology," *Lancet* (1895), 1: 589–596, 657–665.

23. Andrew Barlow [grandson], "Sir Thomas Barlow, Bt.," *Three Selected Lectures and a Biographical Sketch* (London: Dawsons of Pall Mall, 1965), 1–17.

24. Thomas Barlow, "Notes on Rheumatism and Its Allies in Childhood," *British Medical Journal* (1883), 2: 509–514. For Holt's opinions, see H. D. Chapin, "Rheumatism of Early Life," *Boston Medical and Surgical Journal* (1886), 114: 231–233 (discussion).

25. H. D. Chapin, "Rheumatism of Early Life," *Boston Medical and Surgical Journal* (1886), 114: 231–233 (discussion). For views about rheumatic fever and children, see Henry Koplik, "Acute Articular Rheumatism in the Nursing Infant," *New York Medical Journal* (1888), 47: 673–676. See also Angel Money, "Nodular Periostitis in Children's Rheumatism and Heart Disease," *Lancet* (1889), 2: 265; Frank S. Parsons, "Acute Rheumatism in Children," *Journal of the American Medical Association* (1890), 15: 60–63; Constant Picot, *Du rhumatisme aigu et de ses diverses manifestations chez les enfants* (Paris: Adrian Delahaye, 1873); Charles Jules Ernest Cadet de Gassicourt, "Leçons sur traitment du rhumatisme aigu et des maladies rhumatismales du coeur les enfants," *Traité clinique des maladies de l'enfance: leçons professées à l'hôpital sainte-eugenie* (Paris: Octave Doin, 1880–84), 2: 181–259; and Karl Vohsen, "Beiträge

zur Kenntniss des Gelenkrheumatismus im Kindesalter," *Jahrbuch für Kinderheilkunde und Physiche Erziehung* (1883), n.f., 19: 83–104.

26. William Fitzwilliam Milton and W. B. Cheadle, *Northwest Passage by Land. Being the Narrative of an Expedition from Atlantic to the Pacific, Undertaken with the View of Exploring a Route across the Continent to British Columbia through British Territory, by One of the Northern Passes in the Rocky Mountains* (London: Cassell, Petter, and Galpin, 1867).

27. Walter Butler Cheadle [Obit.], *British Medical Journal* (1910), 1: 908–909; and Obit., *Lancet* (1910), 1: 962–965. See also Walter Butler Cheadle, *Occasional Lectures on the Practice of Medicine, Addressed Chiefly to the Students of St. Mary's Medical School, to Which Are Appended the Harveian Lectures on the Rheumatism of Childhood* (London: Smith, Elder, and Co., 1900).

28. Thomas Barlow, "Notes on Rheumatism and Its Allies in Childhood," *British Medical Journal* (1883), 2: 509–514.

29. Judson S. Bury, "Rheumatism in Children," *British Medical Journal* (1883), 2: 516–519 (commentary).

30. H. D. Chapin, "Rheumatism of Early Life," *Boston Medical and Surgical Journal* (1886), 114: 231–233.

31. Angel Money, "Lectures on Rheumatism in Children," *Lancet* (1886), 2: 158–159.

32. Walter Butler Cheadle, *The Various Manifestations of the Rheumatic State as Exemplified in Childhood and Early Life* (London: Smith, Edler, 1889), 5.

33. Ibid.

34 Ibid.

35 R. W. Quinn, "Did Scarlet Fever and Rheumatic Fever Exist in Hippocrates' Time?" *Reviews of Infectious Diseases* (1991), 13: 1243–1244.

CHAPTER 4    *Rheumatic Fever as Sepsis*

1. Alfred Mantle, *The Etiology of Rheumatism Considered from a Bacterial Point of View* (New Castle-upon-Tyne: Havelock, 1886).

2. Arthur Newsholme, "The Milroy Lectures on the Natural History and Affinities of Rheumatic Fever: A Study in Epidemiology," *Lancet* (1895), 1: 589–596, 657–665. See also John M. Eyler, *Sir Arthur Newsholme and State Medicine, 1835–1935* (Cambridge: Cambridge University Press, 1997); and Eyler, "The Sick Poor and the State: Arthur Newsholme on Poverty, Disease, and Responsibility," in *Framing Disease: Studies in Cultural History*, ed. Charles E. Rosenberg and Janet Golden (New Brunswick, N.J.: Rutgers University Press, 1992), 275–296.

3. See also Arthur Newsholme, "The Epidemiology of Rheumatic Fever," *Practitioner* (1901), 66: 11–21.

4. G. B. Longstaff, "A Contribution to the Etiology of Rheumatic Fever," *Transactions of the Epidemiological Society of London* (1904–1905), n.s., 24: 33–83.

5. W. B. Cheadle, "Acute Rheumatism," *British Medical Journal* (1896), 1: 65–74

6. Jefferson C. Crossland, "Tonsillitis as an Initial Symptom of Acute Rheumatism in the Adult," *Journal of the American Medical Association* (1892), 19: 519–520; Sir Willoughby Wade, "Remarks on Tonsillitis as a Factor in Rheumatic Fever," *British Medical Journal* (1896), 1: 829–832; A. Ernest Sanson, "On the Treatment of the Rheumatic Diseases of the Heart in the Early Periods of Their Manifestation: A Retrospect and an Estimate," *Lancet* (1900), 1: 923–925; William Henry Thayer, "Ob-

servations on Rheumatism: Especially as Involving the Tonsils," *New York Medical Journal* (1890), 52: 90–93.

7. F. A. Packard, "On Infection through the Tonsils: Especially in Connection with Acute Articular Rheumatism," *Transactions of the New York Academy of Medicine* (1896–1901), 13: 298–346.

8. Charles F. Kieffer, "The Relation between Tonsillitis and Acute Articular Rheumatism: With Particular Reference to the Prophylaxis of Postanginal Rheumatism, *American Medicine* (1906), 12: 318–322.

9. For a discussion of Koch, his postulates, and precursors, see K. Codell Carter, "Koch's Postulates in Relation to the Work of Jacob Henle and Edwin Klebs," *Medical History* (1985), 29: 353–374; and Carter, "The Development of Pasteur's Concept of Disease Causation and the Emergence of Specific Causes in Nineteenth-Century Medicine," *Bulletin of the History of Medicine* (1991), 65: 528–548. See also Keith Vernon, "Pus, Sewage, Beer, and Milk: Microbiology in Britain, 1870–1940," *History of Science* (1990), 28: 289–325.

10. Charles-Edward Amory Winslow, *The Conquest of Epidemic Disease: A Chapter in the History of Ideas* (1943; Madison: University of Wisconsin Press, 1980); Hubert A. Lechevalier and Morris Solotorovsky, *Three Centuries of Microbiology*, corrected reprint, with additional bibliographical references, of the 1965 edition (New York: Dover Publications, 1974); and William Bulloch, *A History of Bacteriology* (1936; New York: Dover Publications, 1979).

11. Peter C. English, "Diphtheria and Theories of Infectious Disease: Centennial Appreciation of the Critical Role of Diphtheria in the History of Medicine," *Pediatrics* (1985), 76: 1–9.

12. Peter C. English, "Therapeutic Strategies to Combat Pneumococcal Disease: Repeated Failure of Physicians to Adopt Pneumococcal Vaccine, 1900–1945," *Perspectives in Biology and Medicine* (1987), 30: 170–185.

13. For a similar bacteriological enthusiasm, see Peter C. English, *Shock, Physiological Surgery, and George Washington Crile: Medical Innovation in the Progressive Era* (Westport, Conn.: Greenwood Press, 1980), "Science, Shock, and American Surgery: The Growth of Radical Surgery, 1870–1890," pp. 20–46.

14. James Howard Brown, *The Use of Blood Agar for the Study of Streptococci* (New York: Rockefeller Institute for Medical Research, 1919).

15. William Osler, "The Gulstonian Lectures on Malignant Endocarditis," *British Medical Journal* (1885), 1: 467–470, 522–526, 577–579. See David M. Levy, "Centenary of William Osler's 1885 Gulstonian Lectures and Their Place in the History of Bacterial Endocarditis," *Journal of the Royal Society of Medicine* (1985), 78: 1039–1046; and P. R. Fleming, *A Short History of Cardiology*, Wellcome Institute Series in the History of Medicine (Amsterdam: Rodopi, 1997), 134–142.

16. Mantle, *Etiology of Rheumatism*. Years later Mantle discussed his earlier work; see Alfred Mantle, "A History of the Present-Day Accepted Aetiology of Acute Rheumatism," *Practitioner* (1912), 88: 185–192.

17. Pierre Achalme, "Examen bactériologique d'un cas de rhumatisme articulaire aigu: Mort de rhumatisme cérébral," *Comptes rendus hebdomadaires des séances et mémoires de la société de biologie* (1891), 43: 651–656.

18. Dr. Achalme, "Pathogénie du rhumatisme articulaire aigu; examen bactériologique d'un cas terminé par la mort," *Comptes rendus hebdomadaires des séances et mémoires de la société de biologie* (1897), 49: 276–278.

19. J. Thiroloix, "Constatation du microbe trouvé par M. Thiroloix dans le rhumatisme articulaire, a l'autopsie d'un sujet mort de rhumatisme articulaire aigu compliqué d'endopéricardite et de chorée," *Bulletins et mémoires de la société médicale des hôpitaux de Paris* (1897), 3rd series, 14: 1343–1344.

20. J. Thiroloix, "Examen bactériologique du sang de deux malades atteints de rhumatisme articulaire aigu," *Comptes rendus hebdomadaires des séances et mémoires de la société de biologie* (1897), 49: 268.

21. J. Thiroloix, "Bactériologie d'un cas de rhumatisme articulaire aigu," *Comptes rendus hebdomadaires des séances et mémoires de la société de biologie* (1897), 49: 945–946.

22. Anon., "Le Docteur Triboulet," *Chanteclair* (Dec. 1907), 2: 1, 3.

23. Henri Triboulet and Amand Coyon, "Bactériologie comparée des formes compliquées et des formes franches du rhumatisme articulaire aigu," *Bulletins et mémoires de la société médicale des hôpitaux de Paris* (1897), 3rd series, 14: 1458–1462; and Triboulet and Coyon, "Recherches sur la bactériologie du rhumatisme articulaire aigu," *Bulletins et mémoires de la société de médicale des hôpitaux de Paris* (1900), 3rd series, 17: 303–306.

24. P. Achalme, "Recherches sur l'anatomie pathologique de l'endocardite rhumatismale," *Archives de médecine expérimentale et d'anatomie pathologique* (1898), 10: 370–388.

25. Henri Triboulet and Amand Coyon, "Bactériologie du rhumatisme articulaire aigu," *Bulletins et mémoires de la société médicale des hôpitaux de Paris* (1898), 15: 93–96; Triboulet and Coyon, "Bactériologie du rhumatisme articulaire aigu: Endocardite végétante mitrale provoquée chez le lapin par inoculation intra-veineuse d'un cocco-bacille en points doubles extrait du sang du rhumatisme articulaire aigu de l'homme," *Comptes rendus hebdomadaires des séances et mémoires de la société de biologie* (1898), 50: 124–128.

26. Gustav Singer, *Aetiologie und Klinik des Acuten Gelenkrheumatismus* (Vienna: Welhom Braumuller, 1898), table, pp. 122–216.

27. F. Chvostek, "Zur Aetiologie des acuten Gelenkrheumatismus," *Verhandlungen des Congresses für Innere Medizin* (1897), 15: 99–116. For a discussion of Chvostek's work, see James J. Walsh, "Rheumatism and the Prevention of Heart Complications," *Journal of the American Medical Association* (1900), 35: 1535–1538.

28. Editorial, "The Bacteriology of Acute Rheumatism," *Boston Medical and Surgical Journal* (1898), 139: 454–455.

29. A. S. Wohlmann, "Bacteriology of Rheumatic and Allied Diseases," *British Medical Journal* (1899), 2: 1348–1350. For a good historical treatment, see Frederick J. Poynton and Alexander Paine, "The Etiology of Rheumatic Fever," *Lancet* (1900), 2: 861–871.

30. R. Oppenheim and A. Lippmann, "Contribution a l'étude bactériologique du rhumatisme articulaire aigu," *Comptes rendus hebdomadaires des séances et mémoires de la société de biologie* (1900), 52: 180–182.

31. F. J. Poynton and Alexander Paine, "The Etiology of Rheumatic Fever," *Lancet* (1900), 2: 861–871.

32. F. J. Poynton and Alexander Paine, "The Pathogenesis of Rheumatic Fever," *Transactions of the Pathological Society of London* (1900–1901), 52: 10–19; Poynton and Paine, "Some Further Investigations upon Rheumatic Fever," *Lancet* (1901), 1: 1260–1265; Poynton and Paine, "Observations upon the Arthritis Produced in Rabbits by the Intra-venous Inoculation of a Diplococcus Isolated from Cases of Rheumatic Fever," *Transactions of the Pathological Society of London* (1900–1901), 52: 248–253. See also F. J. Poynton and Alexander Paine, *Researches on Rheumatism* (London: J. and A. Churchill, 1913).

33. F. J. Poynton and Alexander Paine, "The Present Position of the Bacteriology of Rheumatic Fever," *British Medical Journal* (1901), 2: 779–781.

34. G. N. Pitt, "A Case of Acute Rheumatism, Minute Vegetations on Mitral Valve, Streptococci in Blood, Infective Emboli in Spleen and Brain: Death from Cerebral Hemorrhage," *Guy's Hospital Gazette* (1901), 15: 513–519.

35. E. W. Ainley Walker and J. Henry Ryffel, "The Pathology of Acute Rheumatism and Allied Conditions," *British Medical Journal* (1903), 2: 659–660.

36. R. M. Beaton and E. W. Ainley Walker, "The Etiology of Acute Rheumatism and Allied Conditions," *British Medical Journal* (1903), 1: 237–239.

37. W. V. Shaw, "Acute Rheumatic Fever and Its Etiology," *Journal of Pathology and Bacteriology* (1904), 9: 158–171.

38. James M. Beattie, "Acute Rheumatism Caused by the 'Diplococcus Rheumaticus,'" *Journal of Pathology and Bacteriology* (1904), 9: 272–277; Beattie, "The 'Micrococcus Rheumaticus': Its Cultural and Other Characters," *British Medical Journal* (1904), 2: 1510–1511.

39. Thomas McCrae, "Acute Articular Rheumatism: A Report of the Cases in the Johns Hopkins Hospital, 1901–1903," *American Medicine* (1903), 6: 221–225.

40. F. J. Poynton, "Remarks on the Infective Nature of Rheumatic Fever, Illustrated by the Study of a Fatal Case," *British Medical Journal* (1904), 1: 1117–1120.

41. F. J. Poynton, "The Parallelism between the Clinical Symptoms and Pathological Lesions of Rheumatic Fever," *International Clinics* (1904), 13th series, 4: 95–111.

42. Rufus I. Cole, "Experimental Streptococcus Arthritis in Relation to the Etiology of Acute Articular Rheumatism," *Journal of Infectious Diseases* (1904), 1: 714–737.

43. James M. Beattie, "Experimental Work in Relation to Micrococcus Rheumaticus and Streptococcus Pyogenes," *Journal of Medical Research* (1905–1906), 14: 399–421; and Beattie, "A Contribution to the Bacteriology of Rheumatic Fever," *British Medical Journal* (1906), 2: 1781–1782.

44. William Osler, "Chronic Infectious Endocarditis," *Quarterly Journal of Medicine* (1908–1909), 2: 219–230. For an excellent statement of knowledge at St. Bartholomew's Hospital, see Thomas J. Horder, "Infective Endocarditis: With Analysis of 150 Cases and with Special Reference to the Chronic Form of the Disease," *Quarterly Journal of Medicine* (1908–1909), 2: 289–324; and Horder, "Lumleian Lecture on Endocarditis," *Lancet* (1926), 1: 695–700, 745–750, and 850–855.

45. Rufus I. Cole, "Aetiology of Acute Articular Rheumatism," *New York Medical Journal* (1906), 83: 534–538.

46. E.W.A. Walker, "On the Micro-organism Isolated from Acute Rheumatism, and Its Relation to Other Members of the Streptococcus Group," *British Medical Journal* (1907), 1: 1233–1236.

47. James M. Beattie, "A Contribution to the Bacteriology of Rheumatic Fever," *Journal of Experimental Medicine* (1907), 9: 186–206; and Beattie, "Further Experiments with a Streptococcus Isolated from Cases of Acute Rheumatism," *Journal of Pathology and Bacteriology* (1910), 14: 432–445.

48. F. J. Poynton, "A Contribution to the Subject of Rheumatism Based upon a Study of 52 Cases in Children under Five Years of Age, and an Analysis of 100 Cases of Fatal Suppurative Pericarditis in Childhood," *Quarterly Journal of Medicine* (1907–1908), 1: 225–238; Poynton and Alexander Paine, "Some Further Investigations and Observations upon the Pathology of Rheumatic Fever," *Lancet* (1910), 1: 1524–1528; and Poynton and Paine, "A Research upon Combined Mitral and Aortic Disease of Rheumatic Origin: A Contribution to the Study of Rheumatic Malignant Endocarditis," *Quarterly Journal of Medicine* (1911–12), 5: 463–494.

49. Lewis A. Conner, "Review of the Bacteriology of Acute Articular Rheumatism," *Journal of the American Medical Association* (1907), 48: 379–381.

50. Charles Hunter Dunn, "The Clinical Aspects of Rheumatic Fever in Childhood, and Their Significance in the Question of Specific Etiology," *Journal of the American Medical Association* (1907), 48: 493–501; J. Ross Snyder, "Rheumatism of Childhood," *Journal of the American Medical Association* (1907), 48: 490–493; Ludwig M. Loeb, "The Bacteriology of Acute Rheumatism," *Archives of Internal Medicine* (1908), 2: 266–276.

51. Poynton and Paine, "Some Further Investigations." See also F. J. Poynton and Alexander Paine, *Researches on Rheumatism* (London: J. and A. Churchill, 1913).

52. J. Thiroloix and Georges Rosenthal, "Biosepticémie à bacille d'Achalme au cours d'une attaque de rhumatisme articulaire aigu," *Bulletins et mémoires de la société médicale des hôpitaux de Paris* (1907), 3rd series, 24: 879–885.

53. Triboulet and Silbert, "À propos du rhumatisme articulaire aigu," *Bulletins et mémoires de la société médicale des hôpitaux de Paris* (1907), 3rd series, 24: 885–893.

54. J. Thiroloix and Georges Rosenthal, "Constatation directe par simple coloration du bacille d'Achalme dans le sang d'une rhumatisante," *Bulletins et mémoires de la société médicale des hôpitaux de Paris* (1907), 3rd series, 24: 969–970; Thiroloix and Rosenthal, "Hémoculture dans le rhumatisme articulaire aigu: Anaéroboise et aérobisation rapide du bacille obtenu: son polymorphisme et sa transformation," *Bulletins et mémoires de la société médicale des hôpitaux de Paris* (1907), 3rd series, 24: 971–982; Thiroloix, "Bacille d'Achalme: Sa plasticité physique et fonctionnelle," *Bulletins et mémoires de la société medical des hôpitaux de Paris* (1907), 3rd series, 24: 1195–1201.

55. Triboulet and Silbert, "À propos de las spécificité bactériologique du rhumatisme," *Bulletins et mémoires de la société médicale des hôpitaux de Paris* (1907), 3rd series, 24: 1091–1107.

56. Georges Rosenthal, "Les rapport de variétés banale et rhumatismale du bacille d'Achalme (bacille anaérobie du rhumatisme articulaire aigu et bacille perfringens) démontrés par l'action identique croisée de sérum T.R.—La culture virus fixe du bacille perfringens," *Comptes rendus hebdomadaires des séances et mémoires de la société de biologie* (1909), 66: 1027–1028.

57. Georges Rosenthal and P. Chazarain-Wetzel, "Recherches sur les cultures croisées de bacillus perfringens et de l'anhémobacille du rhumatisme articulaire aigu," *Archives générales de médecine* (1909), 888–897. For the best review of the situation in 1909, see Rosenthal, "Bactériologie, sérothérapies, et vaccinations du rhumatisme articulaire aigu," *Archives générales de médecine* (1909), 571–625; and Rosenthal and Chazarain-Wetzel, "La culture du bacille perfringens dans les cultures sporulées en eau blanc d'oeuf du bacille anaérobie du rhumatisme aigu; moyen de différenciation des deux variétés du bacille d'Achalme," *Comptes rendus hebdomadaires des séances et mémoires de la société de biologie* (1909), 67: 677–678.

58. J. Thiroloix and J. Debertrand, "Histo-bactériologie d'un cas de rhumatisme articulaire aigu terminé par le mort," *Bulletins et mémoires de la société medical des hôpitaux de Paris* (1909), 3rd series, 26: 1019–1034.

59. F. G. Bosc and Carrieu, "Le virus rhumatisme articulaire aigu n'est pas de nature bactérienne," *Comptes rendus hebdomadaires des séances et mémoires de la société de biologie* (1913), 74: 1165–1167.

60. F. J. Bosc and Carrieu, "Le bacille d'Achalme est un saprophyte banal, hôte habituel de la peau des rhumitisants et dépourvu de toute spécificité pour le rhumatisme,"

*Comptes rendus hebdomadaires des séances et mémoires de la société de biologie* (1913), 74: 1229–1230.

61. P. Achalme, "À propos du bacille du rhumatisme articulaire aigu," *Comptes rendus hebdomadaire des séances et mémoires de la société de biologie* (1913), 75: 82–84.

62. Tinsley Randolph Harrison and S. A. Levine, "Notes on the Regional Distribution of Rheumatic Fever and Rheumatic Heart Disease in the United States," *Southern Medical Journal* (1924), 17: 914–915.

63. J. Thiroloix, "Étude bactériologique d'un cas de rhumatisme articulaire aigu," *Comptes rendus hebdomadaires des séances et mémoires de la société de biologie* (1897), 49: 882–884.

64. Henri Triboulet and Amand Coyon, "Bactériologie du rhumatisme articulaire aigu," *Bulletins et mémoires de la société médicale des hôpitaux de Paris* (1898), 3rd series, 15: 93–96; Triboulet and Coyon, "Bactériologie du rhumatisme articulaire aigu: Endocardite végétante mitrale provoquée chez le lapin par inoculation intra-veineuse d'un cocco-bacille en points doubles extrait du sang du rhumatisme articulaire aigu de l'homme," *Comptes rendus hebdomadaires des séances et mémoires de la société de biologie* (1898), 50: 124–128.

65. Poynton and Paine, "Etiology of Rheumatic Fever."

66. Poynton and Paine, "Some Further Investigations."

67. Poynton and Paine,"Observations upon the Arthritis Produced in Rabbits."

68. Rufus I. Cole, "Experimental Streptococcus Arthritis in Relation to the Etiology of Acute Articular Rheumatism," *Journal of Infectious Diseases* (1904), 1: 714–737; and Cole, "Aetiology of Acute Articular Rheumatism," *New York Medical Journal* (1906), 83: 534–538.

69. Leonard G. Wilson, "The Early Recognition of Streptococci as Causes of Disease" *Medical History* (1987), 31: 403–414.

70. Beattie, "Experimental Work in Relation to Micrococcus Rheumaticus and Streptococcus Pyogenes"; Beattie, "A Contribution to the Bacteriology of Rheumatic Fever"; Beattie and A. G. Yates, "The Bacteriology of Rheumatism: Further Evidence in Favour of the Causal Relation of Streptococci," *Journal of Pathology and Bacteriology* (1912–13), 17: 538–551; and Beattie and Yates, "The Streptococcus in Rheumatism," *Journal of Pathology and Bacteriology* (1912–13), 17: 416–418.

71. Oscar M. Schloss, "The Injection of Rhesus Monkeys with Blood from Patients with Rheumatic Fever," *Journal of the American Medical Association* (1912), 59: 1946.

72. Leila Jackson, "Experimental Streptococcal Arthritis in Rabbits: A Second Study Dealing with Streptococci from the Milk Epidemic of Sore Throat in Chicago, 1911–12," *Journal of Infectious Diseases* (1913), 12: 364–385.

73. Harold Kniest Faber, "Experimental Arthritis in the Rabbit: A Contribution to the Pathogeny of Arthritis in Rheumatic Fever," *Journal of Experimental Medicine* (1915), 22: 615–628; E. C. Rosenow, "The Etiology of Acute Rheumatism, Articular, and Muscular," *Journal of Infectious Diseases* (1914), 14: 61–80; M. A. Rothschild and William Thalhimer, "Experimental Arthritis in the Rabbit, Produced with Streptococcus Mitis," *Journal of Experimental Medicine* (1914), 19: 444–449.

74. Obit., *Journal of the American Medical Association* (1953), 153: 967.

75. Homer F. Swift and Ralph A. Kinsella, "Bacteriologic Studies in Acute Rheumatic Fever," *Archives of Internal Medicine* (1917), 19: 381–396. For a restatement of his research nearly twenty years after the original publication, see F. John Poynton, "A Contribution to the Study of Acute Rheumatism," *British Medical Journal* (1919), 1: 371–372.

76. Homer F. Swift and Ralph H. Boots, "The Question of Sensitization with Non-Hemolytic Streptococci," *Journal of Experimental Medicine* (1923), 38: 573–589.

77. Samuel West, "Analysis of Forty Cases of Rheumatic Fever," *St. Bartholomew's Hospital Reports* (1878), 14: 221–233.

78. Obit., *Lancet* (1904), 2: 1256–1257; and Obit., *British Medical Journal* (1904), 2: 1196.

79. Angel Money, "Rheumatic Nodules," *British Medical Journal* (1883), 1: 622.

80. Ludolf Krehl, "Beitrag zur Pathologie der Herzklappenfehler," *Deutsches Archiv für Klinische Medicin* (1890), 46: 454–477; Ernest Romberg, "Über die Bedeutung des Herzmuskels für die Symptome und den Verlauf der acuten Endocarditis und der Chronischen Klappenfehler," *Deutsches Archiv für Klinische Medicin* (1894), 53: 141–188.

81. Ludwig Aschoff, "Zur Myocarditisfrage," *Verhandlungen der deutschen pathologischen Gesellschaft* (1904), 8: 46–53. For a translation, Frederick A. Willius and Thomas Keys, *Classics of Cardiology* (Malaar, Fla.: Robert W. Krieger Co., 1983), vol. 2, pp. 733–739; and Aschoff, "A Discussion of Some Aspects of Heart-Block," *British Medical Journal* (1906), 2: 1103–1107.

82. Carey Coombs, "The Histology of Rheumatic Carditis and Other Rheumatic Phenomena," *British Medical Journal* (1911), 1: 620. See also Carey F. Coombs, *Rheumatic Heart Disease*, intro. F. J. Poynton (Bristol: John Wright and Sons, 1924).

83. William Thalhimer and M. A. Rothschild, "On the Significance of the Submiliary Myocardial Nodules of Aschoff in Rheumatic Fever," *Journal of Experimental Medicine* (1914), 19: 417–428.

84. Carey Coombs, Reginald Miller, and E. H. Kettle, "The Histology of Experimental Rheumatism," *Lancet* (1912), 2: 1209–1212.

85. William Lintz, "Rheumatic Carditis," *Journal of the American Medical Association* (1912), 58: 615–618.

86. Oscar M. Schloss and Nellis B. Foster, "Experimental Streptococcic Arthritis in Monkeys," *Journal of Medical Research* (1913), 29: 9–22.

87. William Thalhimer and M. A. Rothschild, "Experimental Focalized Myocardial Lesions Produced with Streptococcus Mitis," *Journal of Experimental Medicine* (1914), 19: 429–442.

88. R. C. Whitman and A. C. Eastlake, "Rheumatic Myocarditis: A Histogenic Study of the Type of Cells of the Aschoff Body," *Archives of Internal Medicine* (1920), 26: 601–611; and Joseph H. Pratt, "Acute Rheumatic Myocarditis," *Medical Clinics of North America* (1922), 5: 1305–1318.

89. C. Philip Miller, Jr., "Attempts to Transmit Rheumatic Fever to Rabbits and Guinea Pigs," *Journal of Experimental Medicine* (1924), 40: 525–541.

90. Homer F. Swift, "The Pathogenesis of Rheumatic Fever," *Journal of Experimental Medicine* (1924), 39: 497–508; David Riesman, "Acute Rheumatic Fever and Its Variants in Childhood and Adolescence," *Journal of the American Medical Association* (1921), 76: 1377–1380; and B. J. Clawson, "Studies on the Etiology of Acute Rheumatic Fever," *Journal of Infectious Diseases* (1925), 36: 444–456.

CHAPTER 5    *Clinical Management*

1. A small sample of articles showing Cheadle's influence includes: A. Ernest Sansom, "A Clinical Lecture on the Nature of True Rheumatism," *Clinical Journal of London* (1892–93), 1: 81–83; Thomas Churton, "On the Localising Factors in Rheumatic Fever and Chorea," *Transactions of the Medical Society (London)*, (1897–98), 21: 29–

41; Stephen MacKenzie, "On the Various Forms of Rheumatism Especially in Reference to Age and Sex," *Edinburgh Medical Journal* (1897), n.s., 1: 32–37, 139–147; John F. H. Broadbent, "Rheumatic Affections of the Heart in Childhood and Early Adolescence," *Edinburgh Medical Journal* (1898), n.s., 3: 473–480; Philip F. Barbour, "Rheumatism in Children," *Pediatrics* (1898), 6: 289–297; F. J. Poynton and Alexander Paine, "The Infectivity of Acute Rheumatism: With Especial Reference to the Chronic Type of the Disease," *Clinical Journal of London* (1901), 18: 41–44; Archibald E. Garrod, "The Clinical and Pathological Relations of the Chronic Rheumatic and Rheumatoid Affections to Acute Infective Rheumatism," *Lancet* (1901), 1: 774–777; Alfred Friedlander, "Rheumatism in Childhood," *Pediatrics* (1903), 15: 513–520; Joseph M. Patton, "Etiology and Prophylaxis of the Cardiac Manifestations of Articular Rheumatism," *Journal of the American Medical Association* (1903), 40: 83–87; Sir Dyce Duckworth, "The Varied Manifestations of Rheumatic Infection," *St. Bartholomew's Hospital Journal* (1904–1905), 12: 111–114; F. J. Poynton, "The Influence of School Life Upon Rheumatic Children," *Journal of Preventive Medicine* (1905), 13: 406–415; Alex D. Blackader, "Rheumatism in Children," *British Medical Journal* (1906), 2: 925–927; C. O. Hawthorne, "The Protection of Rheumatic Children," *British Journal of Children's Diseases* (1907), 4: 85–88; Norman Moore, "Lumleian Lectures on Rheumatic Fever and Valvular Disease," *Lancet* (1909), 1: 1159–1164, 1227–1230, 1297–1301; Herman B. Sheffield, "Rheumatismus Acutus. Rheumatic Fever. Polyarthritis Acuta," *Pediatrics* (1910), 22: 276–281; F. J. Poynton, "A Lecture on the Complications of Rheumatism in Childhood," *British Medical Journal* (1911), 2: 253–256; and W. G. MacCallum, "Rheumatism: The Harrison Lecture," *Journal of the American Medical Association* (1925), 84: 1545–1551.

2. T. Duckett Jones, "The Diagnosis of Rheumatic Fever," *Journal of the American Medical Association* (1944), 126: 481–484.

3. Carey Coombs, "Some Clinical Aspects of the Rheumatic Infection," *Lancet* (1904), 1: 565–568.

4. Oscar M. Schloss, "The Association of 'Rheumatic Fever' and the Erythema Group of Skin Disease: With a Report of Four Cases," *American Journal of the Medical Sciences* (1910), 140: 226–239.

5. Stephen MacKenzie, "On the Relationship of Purpura Rheumatica to Erythema Exudativum Multiforme," *British Journal of Dermatology* (1896), 8: 116–129; and Murray H. Bass, "The Cutaneous Manifestations of Acute Rheumatic Fever in Childhood," *Medical Clinics of North America* (1918), 2: 201–214.

6. George Frederick Still, "On a Form of Chronic Joint Disease in Children," *Medico-Chirurgical Transactions* (1896–97), 80: 47–59.

7. George Parker, "On the Diagnosis of Certain So-called Rheumatic Diseases from Each Other and from Rheumatism," *Lancet* (1897), 1: 1735–1738; Thomas F. Harrington, "Differential Diagnosis of Rheumatism and the Arthrites," *Boston Medical and Surgical Journal* (1904), 150: 85–90; Joseph Brennemann, "The Incidence and Significance of the Rheumatic Nodules in Children," *American Journal of Diseases of Children* (1919), 18: 179–186; James B. Herrick, "Differential Diagnosis of Rheumatoid Joint Affections," *Journal of the American Medical Association* (1907), 48: 381–383, 391–393.

8. Mary F. Williams, "Rheumatic Conditions in School-Children," *Lancet* (1928), 1: 720–721.

9. Max Seham and Eunice H. Hilbert, "Muscular Rheumatism in Childhood," *American Journal of Diseases of Children* (1933), 46: 826–853.

10. M. J. Shapiro, "Differential Diagnosis of Nonrheumatic 'Growing Pains' and Subacute Rheumatic Fever," *Journal of Pediatrics* (1939), 14: 315–322; and J. C. Hawksley, "The Nature of Growing Pains and Their Relation to Rheumatism in Children and Adolescents," *British Medical Journal* (1939), 1: 155–157.

11. E. M. Brockbank, "'Growing Pains' as a Symptom of Rheumatism," *British Medical Journal* (1900), 1: 1020–1021.

12. P. B. Bennie, "Growing Pains," *Archives of Pediatrics* (1894), 11: 337–347.

13. David B. Lees and Frederick J. Poynton, "Rheumatic Dilatation of the Heart in the Rheumatism and Chorea of Childhood," *Proceedings of the Royal Medical and Chirurgical Society of London* (1897–98), 3rd series, 10: 188–193.

14. D. B. Lees, "A Discussion on Rheumatic Heart Disease in Children," *British Medical Journal* (1898), 2: 1129–1134.

15. Delancey Rochester, "The Heart in Acute Rheumatism," *Journal of the American Medical Association* (1900), 35: 1538–1543; Alexander Lambert, "Cardiac Complications of Acute Rheumatism," *Journal of the American Medical Association* (1908), 50: 741–743; and Theodore Fisher, "Rheumatic Myocarditis," *British Medical Journal* (1902), 2: 949–950.

16. David B. Lees, "Discussion on the Diagnosis and Treatment of Early Cardiac Complications of Rheumatism," *British Medical Journal* (1912), 2: 929–936.

17. F. J. Poynton, "Observations on the Nature and Symptoms of Cardiac Infection in Childhood," *British Medical Journal* (1918), 2: 1–4.

18. F. J. Poynton, "Clinical Evidences of Myocardial Damage in Rheumatic Fever," *International Clinics* (1903), 3 (ser. 13): 226–241.

19. Carey Coombs, "The Myocardial Lesions of the Rheumatic Infection," *British Medical Journal* (1907), 2: 1513–1514.

20. I. E. Atkinson, "Bradycardia (Bradysphygmie-Ozanam) in Acute Rheumatism," *Transactions of the Association of American Physicians* (1891), 6: 292–304.

21. Pierre Achalme, "Sur un signe de diagnostic précoce des attaques et des rechutes de rhumatisme articulaire aigu," *Archives générales de médecine* (1902), 8: 257–267.

22. For histories of the electrocardiogram, see W. Bruce Fye, "A History of the Origin, Evolution, and Impact of Electrocardiography," *American Journal of Cardiology* (1994), 73: 937–949; Joel D. Howell, "Early Use of X-ray Machines and Electrocardiographs at the Pennsylvania Hospital, 1897–1927," *Journal of the American Medical Association* (1986), 255: 2320–2323; John Burnett, "The Origins of the Electrocardiograph as a Clinical Instrument," *The Emergence of Modern Cardiology*, ed. W. F. Bynum, C. Lawrence, and V. Nutton (London: Wellcome Institute for the History of Medicine), *Medical History* (1985), suppl., 5: 53–76; Mark E. Silverman, "From Rebellious Palpitations to the Discovery of Auricular Fibrillation: Contributions of MacKenzie, Lewis, and Einthoven," *American Journal of Cardiology* (1994), 73: 384–389; and James K. Cooper, "Electrocardiography 100 Years Ago: Origins, Pioneers, and Contributors," *New England Journal of Medicine* (1986), 315: 461–464.

23. G. A. Sutherland, "Auricular Flutter in Acute Rheumatic Carditis," *British Journal of Children's Diseases* (1914), 11: 337–345.

24. Selian Neuhof, "A Case of Independent Ventricular Activity Occurring during Acute Articular Rheumatism," *Archives of Internal Medicine* (1915), 15: 169–176.

25. Paul D. White, "Acute Heart Block Occurring as the First Sign of Rheumatic Fever," *American Journal of the Medical Sciences* (1916), 152: 589–591.

26. John Parkinson, A. Hope Gosse, and E. B. Gunson, "The Heart and Its Rhythm in Acute Rheumatism," *Quarterly Journal of Medicine* (1919–20), 13: 363–379.

27. Alfred E. Cohn and Homer F. Swift, "Electrocardiographic Evidence of Myocardial Involvement in Rheumatic Fever," *Journal of Experimental Medicine* (1924), 39: 1–35.

28. Howell, "Early Use of X-ray Machines and Electrocardiographs."

29. Ruth Tunnicliff, "The Opsonic Index in Acute Articular Rheumatism," *Journal of Infectious Diseases* (1909), 6: 346–360.

30. Homer F. Swift, C. Philip Miller, and Ralph H. Boots, Jr., "The Leucocyte Curve as an Index of the Infection in Rheumatic Fever," *Journal of Clinical Investigation* (1924), 1: 197–215.

31. William Ewart, "The Treatment of Rheumatism: With Special Reference to Prophylaxis and Its Cardiac Compilations," *Lancet* (1900), 1: 761–768.

32. Rosemary Stevens, *In Sickness and in Wealth: American Hospitals in the Twentieth Century* (New York: Basic Books, 1989), 105, 139, and 172. The history of tonsillectomy is remarkably silent on such a common procedure. See J. McAuliffe Curtin, "The History of Tonsil and Adenoid Surgery," *Otolaryngologic Clinics of North America* (1987), 20: 415–419.

33. Quoted in Floyd M. Crandall, "The Management of Rheumatic Children," *Transactions of the American Pediatric Society* (1902),14: 68–69.

34. Quoted in ibid., 69.

35. William Osler, *The Principles and Practice of Medicine: Designed for the Use of Practitioners and Students of Medicine* (New York: D. Appleton & Co., 1892), 333.

36. Edmund D. Spear, "Luschka's Tonsil: The Site of Infection in Articular Rheumatism," *Boston Medical and Surgical Journal* (1903), 149: 359.

37. Joseph M. Patton, "Rheumatic Carditis in Children," *Archives of Pediatrics* (1907), 24: 674–682.

38. William P. Lucas and Mark H. Wentworth, "The Treatment of Rheumatic Endocarditis: From an Outpatient Department Standpoint," *American Journal of Diseases of Children* (1914), 7: 41–47.

39. T. H. Halsted, "The Tonsil in Its Relation to Rheumatic Infections," *New York State Journal of Medicine* (1915), 15: 438–442; William E. Preble, "Focal Infection and Rheumatism," *Boston Medical and Surgical Journal* (1918), 178: 82–86; and Martin O. Raven, "Rheumatic Carditis: Some Principles Governing Its Prevention and Early Treatment," *Lancet* (1923), 2: 1227–1233.

40. E. Fletcher Ingals, "The Relation of Tonsillitis to Rheumatism," *Laryngoscope* (1907), 17: 712–717.

41. S. J. Crowe, S. Shelton Watkins, and Alma S. Rothholz, "Relation of Tonsillar and Nasopharyngeal Infections to General Systemic Disorders," *Johns Hopkins Hospital Bulletin* (1917), 28: 1–63; and Roland Hammond, "The Teeth and Tonsils or Causative Factors in Arthritis," *American Journal of the Medical Sciences* (1918), 156: 541–553.

42. G. H. Hunt and A. A. Osman, "The Results of Tonsillectomy in Acute Rheumatism in Children," *Guy's Hospital Reports* (1923), 4th series, 73: 383–387.

43. F. J. Poynton, "Discussion on Rheumatic Infection in Childhood: Early Diagnosis and Preventive Treatment," *British Medical Journal* (1925), 2: 788–796.

44. "Report of the Bureau for Medical Inspection of Schools," *Biennial Report of the North Carolina State Board of Health* (1919–20), 18: 50–52; (1921–22), 19: 33–35; (1923–24), 20: 54–56; (1925–26), 21: 40–41.

45. For example, see Peter C. English, "Therapeutic Strategies to Combat Pneumococcal Disease: Repeated Failure of Physicians to Adopt Pneumococcal Vaccine, 1900–1945," *Perspectives in Biology and Medicine* (1987), 30: 170–185.

46. M. Boucheron, "Sérothérapie dans certains rhumatismes à streptocoques et dans certaines iritis rhumatismales," *Comptes rendus hebdomadaires des séances et mémoires de la société de biologie* (1897), 49: 347–349; and Boucheron, "Sérothérapie antistreptococcique dans certains rhumatismes à streptocoques," *Comptes rendus hebdomadaires des séances et mémoires de la société de biologie* (1897), 49: 917–919.

47. R. J. Chipman, "Case of Acute Articular Rheumatism with Pyaemic Temperature, Treated by Anti-Streptococcic Serum," *Medical Record* (1902), 61: 167.

48. Dr. Menzer, "Zur Frage der Streptokokkenserumbehandlung des acuten und chronischen Gelenkrheumatismus," *Berliner Klinische Wochenschrift* (1904), 41: 75; E. G. Brackett, "Serum Treatment in Multiple Infectious Arthritis," *Boston Medical and Surgical Journal* (1905), 152: 457–461; and N. S. Davis, "The Treatment of Rheumatism by Specifics," *Journal of the American Medical Association* (1907), 49: 2053–2059.

49. J. Thiroloix and Georges Rosenthal, "Pouvoir préventif et curateur expérimental du sérum des chevaux vaccines contre la bactérie anaérobie de l'hémobioculture rhumatismale (sérum T. R.)," *Comptes rendus hebdomadaires des séances et mémoires de la société de biologie* (1909), 66: 46–47; Rosenthal, "Rôle prépondérant du microbe, rôle effacé de la toxine dans l'infection mortelle du cobaye par l'anhémobacille du rhumatisme articulaire aigu," *Comptes rendus hebdomadaires des séances et mémoires de la société de biologie* (1912), 72: 764–765; and M. Fernand Widal, "Sur un travail du Dr. Georges Rosenthal, intitulé: La sérothérapie du rhumatisme articulaire aigu et le Wright vaccin du rhumatisme," *Bulletin de l'académie de médecine* (1910), 64: 8–10; Thiroloix and Rosenthal, "Recherches sur la vaccination contre le bacille d'Achalme (variété rhumatismale): Vaccination massive du lapin par les cultures aérobisées," *Comptes rendus hebdomadaires des séances et mémoires de la société de biologie* (1908), 64: 360–361; and Rosenthal, "Conditions d'innocuité et le réveil de la spore de l'anhémobacille du rhumatisme articulaire aigu," *Comptes rendus hebdomadaires des séances et mémoires de la société de biologie* (1913), 74: 1104–1106.

50. Russell L. Cecil, " A Report on Forty Cases of Acute Arthritis Treated by Intravenous Injection of Foreign Protein," *Archives of Internal Medicine* (1917), 20: 951–963.

51. H. Warren Crowe, "Some Causes of Failure in the Vaccine Treatment of Arthritis, Rheumatism, and Neuritis," *Lancet* (1919), 2: 637–639; and Hazel H. Chodak Gregory, "Notes on the Vaccine Treatment of Acute Rheumatism," *British Journal of Children's Diseases* (1924), 21: 131–138.

52. Ralph Stockman, "The Action of Salicylic Acid and Chemically Allied Bodies in Rheumatic Fever," *British Medical Journal* (1913), 1: 597–600; P. J. Hanzlik, R. W. Scott, C. M. Weidenthal, and Joseph Fetterman, "Cinchophen, Neocinchophen, and Novaspirin in Rheumatic Fever: Comparative Therapeutic Efficiency, Toxicity and Renal Functional Effects," *Journal of the American Medical Association* (1921), 76: 1728–1734; J. K. Fowler, "On the Treatment of Acute Rheumatism with Salicylic Acid," *Lancet* (1881), 2: 1120–1121.

53. T. Gilbart-Smith, "Cardiac Complications in Acute Rheumatism: Prior to and Subsequent to the Inroduction of the Salicyl Compounds," *Lancet* (1882), 1: 135–137; and Donald W. C. Hood, "Statistics in Connexion with the Treatment of Acute Rheumatism by the Salicylates, Being an Analysis of 1200 Cases at Guy's Hospital," *Lancet* (1881), 2: 1119–1120.

54. Walter B. Cheadle, "The Diagnosis and Treatment of Acute Rheumatism in Children," *Treatment* (1897), 1: 97–100.

55. F. J. Poynton, "A Lecture on Combined Aortic and Mitral Disease in Rheumatic Children," *British Medical Journal* (1905), 2: 837–840; and Poynton, "Observations upon Nervous Manifestations in the Rheumatism of Childhood," *British Journal of Children's Diseases* (1912), 9: 49–65.

56. David B. Lees, "Discussion on the Diagnosis and Treatment of Early Cardiac Complications of Rheumatism," *British Medical Journal* (1912), 2: 929–936.

57. Homer F. Swift, "Rheumatic Fever," *Medical Clinics of North America* (1917), 1: 641–658

58. Paul D. White, "Observations on Rheumatic Fever at United States Base Hospital no. 6 A.E.F., in the Spring of 1918," *American Journal of the Medical Sciences* (1920), 159: 702–704.

59. Reginald Miller, "The Theory of Salicylate Therapy in Rheumatic Infection," *Lancet* (1915), 1: 175–178.

60. Henry B. Favill, "Treatment of Acute Rheumatism," *Journal of the American Medical Association* (1899), 32: 1017–1020; Reginald Miller, "The 'Specific' Use of Salicylate in Acute Rheumatism: A Consideration of Practical Objections," *Quarterly Journal of Medicine* (1913), 6: 519–540; James J. Walsh, "The Salicylates in Acute Rheumatism," *Journal of the American Medical Association* (1903), 40: 217–218; Ralph Stockman, "A Clinical Lecture on the Action of Salicylates in Acute Rheumatism," *British Medical Journal* (1906), 2: 1439–1442; Joseph L. Miller, "The Specific Action of Salicylate in Acute Articular Rheumatism," *Journal of the American Medical Association* (1914), 63: 1107–1110; and Paul J. Hanzlik, R. W. Scott, P. C. Gauchat, "The Salicylates. X. The Specificity of Salicylate in Rheumatic Fever," *Journal of Laboratory and Clinical Medicine* (1918–19), 4: 112–122.

61. David John Davis, "The Effect of Sodium Salicylate on Various Types of Experimental Arthritis," *Archives of Internal Medicine* (1915), 15: 555–557.

62. Bernard Fantus, Walter E. Simmonds, and Josiah J. Moore, "The Effect of Salicylates on Experimental Arthritis in Rabbits," *Archives of Internal Medicine* (1917), 19: 529–537.

63. Homer F. Swift, "The Treatment of Rheumatic Fever," *Boston Medical and Surgical Journal* (1922), 187: 331–337; Swift and Ralph H. Boots, "Influence of Sodium Salicylate upon the Arthritis of Rabbits Inoculated with Non-hemolytic Streptococci," *Journal of Experimental Medicine* (1923), 37: 553–584; and Ralph H. Boots and C. Philip Miller, "A Study of Neocinchophen in the Treatment of Rheumatic Fever," *Journal of the American Medical Association* (1924), 82: 1028–1036.

## CHAPTER 6    *Allergy, Heredity, Environment*

1. Philip S. Hench assembled annual bibliographies, "The Present Status of the Problem of Rheumatism: A Review of Recent American and English Literature on 'Rheumatism' and Arthritis," beginning in 1935 in the *Annals of Internal Medicine*. These reviews cited between 400 and 1,100 articles and books each year, proving a rich source on research for this period. *Annals of Internal Medicine* (1935), 8: 1315–1374; (1936), 9: 883–982; (1936), 10: 754–909; (1938), 11: 1089–1247; (1939), 12: 1005–1104; (1940), 13: 1655–1739, 1837–1990; (1941), 14: 1383–1448; (1941), 15: 1002–1108.

2. Homer F. Swift, C. L. Derick, and C. H. Hitchcock, "Bacterial Allergy (hyperergy) to Nonhemolytic Streptococci," *Journal of the American Medical Association* (1928), 90: 906–908.

3. Homer F. Swift, "Rheumatic Fever," *American Journal of the Medical Sciences* (1925), 170: 631–647.

4. Homer F. Swift, C. L. Derick, and C. H. Hitchcock, "Rheumatic Fever as a Manifestation of Hypersensitiveness (Allergy or Hyperergy) to Streptococci," *Transactions of the Association of American Physicians* (1928), 43: 192–202.

5. Homer F. Swift, "Rheumatic Fever," *Journal of the American Medical Association* (1929), 92: 2071–2083.

6. C. L. Derick and Homer F. Swift, "Reactions to Non-Hemolytic Streptococci: I. General Tuberculin-like Hypersensitiveness, Allergy, or Hyperergy Following the Secondary Reaction," *Journal of Experimental Medicine* (1929), 49: 615–636; C. H. Hitchcock and Swift, "Studies on Indifferent Streptococci: III. The Allergizing Capacity of Different Strains," *Journal of Experimental Medicine* (1929), 49: 637–647; C. L. Derick, C. H. Hitchcock, and Homer F. Swift, "An Address on the Allergic Conception of Rheumatic Fever," *Canadian Medical Association Journal* (1929), 20: 349–355; and Ronald A. MacDonald, "Streptococcal Allergy in Acute Rheumatic Infection," *Archives of Disease in Childhood* (1930), 5: 60–72.

7. Homer F. Swift and C. L. Derick, "II: Reactions of Rabbits to Non-Hemolytic Streptococci: Skin Reactions in Intravenously Immunized Animals," *Journal of Experimental Medicine* (1929), 49: 883–897.

8. B. J. Clawson, "Experimental Streptococcic Inflammation in Normal, Immune, and Hypersensitive Animals," *Archives of Pathology* (1930), 9: 1141–1153.

9. Homer F. Swift, C. H. Hitchcock, C. L. Derick, and Currier McEwen, "Intravenous Vaccinations with Streptococci in Rheumatic Fever," *American Journal of the Medical Sciences* (1931), 181: 1–11; and B. J. Clawson, "Experiments Relative to a Possible Basis for Vaccine Therapy in Acute Rheumatic Fever," *Journal of Infectious Diseases* (1931), 49: 90–97.

10. May G. Wilson and Homer F. Swift, "Intravenous Vaccination with Hemolytic Streptococci: Its Influence on the Incidence of Recurrence of Rheumatic Fever in Children," *American Journal of Diseases of Children* (1931), 42: 42–51; Wilson, Marion G. Josephi, and Dorothy M. Lang, "Intravenous Vaccination with Streptococci: Its Influence on the Incidence of Recurrence of Rheumatic Fever in Children," *American Journal of Diseases of Children* (1933), 46: 1329–1337; at the Hospital for Sick Children, Great Ormond Street, W.R.F. Collis conducted similar tests with similarly mixed results: Collis and Wilfrid Sheldon, "Intravenous Vaccines of Haemolytic Streptococci in Acute Rheumatism in Childhood," *Lancet* (1932), 2: 1261–1264.

11. Homer F. Swift, May G. Wilson, and E. W. Todd, "Skin Reactions of Patients with Rheumatic Fever to Toxic Filtrates of Streptococcus," *American Journal of Diseases of Children* (1929), 37: 98–111; Clifford L. Derick and Marshall N. Fulton, "Skin Reactions of Patients and Normal Individuals to Protein Extracts of Streptococci," *Journal of Clinical Investigation* (1931), 10: 121–138; and Walter K. Myers, Chester S. Keefer, and Theodore W. Oppel, "Skin Reactions to Nucleoproteins of Streptococcus Scarlatinae in Patients with Rheumatoid Arthritis and Rheumatic Fever," *Journal of Clinical Investigation* (1933), 12: 279–289. See also Swift, Hitchcock, Derick, and McEwen, "Intravenous Vaccination with Streptococci in Rheumatic Fever"; and M. P. Schultz and Homer F. Swift, "Reaction of Rabbits to Streptococci: Compara-

tive Sensitizing Effect of Intracutaneous and Intravenous Inocula of Minute Doses," *Journal of Experimental Medicine* (1932), 55: 591–607.

12. George E. Murphy and Homer F. Swift, "Induction of Cardiac Lesions, Closely Resembling Those of Rheumatic Fever, in Rabbits Following Repeated Skin Infections with Group A Streptococci," *Journal of Experimental Medicine* (1949), 89: 687–698; and Robert J. Glaser, Wilbur A. Thomas, Stephen I. Morse, and James E. Darnell, "The Incidence and Pathogenesis of Myocarditis in Rabbits after Group A Streptococcal Pharyngeal Infections," *Journal of Experimental Medicine* (1956), 103: 173–188.

13. Homer F. Swift, "Rheumatic Heart Disease: Pathogenesis and Etiology in Their Relation to Therapy and Prophylaxis," *Medicine* (1940), 19: 417–440; Swift, "The Relationship of Streptococcal Infections to Rheumatic Fever," *American Journal of Medicine* (1947), 2: 168–189; and Swift, "The Etiology of Rheumatic Fever," *Annals of Internal Medicine* (1949), 31: 715–738. For assessments of the allergic theory of rheumatic fever, see Edward E. Fischel, "The Role of Allergy in the Pathogenesis of Rheumatic Fever," *American Journal of Medicine* (1949), 7: 772–793; and Jerry K. Aikawa, "Hypersensitivity and Rheumatic Fever," *Annals of Internal Medicine* (1954), 41: 576–604. For further evaluations of attempts to produce cardiac lesions, see Arnold R. Rich and John E. Gregory, "Experimental Evidence that Lesions with the Basic Characteristics of Rheumatic Carditis Can Result from Anaphylactic Hypersensitivity," *Bulletin of the Johns Hopkins Hospital* (1943), 73: 239–255; Rich and Gregory, "Further Experimental Cardiac Lesions of the Rheumatic Type Produced by Anaphylactic Hypersensitivity," *Bulletin of the Johns Hopkins Hospital* (1944), 75: 115–122; and Sidney D. Kobernick, "Experimental Rheumatic Carditis, Periarteritis Nodosa, and Glomerulonephritis," *American Journal of the Medical Sciences* (1952), 224: 329–342.

14. Abram Joseph Abeloff and Irwin Philip Sobel, "The Communicability of Rheumatic Disease," *Archives of Pediatrics* (1926), 43: 576–584.

15. May G. Wilson, Claire Lingg, and Geneva Croxford, "Statistical Studies Bearing on Problems in the Classification of Heart Disease: III. Heart Disease in Children," *American Heart Journal* (1928), 4: 164–196.

16. May G. Wilson, "The Natural History of Rheumatic Fever in the First Three Decades," *Journal of Pediatrics* (1937), 10: 456–465 (459).

17. John R. Paul and Robert Salinger, "The Spread of Rheumatic Fever through Families," *Journal of Clinical Investigation* (1931), 10: 33–51 (37, 43); Paul, "Age Susceptibility to Familial Infection in Rheumatic Fever," *Journal of Clinical Investigation* (1931), 10: 53–60.

18. May G. Wilson and Morton D. Schweitzer, "Rheumatic Fever as a Familial Disease: Environment, Communicability, and Heredity in Their Relation to the Observed Familial Incidence of the Disease," *Journal of Clinical Investigation* (1937), 16: 555–570; and Wilson, "Heredity and Rheumatic Disease, *American Journal of Medicine* (1947), 2: 190–198.

19. May G. Wilson, *Rheumatic Fever: Studies of the Epidemiology, Manifestations, Diagnosis, and Treatment of the Disease During the First Three Decades* (New York: Commonwealth Fund, 1940), 35.

20. Ibid.

21. Wilson and Schweitzer, "Rheumatic Fever as a Familial Disease"; Wilson, "Natural History of Rheumatic Fever."

22. May G. Wilson, Morton Schweitzer, and Rose Lubschez, "The Familial Epidemiology of Rheumatic Fever: Genetic and Epidemiologic Studies: I. Genetic Studies," *Journal of Pediatrics* (1943), 22: 468–492; Wilson, Schweitzer, and Lubschez, "II. Epidemiological Studies," *Journal of Pediatrics* (1943), 22: 581–611; Wilson, Lubschez, and Schweitzer, "The Integration of Genetic and Epidemiological Methods of Analysis in Rheumatic Fever," *Science* (1943), 97: 335–336; Wilson, "Hereditary Susceptibility in Rheumatic Fever: The Potential Rheumatic Family," *Journal of the American Medical Association* (1944), 124: 1188–1189; Wilson and Lubschez, "Recurrence Rates in Rheumatic Fever: The Evaluation of Etiologic Concepts and Consequent Preventive Therapy," *Journal of the American Medical Association* (1944), 126: 477–480.

23. May G. Wilson, "Susceptibility of the Host in Rheumatic Fever," *Medical Clinics of North America* (1946), 30: 534–539; Wilson, "Heredity and Rheumatic Disease," *American Journal of Medicine* (1947), 2: 190–198. For additional familial studies, see Ross L. Gauld, Antonio Ciocco, and Frances E. M. Read, "Further Observations on the Occurrence of Rheumatic Manifestations in the Families of Rheumatic Patients," *Journal of Clinical Investigation* (1939), 18: 213–217; Read and Gauld, "Studies in Rheumatic Disease: The Familial Aggregation of Rheumatic Disease: Tabulation of Basic Data Relative to the Occurrence of Rheumatic Manifestations of 96 Rheumatic Index Cases and Their Near Relatives," *American Journal of Hygiene* (1940), 31 (sect. A): 124; Arthur Rosenblum and Ruth L. Rosenblum, "A Study of Seventy Rheumatic Families," *American Heart Journal* (1942), 23: 71–83.

24. John R. Paul and P. A. Leddy, "The Social Incidence of Rheumatic Heart Disease: A Statistical Study in Yale University Students," *American Journal of the Medical Sciences* (1932), 184: 597–610.

25. John R. Paul, Elizabeth R. Harrison, R. Salinger, and G. K. DeForest, "The Social Incidence of Rheumatic Heart Disease: A Statistical Study in New Haven School Children," *American Journal of the Medical Sciences* (1934), 188: 301–309.

26. John R. Paul, "Environmental Factors in Rheumatic Fever," *Transactions of the Association of American Physicians* (1940), 55: 290–293. In 1930 and 1943, Paul summarized the vast number of studies that looked at various epidemiological factors; see John R. Paul, *The Epidemiology of Rheumatic Fever: A Preliminary Report with Special Reference to Environmental Factors in Rheumatic Heart Disease and Recommendations for Future Investigations* (New York: Metropolitan Life Insurance Company, 1930), 49–50.

27. G. H. Daniel, "Social and Economic Conditions and the Incidence of Rheumatic Heart Disease," *British Heart Journal* (1944), 6: 103–104.

28. Paul, *The Epidemiology of Rheumatic Fever*, 44–45.

29. Arnold G. Wedum and Bernice G. Wedum, "Rheumatic Fever in Cincinnati in Relation to Rentals, Crowding, Density of Population, and Negroes," *American Journal of Public Health* (1944), 34: 1065–1070.

30. Robert L. Jackson, Helen G. Kelly, Cecilia Healy Rohret, and Julia M Duane, "Rheumatic Fever Recurrences in Children without Sulfonamide Prophylaxis: An Evaluation of Environmental Factors," *Journal of Pediatrics* (1947), 31: 390–402.

31. A. P. Thomson, "A Study of the Distribution of Rheumatic Infection in Children in Birmingham," *Archives of Diseases in Childhood* (1928), 3: 20–27.

32. Matthew Young, "A Preliminary Study of the Epidemiology of Rheumatic Fever," *Journal of Hygiene* (1921), 20: 248–257.

33. M. Greenwood, Jr., and Theodore Thompson, "On Meteorological Factors in the Aetiology of Acute Rheumatism," *Journal of Hygiene* (1907), 7: 171–181.

34. James M. Faulkner and Paul D. White, "The Incidence of Rheumatic Fever, Chorea, and Rheumatic Heart Disease: With Especial Reference to Its Occurrence in Families," *Journal of the American Medical Association* (1924), 83: 425–426.

35. Ibid.; and David Seegal and Beatrice Carrier Seegal, "Studies in the Epidemiology of Rheumatic Fever: Annual Incidence in Some Hospitals in the United States, Its Possessions, and Canada," *Journal of the American Medical Association* (1927), 89: 11–17.

36. Tinsley Randolph Harrison and S. A. Levine, "Notes on the Regional Distribution of Rheumatic Fever and Rheumatic Heart Disease in the United States," *Southern Medical Journal* (1924), 17: 914–915.

37. F. John Poynton, "The Bradshaw Lecture on the Prevention of Acute Rheumatism," *Lancet* (1924), 2: 1000–1003.

38. Arnold G. Wedum and Bernice G. Wedum, "Rheumatic Infections in Cincinnati Hospitals: A Study of 3475 Admissions from 1930 to 1940; Comparison with Incidence in Philadelphia Hospitals from 1930 to 1934," *American Journal of Diseases of Children* (1944), 67: 182–188; and Paul, The *Epidemiology of Rheumatic Fever*, 38.

39. Eric L. Cooper, "A Note on the Incidence of Rheumatic Infections in Australia," *Medical Journal of Australia* (1935), 1: 714–715.

40. David Seegal, Emily Beatrice Carrier Seegal, and Elizabeth L. Jost, "A Comparative Study of the Geographic Distribution of Rheumatic Fever, Scarlet Fever and Acute Glomerulonephritis in North America," *American Journal of the Medical Sciences* (1935), 190: 383–389.

41. E. W. Bitzer and Geo L. Cook, "A Clinical Investigation of Incidence of Rheumatic Heart Disease in a Subtropical Climate," *Southern Medical Journal* (1934), 27: 503–507; and E. Sterling Nichol, "Geographical Distribution of Rheumatic Fever and Rheumatic Heart Disease in the United States," *Journal of Laboratory and Clinical Medicine* (1935–36), 21: 588–596.

42. Amos Christie, "Rheumatic Fever in Northern California," *American Heart Journal* (1936), 12: 153–161; these conclusions were largely confirmed in David B. Davis and Sidney Rosen, "Rheumatic Fever and Rheumatic Heart Disease in Los Angeles Children: A Hospital Study," *Journal of Pediatrics* (1944), 24: 502–513.

43. John R. Paul and George L. Dixon, "Climate and Rheumatic Heart Disease: A Survey among American Indian School Children in Northern and Southern Localities," *Journal of the American Medical Association* (1937), 108: 2096–2100.

44. J. Tertius Clarke, "The Geographical Distribution of Rheumatic Fever," *Journal of Tropical Medicine and Hygiene* (1930), 33: 249–258.

45. Ernest P. Boas, "Rheumatic Fever in Adult Porto Rican Immigrants," *American Journal of the Medical Sciences* (1931), 182: 25–34.

46. E. García Carrillo, "Rheumatic Carditis in a Tropical Country," *American Heart Journal* (1942), 23: 170–174; Sigmund L. Wilens, H. John M. Pearce, and Marcial Fallas Diaz, "The Relative Incidence of Rheumatic Valve Disease in New York and Costa Rica and Its Bearing on the Rheumatic Origin of Calcareous Aortic Stenosis," *American Heart Journal* (1945), 30: 573–579.

47. Philip H. Hartz and Ary van der Sar, "Occurrence of Rheumatic Carditis in the Native Population of Curaçao, Netherlands West Indies," *Archives of Pathology* (1946), 41: 32–36; Maurice Hargrove, Lamont Whittier, and Elmer R. Smith, "Rheumatic

Fever on the Isthmus of Panama," *Journal of the American Medical Association* (1946), 130: 488–490; Harold D. Levine, "Rheumatic Heart Disease in New Guinea: Including a Cardiovascular Survey of 200 Native Papuans," *Annals of Internal Medicine* (1946), 24: 826–836; and J. Robles Gil, "Incidence and Clinical Features of Rheumatic Fever in Mexico City," *American Heart Journal* (1947), 33: 713–714.

48. Ross L. Gauld and Frances E. M. Read, "Studies of Rheumatic Disease. III. Familial Association and Aggregation in Rheumatic Disease," *Journal of Clinical Investigation* (1940), 19: 393–398.

49. James Craig Small, "Rheumatic Fever: Part I: Streptococcus Cardioarthritidis in Rheumatic Fever," *Annals of Internal Medicine* (1928), 1: 1004–1006; Small, "Rheumatic Fever I: Observations Bearing on the Specificity of Streptococcus Cardioarthritidis in Rheumatic Fever and Sydenham's Chorea," *American Journal of the Medical Sciences* (1928), 175: 638–649; and Small, "Rheumatic Fever II: The Present Development of the Biologic Products of Streptococcus, Cardioarthritidis and Their Application in the Treatment of Rheumatic Diseases," *American Journal of the Medical Sciences* (1928), 175: 650–675.

50. Hans Zinnser and H. Yu, "The Bacteriology of Rheumatic Fever and the Allergic Hypothesis," *Archives of Internal Medicine* (1928), 42: 301–309.

51. D. Murray Angevine, Sydney Rothbard, and Russell L. Cecil, "Cultural Studies on Rheumatoid Arthritis and Rheumatic Fever," *Annals of the Rheumatic Diseases* (1942), 3: 101–106.

52. Anna Wessels Williams, *Streptococci in Relation to Man in Health and Disease* (Baltimore: Williams and Wilkins Co, 1932).

53. Rebecca C. Lancefield, "A Serological Differentiation of Human and Other Groups of Hemolytic Streptococci," *Journal of Experimental Medicine* (1933), 57: 571–595.

54. Rebecca Lancefield, "Specific Relationship of Cell Composition to Biological Activity of Hemolytic Streptococci," *The Harvey Lectures* (1940–41), 36: 251–290.

55. David Nabarro and R. A. MacDonald, "Bacteriology of the Tonsils in Relation to Rheumatism in Children," *British Medical Journal* (1929), 2: 758–759.

56. For an exhaustive survey of the streptococcus in rheumatic fever at the end of the 1920s, see David Thomson and Robert Thomson, "An Historical Survey of Researches on the Rôle of the Streptococci in Acute Articular Rheumatism or Rheumatic Fever," *Annals of the Pickett-Thomson Research Laboratory* (1928), 4: 1–108; Thomson and Thomson, "An Historical Survey of the Researches on the Rôle of Streptococci in Chorea," 4: 109–124; Thomson and Thomson, "The Rôle of the Streptococci in Erythema Nodosum," 4: 125–130; and Thomson and Thomson, "An Historical Survey of Researches of the Rôle of the Streptococci in Carditis," 4: 133–250.

57. Arthur L. Bloomfield [Obit.], *Journal of the American Medical Association* (1962), 181: 562.

58. Arthur L. Bloomfield and Augustus R. Felty, "Bacteriologic Observations on Acute Tonsillitis with Reference to Epidemiology and Susceptibility," *Archives of Internal Medicine* (1923), 32: 483–496.

59. J. Alison Glover, "Milroy Lectures on the Incidence of Rheumatic Diseases," *Lancet* (1930), 1: 499–505; and Glover and Fred Griffith, "Acute Tonsillitis and Some of Its Sequels: Epidemiological and Bacteriological Observations," *British Medical Journal* (1931), 2: 521–527.

60. W.R.F. Collis, "Acute Rheumatism and Haemolytic Streptococci," *Lancet* (1931), 1: 1341–1345; and J. Alison Glover and Fred Griffith, "Acute Tonsillitis and Some of

Its Sequels: Epidemiological and Bacteriological Observations," *British Medical Journal* (1931), 2: 521–527.

61. G. H. Stollerman, "Alvin Coburn, 1899–1975," *Journal of Infectious Diseases* (1976), 133: 595; Alvin F. Coburn and Ruth H. Pauli, "Studies on the Relationship of Streptococcus Hemolyticus to the Rheumatic Process: I. Observations on the Ecology of Hemolytic Streptococcus in Relation to the Epidemiology of Rheumatic Fever," *Journal of Experimental Medicine* (1932), 56: 609–632; Coburn and Pauli, "II. Observations on the Biological Character of Streptococcus Hemolyticus Associated with Rheumatic Disease," *Journal of Experimental Medicine* (1932), 56: 633–650; and Coburn, *The Factor of Infection in the Rheumatic State* (Baltimore: Williams and Wilkins, 1931), 30.

62. Coburn, *The Factor of Infection in the Rheumatic State*, 47–48.

63. Ibid., 65.

64. Ibid., 102–103.

65. Ibid., 165–166.

66. Ibid., 195.

67. Ibid., 213–214.

68. Alvin F. Coburn and Ruth H. Pauli, "Studies on the Relationship of the Streptococcus Hemolyticus to the Rheumatic Process: III. Observations on the Immunological Responses of Rheumatic Subjects to Hemolytic Streptococcus," *Journal of Experimental Medicine* (1932), 56: 651–676; and Coburn, *The Factor of Infection in the Rheumatic State*, 233.

69. Charles H. Hitchcock and Homer F. Swift, "The Agglutinating Properties of Exudates from Patients with Rheumatic Fever," *Journal of Clinical Investigation* (1933), 12: 673–681.

70. Coburn, *The Factor of Infection in the Rheumatic State*, 272.

71. Ibid., 267.

72. Bernard Schlesinger and A. Gordon Signy, "Precipitin Reactions in the Blood of Rheumatic Patients Following Acute Throat Infections," *Quarterly Journal of Medicine* (1933), 2: 255–266.

73. Wilfrid Sheldon, "On Acute Rheumatism Following Tonsillitis," *Lancet* (1931), 1: 1337–1341; W.R.F. Collis, "Discussion on Some Problems Concerning the Prevention and Treatment of Acute Rheumatic Infection," *Proceedings of the Royal Society of Medicine* (1932), 25: 1631–1642; Collis, "Acute Rheumatism and Haemolytic Streptococci"; and Collis, "The Contagious Factor in the Etiology of Rheumatic Fever," *American Journal of Diseases of Children* (1932), 44: 485–493.

74. W. H. Bradley, "Epidemiology of Streptococcal Infections," *Guy's Hospital Reports* (1937), 87: 372–390; Scott Thomson and A. J. Glazebrook, "Infectious Diseases in a Semi-Closed Community," *Journal of Hygiene* (1941), 41: 570–615; C. A. Green, "Epidemiology of Haemolyltic Streptococcal Infection in Relation to Acute Rheumatism: I. Haemolytic Streptococcal Epidemic and First Appearance of Rheumatism in a Training Centre," *Journal of Hygiene* (1942), 42: 365–370.

75. Sol P. Ditkowsky, Edward Stevenson, and Joseph M. Campbell, "An Epidemic of Rheumatic Fever in a Children's Institution: Following an Outbreak of Acute Tonsillitis," *Journal of the American Medical Association* (1943), 121: 991–995.

76. E. W. Todd, "Antihaemolysin Titres in the Haemolytic Streptococcal Infections and Their Significance in Rheumatic Fever," *British Journal of Experimental Pathology* (1932), 13: 248–259.

77. Alvin F. Coburn and Ruth H. Pauli, "Studies on the Immune Response of the Rheumatic Subject and Its Relationship to Activity of the Rheumatic Process: I. The Determination of Antistreptolysin Titer," *Journal of Experimental Medicine* (1935), 62: 129–136; Coburn and Pauli, "II. Observations on an Epidemic of Influenza Followed by Hemolytic Streptococcus Infections in a Rheumatic Colony," *Journal of Experimental Medicine* (1935), 62: 137–158; and Coburn and Pauli, "III. Observations on the Reactions of a Rheumatic Group to an Epidemic Infection with Hemolytic Streptococcus of a Single Type," *Journal of Experimental Medicine* (1935), 62: 159–178. See also Walter K. Myers and Chester S. Keefer, "Antistreptolysin Content of the Blood Serum in Rheumatic Fever and Rheumatoid Arthritis," *Journal of Clinical Investigation* (1934), 13: 155–167; Joseph J. Bunim and Currier McEwen, "The Antistreptolysin Titer in Rheumatic Fever, Arthritis, and Other Diseases," *Journal of Clinical Investigation* (1940), 19: 75–82; and C. A. Green, "Observations on the Antistreptolysin O Titre in Relation to the Mechanism of Acute Rheumatic Fever," *Journal of Pathology and Bacteriology* (1941), 53: 223–241.

78. E. W. Todd, Alvin F. Coburn, and A. Bradford Hill, "Antistreptolysin S Titres in Rheumatic Fever," *Lancet* (1939), 2: 1213–1217.

79. Walter K. Myers, Chester S. Keefer, and William F. Holmes, Jr., "The Resistance to Fibrinolytic Activity of the Hemolytic Streptococcus with Special Reference to Patients with Rheumatic Fever and Rheumatoid [Atrophic], Arthritis," *Journal of Clinical Investigation* (1935), 14: 119–123; and C. Bruce Perry, "The Relationship between Acute Rheumatism and Streptococcal Antifibrinolysin," *Archives of Disease in Childhood* (1939), 14: 32–39.

80. Homer F. Swift and B. E. Hodge, "Type-Specific Anti-M Precipitins in Rheumatic and Non-Rheumatic Patients with Hemolytic Streptococcal Infections," *Proceedings of the Society of Experimental Biology and Medicine* (1936), 34: 849–854; Leo M. Taran, James M. Jablon, and Helen N. Weyr, "Immunologic Studies in Rheumatic Fever: I. Cutaneous Response to Type-Specific Proteins of the Hemolytic Streptococcus. A. Response to Combinations of 'M' Protein from Selected Types of Hemolytic Streptococci," *Journal of Immunology* (1944), 49: 209–222; and Taran, Jablon, and Weyr, "B. Response to 'Purified M' Proteins from Forty Known Types of the Hemolytic Streptococcus—Group A," *Journal of Immunology* (1945), 51: 53–64.

81. George J. Friou and Herbert A. Wenner, "On the Occurrence in Human Serum of an Inhibitory Substance to Hyaluronidase Produced by a Strain of Hemolytic Streptococcus," *Journal of Infectious Diseases* (1947), 80: 185–193.

82. John R. Mote and T. Duckett Jones, "Studies of Hemolytic Streptococcal Antibodies in Control Groups, Rheumatic Fever, and Rheumatoid Arthritis: I The Incidence of Antistreptolysin 'O,' Antifibrinolysin, and Hemolytic Streptococcal Precipitating Antibodies in the Sera of Urban Control Groups," *Journal of Immunology* (1941), 41: 35–60; and Mote and Jones, "II. The Frequency of Antistreptolysin 'O,' Antifibrinolysin, and Precipitating-Antibody Responses in Scarlet Fever, Hemolytic Streptococcal Infections, and Rheumatic Fever," *Journal of Immunology* (1941), 41: 61–85.

83. See Alf Westergren, "Studies of the Suspension Stability of the Blood in Pulmonary Tuberculosis," *Acta Medica Scandinavica* (1921), 54: 247–282; and M. M. Wintrobe and J. Walter Landsberg, "A Standardized Technique for the Blood Sedimentation Rate," *American Journal of the Medical Sciences* (1935), 189: 102–115.

84. A. Carlton Ernstene, "Erythrocyte Sedimentation, Plasma Fibrinogen, and Leukocytosis as Indices of Rheumatic Infection," *American Journal of the Medical Sciences* (1930), 180: 12–24; Wilfrid W. Payne, "Acute Rheumatism and the Sedimentation

Rate," *Lancet* (1932), 1: 74–75; William Elghammer, "Erythrocyte Sedimentation Rate in Rheumatic Infection," *Archives of Pediatrics* (1934), 51: 281–287; W. W. Payne and Bernard Schlesinger, "A Study of the Sedimentation Rate in Juvenile Rheumatism," *Archives of Disease in Childhood* (1935), 10: 403–414; for a description of a "micro" method of determining the sedimentation rate, so important for pediatrics, see Bernard Schlesinger, "The Blood Sedimentation Rate in Rheumatic Fever," *Practitioner* (1946), 157: 38–44.

85. Alvin F. Coburn and E. M. Kapp, "Observations on the Development of the High Blood Sedimentation Rate in Rheumatic Carditis," *Journal of Clinical Investigation* (1936), 15: 715–723.

86. Alvin F. Coburn, "Observations on the Mechanism of Rheumatic Fever," *Lancet* (1936), 2: 1025–1030.

87. See Chapter 8.

88. John R. Paul, "The Epidemiology of Rheumatic Fever," *American Journal of Medicine* (1947), 2: 66–75.

89. Paul, *The Epidemiology of Rheumatic Fever*, 9.

90. Homer F. Swift, "Rheumatic Heart Disease: Pathogenesis and Etiology in Their Relation to Therapy and Prophylaxis," *Medicine* (1940), 19: 417–440.

91. Homer F. Swift, "Rheumatic Fever," *American Journal of the Medical Sciences* (1925), 170: 631–647; and Swift, "The Nature of Rheumatic Fever," *Journal of Laboratory and Clinical Medicine* (1935–36), 21: 551–563.

92. Homer F. Swift, "Rheumatic Fever," *Journal of the American Medical Association* (1929), 92: 2071–2083.

93. T. Duckett Jones, "Rheumatic Fever," *New England Journal of Medicine* (1932), 207: 529–530.

94. John R. Paul, "The Epidemiology of Rheumatic Fever," *American Journal of Public Health* (1941), 31: 611–618.

95. Alvin F. Coburn and Lucile V. Moore, "Nutrition as a Conditioning Factor in the Rheumatic State," *American Journal of Diseases of Children* (1943), 65: 744–756.

CHAPTER 7    *From Acute to Chronic*

1. W.S.C. Copeman, *The Treatment of Rheumatism in General Practice* (London: Edward Arnold and Co., 1933).

2. Alfred S. Reinhart, "Evolution of the Clinical Concept of Rheumatic Fever," *New England Journal of Medicine* (1931), 204: 1194–1199.

3. Halbert L. Dunn and O. F. Hedley, "Statistics on Deaths from Rheumatic Heart Disease," *Journal of the American Medical Association* (1938), 110: 1413–1415.

4. George A. Allan, "The Prevention of Rheumatic Heart Disease," *Journal of the Royal Sanitary Institute of London* (1925–26), 46: 179–184.

5. W. S. Church, "An Examination of Nearly Seven Hundred Cases of Acute Rheumatism: Chiefly with a View to Determining the Frequency of Cardiac Affections, and Especially Pericarditis, at the Present Time," *Saint Bartholomew's Hospital Reports* (1887), 23: 269–287.

6. Thomas McCrae, "Acute Articular Rheumatism: The Statistics of a Series of 270 Cases from the Service of Dr. Osler in the Johns Hopkins Hospital," *Journal of the American Medical Association* (1903), 40: 211–216.

7. Alexander Lambert, "The Incidence of Acute Rheumatic Fever at Bellevue Hospital," *Journal of the American Medical Association* (1920), 74: 993–995.

8. Reginald M. Atwater, "Studies in the Epidemiology of Acute Rheumatic Fever and Related Diseases in the United States, Based on Mortality Statistics," *American Journal of Hygiene* (1927), 7: 343–369.

9. Homer F. Swift, "Rheumatic Fever," *American Journal of the Medical Sciences* (1925), 170: 631–647.

10. James Alison Glover [Obit.], *Lancet* (1963), 2: 693.

11. J. Alison Glover, "Milroy Lectures on the Incidence of Rheumatic Diseases," *Lancet* (1930), 1: 499–505; Glover, "Rheumatic Fever," *Lancet* (1939), 1: 465–468; Glover, "War-time Decline of Acute Rheumatism," *Lancet* (1943), 2: 51–52; Glover, "The Decline of Mortality from Rheumatic Fever," *Monthly Bulletin of the Ministry of Health and Emergency Health Services* (1946), 5: 222–229; M. T. Morgan, "Le rhumatisme en Angleterre et du pays de galles," *Bulletin de l'Office internationale d'hygiène publique* (1937), 29: 1427–1437; and Francis Bach, "On the Incidence of Rheumatic Fever," *British Journal of Children's Diseases* (1931), 28: 198–207.

12. Francis Bach, N. Gray Hill, T. Warwick Preston, and Charles E. Thornton, "Juvenile Rheumatism in London," *Annals of the Rheumatic Diseases* (1939), 1: 210–241.

13. J. Alison Glover, "Acute Rheumatism in Military History," *Proceedings of the Royal Society of Medicine* (1946), 39: 113–118; and Glover, "Acute Rheumatism," *Annals of the Rheumatic Diseases* (1946), 5: 126–130.

14. D. J. Davis, "Collective Inquiry on Rheumatism among Children and Adolescents," *School Hygiene* (1915), 6: 17–22.

15. Frederick J. Poynton and James Kerr, "Rheumatic Infection in Relation to School Life (Discussion)," *School Hygiene* (1915), 6: 1–16.

16. Carey F. Coombs, "The Diagnosis and Treatment of Rheumatic Heart Disease in Its Early Stages," *British Medical Journal* (1930), 1: 227–230.

17. Thomas T. Mackie, "Rheumatic Fever: An Analytical Study of Three Hundred and Ninety-Three Cases of Rheumatic Fever and Eighty-Nine Cases of Chorea," *American Journal of the Medical Sciences* (1926), 172: 199–221.

18. N. Gray Hill, "The Aetiology of Juvenile Rheumatism," *British Journal of Children's Diseases* (1930), 27: 161–181.

19. E. C. Warner, "Modern Views on Rheumatism in Childhood," *Lancet* (1930), 2: 719–723.

20. M. J. Shapiro, "The Natural History of Childhood Rheumatism in Minnesota," *Journal of Laboratory and Clinical Medicine* (1936), 21: 564–574. For a view from Johns Hopkins, see Ross L. Gauld and Frances E. M. Read, "Studies in Rheumatic Disease: V. The Age of Onset of Primary Rheumatic Attack," *Journal of Clinical Investigation* (1940), 19: 729–734.

21. O. F. Hedley, "Incidence of Rheumatic Heart Disease among College Students in the United States," *Public Health Reports* (1938), 53: 1635–1647. For additional American surveys, see Robert W. Quinn, "The Incidence of Rheumatic Fever and Heart Disease in School Children in Dublin, Georgia, with Some Epidemiological and Sociological Observations," *American Heart Journal* (1946), 32: 234–242; and Quinn, "Epidemiologic Study of Seven Hundred and Fifty-Seven Cases of Rheumatic Fever," *Archives of Internal Medicine* (1947), 80: 709–727.

22. Shapiro, "Natural History of Childhood Rheumatism in Minnesota."

23. Rachel Ash, "Prognosis of Rheumatic Infection in Childhood: A Statistical Study," *American Journal of Diseases of Children* (1936), 52: 280–295.

24. Leo M. Taran, "Rheumatic Cardiac Disease in Childhood: A Statistical Study," *American Journal of Diseases of Children* (1935), 50: 840–852.

25. T. Duckett Jones, "Heart Disease in Childhood," *American Journal of Public Health* (1938), 28: 637–643; and Elvira M. Deliee, Katharine G. Dodge, and Currier McEwen, "The Prognostic Significance of Age of Onset in Initial Attacks of Rheumatic Fever," *American Heart Journal* (1943), 26: 681–684.

26. Irving S. Wright, "Experiences with Rheumatic Fever in the Army," *Bulletin of the New York Academy of Medicine* (1945), 21: 419–432.

27. Robert C. Manchester, "Rheumatic Fever in Naval Enlisted Personnel: I. An Analysis of the Major Manifestations Observed, the Factors Involved in Its Occurrence and Cardiac Residua," *Archives of Internal Medicine* (1946), 77: 317–331.

28. H. Stuart Barber, "Rheumatic Fever in the R.A.F.: Results of Treatment at a Convalescent Centre," *British Medical Journal* (1946), 2: 83–84.

29. John Parkinson and Ronald Hartley, "Early Diagnosis of Rheumatic Valvular Disease in Recruits," *British Heart Journal* (1946), 8: 212–232. See also Benedict F. Massell and T. Duckett Jones, "Some Practical Aspects of the Rheumatic Fever Problem Which Have Important Bearing in Military Medicine," *American Heart Journal* (1944), 27: 575–587; and William P. Holbrook and Arie C. van Ravenswaay, "The Military Aspects of Acute Rheumatic Fever," *Military Surgeon* (1945), 96: 388–391.

30. John Staige Davis, Jr., "Incidence of Rheumatic Fever in New York City Hospitals," *American Journal of the Medical Sciences* (1933), 186: 180–191.

31. Lucille R. Farquhar and John R. Paul, "Rheumatic Fever in New Haven, Connecticut: A Survey of Recent Hospital Admissions," *Public Health Reports* (1940), 55: 1903–1913.

32. O. F. Hedley, "Rheumatic Heart Disease in Philadelphia Hospitals: A Study of 4653 Cases of Rheumatic Heart Disease, Rheumatic Fever, Sydenham's Chorea, and Subacute Bacterial Endocarditis Involving 5921 Admissions to Philadelphia Hospitals, from January 1, 1930 to December 31, 1934," *Public Health Reports* (1940), 55: 1599–1619. See also Bernice G. Wedum, Arnold G. Wedum, and A. L. Beaghler, "Prevalence of Rheumatic Heart Disease in Denver School Children," *American Journal of Public Health* (1945), 35: 1271–1276.

33. O. F. Hedley, "Mortality from Rheumatic Heart Disease in Philadelphia during 1936," *Public Health Reports* (1937), 52: 1907–1923.

34. May Georgiana Wilson, *Rheumatic Fever: Studies of the Epidemiology, Manifestations, Diagnosis, and Treatment of the Disease During the First Three Decades* (New York: Commonwealth Fund, 1940); and John Rodman Paul, *The Epidemiology of Rheumatic Fever and Some of Its Public Health Aspects*, 2nd ed (New York: Metropolitan Life Insurance Co., 1943).

35. Homer F. Swift, "The Chronicity of Rheumatic Fever," *New England Journal of Medicine* (1934), 211: 197–203.

36. C. F. Ehlertsen, "The Late Prognosis in Rheumatic Fever," *Acta Medica Scandinavica* (1942), 112: 353–392.

37. Bernard Schlesinger, "The Public Health Aspect of Heart Disease in Childhood," *Lancet* (1938), 1: 593–599, 649–655.

38. William D. Stroud and Paul H. Twaddle, "Fifteen Years' Observation of Children with Rheumatic Heart Disease," *Journal of the American Medical Association* (1940), 114: 629–634.

39. T. Duckett Jones and Edward F. Bland, "Rheumatic Fever and Heart Disease: Completed Ten-Year Observations on 1000 Patients," *Transactions of the Association of American Physicians* (1942), 57: 267–270; and Jones, "Rheumatic Fever," *Transactions of the Association of Life Insurance Medical Directors of America* (1947), 30: 9–30.

40. Homer F. Swift, "Public Health Aspects of Rheumatic Heart Disease: Incidence and Measures for Control," *Journal of the American Medical Association* (1940), 115: 1509–1518; and Swift, "Features Which Suggest Public Health Considerations of Rheumatic Fever," *Bulletin of the New York Academy of Medicine* (1940), 16: 501–513. See also Alexander T. Martin, "Twenty Years' Observation of 1438 Children with Rheumatic Heart Disease: Analytic Study Following Convalescent Care from 1921 to 1941," *Journal of the American Medical Association* (1941), 117: 1663–1670.

41. Harry S. Mustard, "Rheumatic Fever in the Perspective of Public Health," *American Journal of Medicine* (1947), 2: 609–617.

42. David D. Rutstein, "Need for a Public Health Program in Rheumatic Fever and Rheumatic Heart Disease," *American Journal of Public Health* (1946), 36: 461–467; T. Duckett Jones, "Chronically Ill Cardiac Children in Institutions and Foster Homes," *American Journal of Public Health* (1941), 31: 813–818; and Homer F. Swift and Alfred E. Cohn, "Cardiac Diseases, Infectious and Non-Infectious, in Relation to Public Health," *Transactions and Studies of the College of Physicians of Philadelphia* (1938), 6: 197–227.

43. Paul D. White, "The Convalescent Care of Children with Heart Disease due to Rheumatic Fever: A Survey of the Problem of the Care of Children with Rheumatic Heart Disease," *New England Journal of Medicine* (1941), 224: 627–628.

44. Bernice G. Wedum and Arnold G. Wedum, "A Method for Determining the Number of Beds Required for Convalescent Care of Rheumatic Infections," *American Journal of Public Health* (1942), 32: 1237–1241.

45. O. F. Hedley, "Facilities in the United States for the Special Care of Children with Rheumatic Heart Disease," *Public Health Reports* (1941), 56: 2321–2341.

46. Other members of the advisory board were Albert D. Kaiser (Rochester, N.Y.), Clifford G. Grulee (Evanston, Ill.), and Henry Helmholz (Rochester, Minn.).

47. Betty Huse, "Care of Children with Heart Disease in the Crippled Children's Program under the Social Security Act," *American Journal of Public Health* (1941), 31: 809–812; Huse, "General Statement Regarding State Rheumatic Fever Programs," *Journal of Pediatrics* (1945), 26: 245–249. In Britain the Education Act of 1944 declared victims of rheumatic fever "handicapped" and needing special education. See Royal College of Physicians, "Rheumatic Fever: A Review," *Lancet* (1947), 1: 606–610; and Alexander T. Martin, "Rheumatic Fever and the American Academy of Pediatrics—General Purpose and Scope," *Journal of Pediatrics* (1945), 26: 209–210.

48. Clark H. Hall, "The Rheumatic Fever Program in Oklahoma," *Journal of Pediatrics* (1945), 26: 259–261.

49. Louise F. Galvin, "The Rheumatic Fever Program in Virginia," *Journal of Pediatrics* (1945), 26: 255–258.

50. Benjamin Sacks, "The Pathology of Rheumatic Fever: A Critical Review," *American Heart Journal* (1925–26), 1: 750–772; and B. J. Clawson, "The Aschoff Nodule," *Archives of Pathology* (1929), 8: 664–685.

51. Alwin M. Pappenheimer and William C. Von Glahn, "A Case of Rheumatic Aortitis with Early Lesions in the Media," *American Journal of Pathology* (1926), 2: 15–17; Von Glahn and Pappenheimer, "Specific Lesions of Peripheral Blood Vessels and Rheumatism," *American Journal of Pathology* (1926), 2: 235–249; and Von Glahn, "Auricular Endocarditis of Rheumatic Origin," *American Journal of Pathology* (1926), 2: 1–14.

52. Ludwig Aschoff, "The Rheumatic Nodules in the Heart," *Annals of the Rheumatic Diseases* (1939), 1: 161–166.

53. Homer F. Swift, "Factors Favoring the Onset and Continuation of Rheumatic Fever," *American Heart Journal* (1930–31), 6: 625–636.

54. Homer F. Swift, "The Pathogenesis of Rheumatic Fever," *Journal of Experimental Medicine* (1924), 39: 497–508; and Sacks, "Pathology of Rheumatic Fever."

55. Alvin F. Coburn, "Relationship of the Rheumatic Process to the Development of Alterations in Tissues, " *American Journal of Diseases of Children* (1933), 45: 933–972; see also Clough Turrill Burnett, "Rheumatic Heart Disease: A Review," *Annals of Internal Medicine* (1932), 5: 1337–1356. A study in Boston showed more endocardial disease than myocardial, but it concurred that deaths from heart disease in rheumatic fever occurred decades after the initial bout with the disease. See David Davis and Soma Weiss, "Rheumatic Heart Disease: I. Incidence and Rôle in the Causation of Death. A Study of 5215 Consecutive Necropsies," *American Heart Journal* (1931–32), 7: 146–156; and Davis and Weiss, "Rheumatic Heart Disease: II. Incidence and Distribution of the Age of Death," *American Heart Journal* (1932–33), 8: 182–189.

56. Clarence L. Laws and Samuel A. Levine, "Clinical Notes on Rheumatic Heart Disease with Special Reference to the Cause of Death," *American Journal of the Medical Sciences* (1933), 186: 833–849.

57. M. A. Rothschild, M. A. Kugel, and Louis Gross, "Incidence and Significance of Active Infection in Cases of Rheumatic Cardiovascular Disease during Various Age Periods, a Clinical and Pathological Study," *American Heart Journal* (1933–34), 9: 586–595. For a spectrum of opinion on this point, see B. J. Clawson, "Rheumatic Heart Disease: An Analysis of 796 Cases," *American Heart Journal* (1940), 20: 454–474; Antonio Jucá and Paul D. White, "The Cause of Death in Rheumatic Heart Disease in Adults," *Journal of the American Medical Association* (1944), 125: 767–769; Norman H. Boyer and Alexander S. Nadas, "The Ultimate Effect of Pregnancy on Rheumatic Heart Disease," *Annals of Internal Medicine* (1944), 20: 99–107; W. G. MacCallum, "Rheumatic Lesions on the Left Auricle of the Heart," *Johns Hopkins Hospital Bulletin* (1924), 35: 329; and William C. von Glahn, "The Pathology of Rheumatism," *American Journal of Medicine* (1947), 2: 76–85.

58. Glover, "The Decline of Mortality from Rheumatic Fever."

59. See for example, Paul Weindling, "From Infections to Chronic Diseases: Changing Patterns of Sickness in the Nineteenth and Twentieth Centuries," in *Medicine in Society: Historical Essays*, ed. Andrew Wear (Cambridge: Cambridge University Press, 1992), 303–316.

CHAPTER 8   *At the Bedside*

1. T. Duckett Jones and John R. Mote, "The Clinical Importance of Infection of the Respiratory Tract in Rheumatic Fever," *Journal of the American Medical Association* (1939), 113: 898–902.

2. Antibiotics, technically speaking, are substances produced by microorganisms which inhibit the growth or kill germs. The sulfonamide family of drugs is based on chemical dyes and, unlike penicillin, is not derived from living micro-organisms. "Antibiotic" was coined in the early 1940s, after the introduction of sulfonamide. In the 1940s and 1950s, physicians often distinguished between sulfonamide and antibiotics, but after the introduction of chemically modified antibiotics in the 1950s, this distinction dropped out of the medical lexicon. See Selman A. Waksman and J. E. Flynn, "History of the Word 'Antibiotic,'" *Journal of the History of Medicine and Allied Sciences* (1973), 28: 284–286.

3. The Pediatrics Section of the American Medical Association held a symposium on "Rheumatic Fever" on 16 June 1944 in Chicago. See *Journal of the American Medical Association* (1944), 126: 477–493; participants included May G. Wilson and Rose Lubchez, "Recurrence Rates in Rheumatic Fever: The Evaluation of Etiologic Concepts and Consequent Preventive Therapy," 477–480; T. Duckett Jones, "The Diagnosis of Rheumatic Fever," 481–484; David D. Rutstein, "The Role of the Cardiac Clinic in the Rheumatic Program," 484–486; Arie C. van Ravenswaay, "The Geographic Distribution of Hemolytic Streptococci: Relationship to the Incidence of Rheumatic Fever," 486–490; Caroline Bedell Thomas, "The Prevention of Recurrences in Rheumatic Subjects," 490–493, discussion by John R. Paul, page 493. See also O. Currier McEwen, "The Management of Rheumatic Fever," *Bulletin of the New York Academy of Medicine* (1943), 19: 679–692; R. R. Struthers, "The Management and Prevention of Rheumatic Fever," *Canadian Medical Association Journal* (1944), 51: 416–422.

4. Harry Keil, "The Rheumatic Erythemas: A Critical Survey," *Annals of Internal Medicine* (1938), 11: 2223–2272.

5. H. M. Hughes, "Digest of One Hundred Cases of Chorea Treated in the Hospital," *Guy's Hospital Reports* (1846), 2nd series, 4: 360–395.

6. Dr. Sée, "De la chorée: Rapports du rhumatisme et des maladies du coeur avec les affections nerveuses et convulsives," *Mémoires de l'Académie nationale de médecine* (1850), 15: 373–525.

7. J. Godwin Greenfield and J. M. Wolfsohn, "The Pathology of Sydenham's Chorea," *Lancet* (1922), 2: 603–606.

8. Franklin G. Ebaugh, "Neuropsychiatric Aspects of Chorea in Children," *Journal of the American Medical Association* (1926), 87: 1083–1088.

9. Lucy Porter Sutton, "The Treatment of Chorea by the Induction of Fever: Preliminary Report," *Journal of the American Medical Association* (1931), 97: 299–301.

10. Edward F. Bland, "Rheumatic Fever: The Way It Was," *Circulation* (1987), 76: 1190–1195.

11. William Osler, *On Chorea and Choreiform Affections* (London: H. K. Lewis and Co., 1894).

12. T. Duckett Jones and Edward F. Bland, "Clinical Significance of Chorea as a Manifestation of Rheumatic Fever," *Journal of the American Medical Association* (1935), 105: 571–577. See also H. L. Wallace, "Chorea: A Short Study of 200 Cases," *Edinburgh Medical Journal* (1933), 40: 417–424.

13. Alvin F. Coburn and Lucile V. Moore, "The Independence of Chorea and Rheumatic Activity," *American Journal of the Medical Sciences* (1937), 193: 1–4 (3).

14. Lucy Porter Sutton and Katharine G. Dodge, "The Relationship of Sydenham's Chorea to Other Rheumatic Manifestations," *American Journal of the Medical Sciences* (1938), 195: 656–666.

15. O. F. Hedley, "Rheumatic Heart Disease in Philadelphia Hospitals: A Study of 4653 Cases of Rheumatic Heart Disease, Rheumatic Fever, Sydenham's Chorea, and Subacute Bacterial Endocarditis Involving 5921 Admissions to Philadelphia Hospitals, from January 1, 1930 to December 31, 1934," *Public Health Reports* (1940), 55: 1599–1619, 1647–1691, 1845–1862; chorea section, 1661–1670.

16. Douglas Hubble, "The Nature of the Rheumatic Child," *British Medical Journal* (1943), 1: 121–125.

17. T. Duckett Jones, "The Diagnosis of Rheumatic Fever," *Journal of the American Medical Association* (1944), 126: 481–484.

18. N. Gray Hill, "On the Value of Tonsillectomy in the Prevention of Acute Rheumatism, Rheumatic Carditis, and Chorea," *Lancet* (1929), 2: 571–572; William H. Robey and Maxwell Finland, "Effect of Tonsillectomy on the Acute Attack of Rheumatic Fever," *Archives of Internal Medicine* (1930), 45: 772–782; Albert D. Kaiser, "Influence of the Tonsils on Rheumatic Infection in Children," *Journal of Laboratory and Clinical Medicine* (1936), 21: 609–617; and Rachel Ash, "Influence of Tonsillectomy on Rheumatic Infection," *American Journal of Diseases of Children* (1938), 55: 63–78.

19. F. J. Poynton, "Discussion on Rheumatic Infection in Childhood: Early Diagnosis and Preventive Treatment," *British Medical Journal* (1925), 2: 788–796.

20. May G. Wilson, "Statistical Studies Bearing on Problems in the Classification of Heart Disease: IV. Tonsillectomy in Its Relation to the Prevention of Rheumatic Heart Disease," *American Heart Journal* (1928–29), 4: 197–209.

21. Warde B. Allan and John W. Baylor, "The Influence of Tonsillectomy upon the Course of Rheumatic Fever and Rheumatic Heart Disease: A Study of 108 Cases," *Bulletin of the Johns Hopkins Hospital* (1938), 63: 111–123.

22. O. F. Hedley surveyed facilities for caring for children with rheumatic fever in 1941, noting that many advocated tonsillectomy as part of the regimen; see Hedley, "Facilities in the United States for the Special Care of Children with Rheumatic Heart Disease," *Public Health Reports* (1941), 56: 2321–2341. Children routinely underwent tonsillectomy at Cook County Hospital in Chicago and Royal Hospital for Sick Children in Glasgow; see Bernard Fantus, ed., "The Therapy of the Cook County Hospital: Therapy of Rheumatic Fever," *Journal of the American Medical Association* (1934), 102: 2100–2101; and Leonard Findlay, James W. MacFarlane, and Mary M. Stevenson, "The Cardiac Clinic and Hospital: Their Value in the Control of Rheumatic Infection," *Archives of Disease in Childhood* (1929), 4: 306–312.

23. Walsh McDermott and David E. Rogers, "Social Ramifications of Control of Microbial Disease," *Johns Hopkins Medical Journal* (1982), 151: 302–312; Marcel H. Bickel, "The Development of Sulfonamides (1932–1938) as a Focal Point in the History of Chemotherapy," *Gesnerus* (1988), 45: 67–86; Harry F. Dowling, *Fighting Infection: Conquests of the Twentieth Century* (Cambridge, Mass.: Harvard University Press, 1977), 105–124; Barron H. Lerner, "Scientific Evidence versus Therapeutic Demand: The Introduction of the Sulfonamides Revisited," *Annals of Internal Medicine* (1991), 115: 315–320; J. D. Abbott, D. M. Jones, M. J. Painter, and S.E.J. Young, "The Epidemiology of Meningococcal Infections in England and Wales, 1912–1983," *Journal of Infection* (1985), 11: 241–257; W. Michael Scheld and Gerald L. Mandell, "Sulfonamides and Meningitis," *Journal of the American Medical Association* (1984), 251: 791–794; and Irvine Loudon, "Puerperal Fever, the Streptococcus, and the Sulphonamides, 1911–1945," *British Medical Journal* (1987), 295: 485–490.

24. Perrin H. Long and Eleanor A. Bliss, "Para-amino-benzene-sulfonamide and Its Derivatives: Experimental and Clinical Observations on Their Use in the Treatment of Beta-Hemolytic Streptococcic Infection: A Preliminary Report," *Journal of the American Medical Association* (1937), 108: 32–37.

25. Homer F. Swift, Johannes K. Moen, and George K. Hirst, "The Action of Sulfanilamide in Rheumatic Fever," *Journal of the American Medical Association* (1938), 110: 426–434.

26. Benedict F. Massell and T. Duckett Jones, "The Effect of Sulfanilamide on Rheumatic Fever and Chorea," *New England Journal of Medicine* (1938), 218: 876–878. For another view of serious side effects from sulfonamide, "cyanosis was [a] common occurrence, and in addition some 40% of those patients . . . suffered from vomiting; it

is felt, however, that these reactions are not contra-indications to the continued use of the drug," in W. A. Hopkins, "The Use of the Sulphonamide Group of Drugs in the Treatment of Tonsillitis due to the Beta-Haemolytic Streptococcus and in Acute Rheumatic Fever," *Annals of the Rheumatic Diseases* (1940–41), 2: 233–246.

27. May G. Wilson, "Susceptibility of the Host in Rheumatic Fever," *Medical Clinics of North America* (1946), 30: 534–539; and Wilson, "Heredity and Rheumatic Disease," *American Journal of Medicine* (1947), 2: 190–198.

28. Caroline Bedell Thomas and Richard France, "A Preliminary Report of the Prophylactic Use of Sulfanilamide in Patients Susceptible to Rheumatic Fever," *Bulletin of the Johns Hopkins Hospital* (1939), 64: 67–77; and Thomas, France, and Franjo Reichsman, "The Prophylactic Use of Sulfanilamide in Patients Susceptible to Rheumatic Fever," *Journal of the American Medical Association* (1941), 116: 551–560.

29. Alvin F. Coburn and Lucile V. Moore, "The Prophylactic Use of Sulfanilamide in Streptococcal Respiratory Infections, with Especial Reference to Rheumatic Fever," *Journal of Clinical Investigation* (1939), 18: 147–155; and Coburn and Moore, "The Prophylactic Use of Sulfanilamide in Rheumatic Subjects," *Medical Clinics of North America* (1940), 24: 633–638.

30. Alvin F. Coburn and Lucile V. Moore, "A Follow-up Report on Rheumatic Subjects Treated with Sulfanilamide," *Journal of the American Medical Association* (1941), 117: 176.

31. David Dudley Stowell and William H. Button, Jr., "Observations on the Prophylactic Use of Sulfanilamide in Rheumatic Patients: With a Report of One Death," *Journal of the American Medical Association* (1941), 117: 2164–2166.

32. Arild E. Hansen, Ralph V. Platou, and Paul F. Dwan, "Prolonged Use of a Sulfonamide Compound in Prevention of Rheumatic Recrudescences in Children, an Evaluation Based on a Four Year Study on Sixty-four Children," *American Journal of Diseases of Children* (1942), 64: 963–976; Charles R. Messeloff and Milton H. Robbins, "The Prophylactic Use of Sulfanilamide in Children with Rheumatic Heart Disease," *Journal of Laboratory and Clinical Medicine* (1942–43), 28: 1323–1327; and Robert H. Feldt, "Sulfanilamide as a Prophylactic Measure in Recurrent Rheumatic Infection: A Controlled Study Involving 131 'Patient-Seasons,'" *American Journal of the Medical Sciences* (1944), 207: 483–488.

33. Caroline Bedell Thomas, "The Prophylactic Treatment of Rheumatic Fever by Sulfanilamide," *Bulletin of the New York Academy of Medicine* (1942), 18: 508–526. See also Ann G. Kuttner and Gertrude Reyersbach, "The Prevention of Streptococcal Upper Respiratory Infections and Rheumatic Recurrences in Rheumatic Children by the Prophylactic Use of Sulfanilamide," *Journal of Clinical Investigation* (1943), 22: 77–85; and Caroline A. Chandler and Helen B. Taussig, "Sulfanilamide as a Prophylactic Agent in Rheumatic Fever," *Bulletin of the Johns Hopkins Hospital* (1943), 72: 42–53.

34. Arthur L. Bloomfield and Lowell A. Rantz, "An Outbreak of Streptococcic Septic Sore Throat in an Army Camp. Clinical and Epidemiologic Observations," *Journal of the American Medical Association* (1943), 121: 315–319.

35. Alvin F. Coburn and Donald C. Young, *The Epidemiology of Hemolytic Streptococcus during World War II in the United States Navy* (Baltimore: Williams and Wilkins Co., 1949), 5–17.

36. Lowell A. Rantz, "Rheumatic Fever," *Internal Medicine in World War II: Infectious Diseases*, ed. John Boyd Coates, Jr. (Washington D.C.: Office of the Surgeon General, 1963), vol. 2, 225–238.

37. W. Paul Holbrook, "The Army Air Forces Rheumatic Fever Control Program," *Journal of the American Medical Association* (1944), 126: 84–87; and Lowell A. Rantz, "Hemolytic Streptococcal Infections," *Preventive Medicine in World War II: Communicable Diseases Transmitted Chiefly through Respiratory and Alimentary Tracts*, ed. John Boyd Coates, Jr. (Washington D.C.: Office of the Surgeon General, 1958), vol. 4, 229–257.

38. Coburn and Young, *The Epidemiology of Hemolytic Streptococcus*, chaps. 6–11, pp. 44–100.

39. Caroline Bedell Thomas, "The Prevention of Recurrences in Rheumatic Subjects," *Journal of the American Medical Association* (1944), 126: 490–493.

40. Edward F. Rosenberg and Philip S. Hench, "Recent Advances in the Treatment of Rheumatic Fever: With Special Reference to Sulfonamide Prophylaxis and Intravenous Salicylate Therapy," *Medical Clinics of North America* (1946), 30: 489–509.

41. Charles H. Slocumb and Howard F. Polley, "Prophylactic Use of Sulfonamide Compounds in the Treatment of Rheumatic Fever," *Medical Clinics of North America* (1944), 28: 838–843.

42. Janet S. Baldwin, "Sulfadiazine Prophylaxis in Children and Adolescents with Inactive Rheumatic Fever," *Journal of Pediatrics* (1947), 30: 284–288.

43. Joseph Berkson's involvement in this debate is discussed in Rosenberg and Hench, "Recent Advances in the Treatment of Rheumatic Fever," 489–509 (494–495).

44. Katharine G. Dodge, Janet S. Baldwin, and Mortimer W. Weber, "The Prophylactic Use of Sulfanilamide in Children with Inactive Rheumatic Fever," *Journal of Pediatrics* (1944), 24: 483–501. See also P. E. Barclay and F. L. King-Lewis, "Prophylactic Use of Sulphonamides in Rheumatic Fever: A Review of Some American Trials," *Lancet* (1945), 2: 751–752.

45. Janet S. Baldwin, "Follow-Up Study in Rheumatic Subjects Previously Treated with Prophylactic Sulfanilamide," *Journal of Pediatrics* (1947), 30: 67–71.

46. Robert F. Watson, Sidney Rothbard, and Homer F. Swift, "The Use of Penicillin in Rheumatic Fever," *Journal of the American Medical Association* (1944), 126: 274–280.

47. Lowell A. Rantz, Wesley W. Spink, Paul Boisvert, and Howard Coggeshall, "The Treatment of Rheumatic Fever with Penicillin," *Journal of Pediatrics* (1945), 26: 576–582 (579). See also Frank P. Foster, George C. McEachern, John H. Miller, Fred E. Ball, Charles S. Higley, and Harry A. Warren, "The Treatment of Acute Rheumatic Fever with Penicillin," *Journal of the American Medical Association* (1944), 126: 281–282.

48. Jessamine R. Goerner, Benedict F. Massell, and T. Duckett Jones, "Use of Penicillin in the Treatment of Carriers of Beta-Hemolytic Streptococci among Patients with Rheumatic Fever," *New England Journal of Medicine* (1947), 237: 576–580.

49. Richard Gubner and Murrill Szucs, "Therapeutic Measures in Rheumatic Fever: A Comparative Study of One Hundred and Fifty Cases," *New England Journal of Medicine* (1945), 233: 652–657.

50. Leonard Findlay, James W. Macfarlane, and Mary M. Stevenson, "The Cardiac Clinic and Hospital: Their Value in the Control of Rheumatic Infection," *Archives of Disease in Childhood* (1929), 4: 306–312.

51. O. F. Hedley, "Facilities in the United States for the Special Care of Children with Rheumatic Heart Disease," *Public Health Reports* (1941), 56: House of the Good Samaritan, 2322–2324, Irvington House, 2325–2327, Children's Heart Hospital, 2328–2329.

52. Leo M. Taran, "Laboratory and Clinical Criteria of Rheumatic Carditis in Children," *Journal of Pediatrics* (1946), 29: 77–89.

53. Bernard Schlesinger, "The Public Health Aspect of Heart Disease in Childhood," *Lancet* (1938), 1: 593–599.

54. Francis Bach, N. Gray Hill, T. Warwick Preston, and Charles E. Thornton, "Juvenile Rheumatism in London," *Annals of the Rheumatic Diseases* (1939), 1: 210–241.

55. O. F. Hedley, "Facilities in the United States for the Special Care of Children with Rheumatic Heart Disease," *Public Health Reports* (1941), 56: 2321–2341.

56. John P. Hubbard and Walter A. Griffin, "Open-Air Sanatorium Care for Patients with Rheumatic Fever and Rheumatic Heart Disease: Preliminary Report," *New England Journal of Medicine* (1940), 223: 968–972.

57. Leo M. Taran, "The Sanatorium Method for the Care of Rheumatic Heart Disease in Children," *Journal of Pediatrics* (1943), 23: 69–78; and Taran, "Problems in Management of Rheumatic Disease in Childhood," *Journal of Pediatrics* (1944), 24: 62–80.

58. Edward F. Bland, "Rheumatic Fever in Childhood, with Especial Reference to a Five-Year Study of Home and Foster-Home Care," *New England Journal of Medicine* (1941), 224: 629–632. For a description of a similar program in the 1950s, see Dennison Young and Manuel Rodstein, "Home Care of Rheumatic Fever Patients," *Journal of the American Medical Association* (1953), 152: 987–990.

59. J. G. Fred Hiss, "A Plan for Rehabilitation for Rheumatic Subjects," *Journal of Pediatrics* (1945), 26: 230–236.

60. R. R. Struthers, "The Management and Prevention of Rheumatic Fever," *Canadian Medical Association Journal* (1944), 51: 416–422.

61. Bland, "Rheumatic Fever in Childhood."

62. O. Currier McEwen, "The Management of Rheumatic Fever," *Bulletin of the New York Academy of Medicine* (1943), 19: 679–692.

63. For one description of hospital schools, see Anon., "The Care of Rheumatic Children: Report by the Cardiac Society and British Paediatric Association," *Archives of Disease in Childhood* (1944), 19: 96–98.

64. Harold F. Robertson, Ralph E. Schmidt, and William Feiring, "The Therapeutic Value of Early Physical Activity in Rheumatic Fever: A Preliminary Report," *American Journal of the Medical Sciences* (1946), 211: 67–73; and Peter V. Karpovich, Merritt P. Starr, Robert W. Kimbro, Charles G. Stoll, and Raymond A. Weiss, "Physical Reconditioning after Rheumatic Fever," *Journal of the American Medical Association* (1946), 130: 1198–1203.

65. Geoffrey Bourne, "The Treatment of Rheumatic Carditis," *Lancet* (1928), 2: 217–220; Evelyn M. Hickmans and Sydney H. Edgar, "The Blood Constituents in Acute Rheumatism before and after Salicylate Treatment," *Archives of Disease in Childhood* (1930), 5: 387–396; Helen B. Taussig, "The Management of Children with Rheumatic Heart Disease (Compensated and Decompensated)," *Medical Clinics of North America* (1935), 18: 1559–1578; and Russell L. Cecil, "The Therapy of Rheumatic Fever," *Journal of the American Medical Association* (1940), 114: 1443–1447.

66. Homer F. Swift, "Factors Favoring the Onset and Continuation of Rheumatic Fever," *American Heart Journal* (1931), 6: 625–636.

67. William D. Reid, "The Prognosis and Treatment of Rheumatic Heart Disease," *New England Journal of Medicine* (1928), 199: 139–143; Ernest P. Boas and Max Ellenberg, "Rheumatic Pericarditis with Effusion Treated with Salicylates," *Journal of the American Medical Association* (1945), 115: 345–348; and George E. Murphy, "Salicylate and Rheumatic Activity: An Objective Clinical-Histologic Study of the Effect of Salicylate on Rheumatic Lesions, Those of Joints and Tendon Sheaths in Particular," *Bulletin of the Johns Hopkins Hospital* (1945), 77: 1–42.

68. Clifton B. Leech, "The Value of Salicylates in Prevention of Rheumatic Manifestations: Report of a Controlled Clinical Study," *Journal of the American Medical Association* (1930), 95: 932–934.

69. Alvin F. Coburn and Lucile V. Moore, "Salicylate Prophylaxis in Rheumatic Fever," *Journal of Pediatrics* (1942), 21: 180–183

70. John Wyckoff, Arthur C. DeGraff, and Solomon Parent, "The Relationship of Auriculo-Ventricular Conduction Time in Rheumatic Fever to Salicylate Therapy," *American Heart Journal* (1929–30), 5: 568–573; and A. M. Master and Alfred Romanoff, "Treatment of Rheumatic Fever Patients with and without Salicylates," *Journal of the American Medical Association* (1932), 98: 1978–1980.

71. Helen B. Taussig, "Acute Rheumatic Fever: The Significance and Treatment of Various Manifestations," *Journal of Pediatrics* (1939), 14: 581–592.

72. Alvin F. Coburn, "Salicylate Therapy in Rheumatic Fever: A Rational Technique," *Bulletin of the Johns Hopkins Hospital* (1943), 73: 435–464.

73. B. V. Jager and R. Alway, "The Treatment of Acute Rheumatic Fever with Large Doses of Sodium Salicylate, with Special Reference to Dose Management and Toxic Manifestations," *American Journal of the Medical Sciences* (1946), 211: 273–285; R. C. Manchester, "Rheumatic Fever in Naval Enlisted Personnel: II. Effectiveness of Intensive Salicylate Therapy in Cases of Acute Infection," *Archives of Internal Medicine* (1946), 78: 170–180; Johan T. Peters, "The Necessity and Possibility of Giving Detoxified Large Oral Doses of Salicylates in the Treatment of Rheumatic Fever in Order to Prevent or Cure the Inflammatory Stage of Carditis," *Acta Medica Scandinavica* (1947), 128: 51–70; and Leo M. Taran, "Treatment of Acute Rheumatic Fever and Acute Rheumatic Heart Disease," *American Journal of Medicine* (1947), 2: 285–295.

74. Katharine Smull, René Wégria, and Jesica Leland, "The Effect of Sodium Bicarbonate on the Serum Salicylate Level: During Salicylate Therapy of Patients with Acute Rheumatic Fever," *Journal of the American Medical Association* (1944), 125: 1173–1175; Wégria and Smull, "Salicylate Therapy in Acute Rheumatic Fever," *Journal of the American Medical Association* (1945), 129: 45–90; and Wégria and Smull, "Salicylate Therapy in Acute Rheumatic Fever," *Journal of Pediatrics* (1945), 26: 211–213.

75. Henry Z. Sable, "Toxic Reactions Following Salicylate Therapy: A Review of the Literature and Clinical Reports," *Canadian Medical Association Journal* (1945), 52: 153–159.

76. John D. Keith and Alan Ross, "Observations on the Salicylate Therapy in Rheumatic Fever," *Canadian Medical Association Journal* (1945), 52: 554–559.

77. Harry A. Warren, C. S. Higley, and F. S. Coombs, "The Effect of Salicylates on Acute Rheumatic Fever," *American Heart Journal* (1946), 32: 311–326.

78. Robert L. Levy and Ross Golden, "Roentgen Therapy of Active Rheumatic Heart Disease: A Summary of Eleven Years' Experience," *American Journal of the Medical Sciences* (1937), 194: 597–601.

79. Geo. C. Griffith and E. P. Halley, "The Treatment of Rheumatic Fever by Roentgen-Ray Irradiation," *Annals of Internal Medicine* (1946), 24: 1039–1042.

80. Sidney P. Schwartz and Morris M. Weiss, "Digitalis Studies on Children with Heart Disease: Effects of Digitalis on the Electrocardiograms of Children with Rheumatic Fever and Chronic Valvular Disease," *American Journal of Diseases of Children* (1929), 38: 699–714; Schwartz and John B. Schwedel, "II. The Effects of Digitalis on the Sinus Rate of Children with Rheumatic Fever and Chronic Valvular Heart

Disease," *American Journal of Diseases of Children* (1930), 39: 298–315; and Schwartz, "III. Auricular Fibrillation in Children with an Early Toxic Digitalis: Manifestations," *American Journal of Diseases of Children* (1930), 39: 549–559. See also Thomas F. Cotton, "The Treatment of Mitral Disease in Children," *British Medical Journal* (1931), 1: 481–482.

81. Lucy Porter Sutton and John Wyckoff, "Digitalis: Its Value in the Treatment of Children with Rheumatic Heart Disease," *American Journal of Diseases of Children* (1931), 41: 801–815.

82. Bernard J. Walsh and Howard B. Sprague, "The Treatment of Congestive Failure in Children with Active Rheumatic Fever," *Journal of the American Medical Association* (1941), 116: 560–562. For an assessment of treatment for heart failure in the 1960s, see Alvan R. Feinstein and Aida C. Arevalo, "Manifestations and Treatment of Congestive Heart Failure in Young Patients with Rheumatic Heart Disease," *Pediatrics* (1964), 33: 661–671.

CHAPTER 9    *Penicillin, Cortisone, and Heart Surgery*

1. In John Parascandola, *The History of Antibiotics: A Symposium* (Madison, Wisc.: American Institute of the History of Pharmacy, 1980); see, in particular, Ernest Chain, "A Short History of the Penicillin Discovery from Fleming's Early Observations in 1929 to the Present Time," pp. 15–29, and W. H. Helfand, H. B. Woodruff, K.M.H. Coleman, and D. L. Cowen, "Wartime Industrial Development of Penicillin in the United States," pp. 31–56. See also Carol L. Moberg and Zanvil A. Cohn, eds., *Launching the Antibiotic Era: Personal Accounts of the Discovery and Use of the First Antibiotics* (New York: Rockefeller University Press, 1990); Parascandola, "The Introduction of Antibiotics into Therapeutics," in *History of Therapy*, ed. Yosio Kawakita, Shizu Sakai, and Yasuo Otsuka (Tokyo: Ishiyaku EuroAmerica, 1990), 261–281; and Harry F. Dowling, *Fighting Infection: Conquests of the Twentieth Century* (Cambridge Mass.: Harvard University Press, 1977).

2. Maclyn McCarty, "Lewis Wannamaker in the Campaign against Rheumatic Fever," *Zentralblatt für Bakteriologie, Mikrobiologie, und Hygiene-Series A* (1985), 260: 151–164.

3. Jessamine R. Goerner, Benedict F. Massell, and T. Duckett Jones, "Use of Penicillin in the Treatment of Carriers of Beta-Hemolytic Streptococci among Patients with Rheumatic Fever," *New England Journal of Medicine* (1947), 237: 576–580.

4. Floyd W. Denny, Lewis W. Wannamaker, William R. Brink, Charles H. Rammelkamp, Jr., and Edward A. Custer, "Prevention of Rheumatic Fever: Treatment of the Preceding Streptococcic Infection," *Journal of the American Medical Association* (1950), 143: 151–153; and Harold B. Houser and George C. Eckhardt, "Recent Developments in the Prevention of Rheumatic Fever," *Annals of Internal Medicine* (1952), 37: 1035–1043.

5. American Heart Association, "Prevention of Rheumatic Fever," *Lancet* (1953), 1: 285–286; similar statements were published in *Journal of the American Medical Association* (1953), 151: 141–143; and *Public Health Reports* (1953), 68: 12–15. For discussion of AHA guidelines, see Edward A. Mortimer, Jr., and Charles H. Rammelkamp, Jr., "Prophylaxis of Rheumatic Fever," *Circulation* (1956), 14: 1144–1152.

6. Frank J. Catanzaro, Chandler A. Stetson, Alton J. Morris, Robert Chamovitz, Charles H. Rammelkamp, Jr., Bernard L. Stolzer, and William D. Perry, "The Role of the Strep-

tococcus in the Pathogenesis of Rheumatic Fever," *American Journal of Medicine* (1954), 17: 749–756. This study was part of a symposium on rheumatic fever and rheumatic heart disease that appeared in this issue of the *American Journal of Medicine*, pages 747–825. For the effect of delay in treatment, see also Loring L. Brock and Alan C. Siegel, "Studies on the Prevention of Rheumatic Fever: The Effect of Time of Initiation of Treatment of Streptococcal Infections on the Immune Response of the Host," *Journal of Clinical Investigation* (1953), 32: 630–632.

7. Robert Chamovitz, Francis J. Catanzaro, Chandler A. Stetson, and Charles H. Rammelkamp, Jr., "Prevention of Rheumatic Fever by Treatment of Previous Streptococcal Infections: I. Evaluation of Benzathine Penicillin G," *New England Journal of Medicine* (1954), 251: 466–471.

8. Paul F. Frank, Gene H. Stollerman, and Lloyd F. Miller, "Protection of a Military Population from Rheumatic Fever: Routine Administration of Benzathine Penicillin G to Healthy Individuals," *Journal of the American Medical Association* (1965), 193: 775–783.

9. Alton J. Morris, Robert Chamovitz, Frank J. Catanzaro, and Charles H. Rammelkamp, Jr., "Prevention of Rheumatic Fever by the Treatment of Previous Streptococcic Infections: Effect of Sulfadiazine," *Journal of the American Medical Association* (1956), 160: 114–116.

10. Benedict F. Massell, George P. Sturgis, Joseph D. Knobloch, Richard B. Streeper, Thomas N. Hall, and Pliny Norcross, "Prevention of Rheumatic Fever by Prompt Penicillin Therapy of Hemolytic Streptococcic Respiratory Infections," *Journal of the American Medical Association* (1951), 146: 1469–1474.

11. J. A. Pitt Evans, "Oral Penicillin in the Prophylaxis of Streptococcal Infection and Rheumatic Relapse," *Proceedings of the Royal Society of Medicine* (1950), 43: 206–208; and A. H. Gale, W. A. Gillespie, and C. B. Perry, "Oral Penicillin in the Prophylaxis of Streptococcal Infection in Rheumatic Children," *Lancet* (1952), 2: 61–63.

12. Kate H. Kohn, Albert Milzer, and Helen Maclean, "Oral Penicillin Prophylaxis of Recurrences of Rheumatic Fever: Interim Report on Method after a Three Year Study," *Journal of the American Medical Association* (1950), 142: 20–25; and Kohn, Milzer, and Maclean, "Prophylaxis of Recurrences of Rheumatic Fever with Penicillin Given Orally: Final Report of a Five Year Study," *Journal of the American Medical Association* (1953), 151: 347–351.

13. American Heart Association, "Prevention of Rheumatic Fever," *Public Health Reports* (1953), 68: 12–15; and Ella Roberts, "Use of Sulfonamides and Penicillin to Prevent Recurrence of Rheumatic Fever: A Twelve Year Study," *American Journal of Diseases of Children* (1953), 85: 643–647.

14. Gene H. Stollerman and Jerome H. Rusoff, "Prophylaxis against Group A Streptococcal Infections in Rheumatic Fever Patients: Use of New Repository Penicillin Preparation," *Journal of the American Medical Association* (1952), 150: 1571–1575; Stollerman, "The Use of Antibiotics for the Prevention of Rheumatic Fever," *American Journal of Medicine* (1954), 17: 757–767; Stollerman, Rusoff, and Ilse Hirschfeld, "Prophylaxis against Group A Streptococci in Rheumatic Fever: The Use of Single Monthly Injections of Benzathine Penicillin G," *New England Journal of Medicine* (1955), 252: 787–792; for a detailed discussion of prophylaxis at Irvington House, see Harrison Wood, Rita Simpson, Alvan Feinstein, Angelo Taranta, Esther Tursky, and Gene Stollerman, "Rheumatic Fever in Children and Adolescents: A Long-term Epidemiological Study of Subsequent Prophylaxis, Streptococcal Infections, and Clinical

Sequelae: I. Description of the Investigative Techniques and of the Population Studied," *Annals of Internal Medicine* (1964), 60: suppl. 5; Raymond C. Haas, Angelo Taranta, Harrison F. Wood, "Effect of Intramuscular Injections of Benzathene Penicillin G on Some Acute-Phase Reactants," *New England Journal of Medicine* (1957), 256: 152–155; for confirmation of the Irvington House studies, see C. B. Perry and W. A. Gillespie, "Intramuscular Benzathine Penicillin in the Prophylaxis of Streptococcal Infection in Rheumatic Children," *British Medical Journal* (1954), 2: 729–730; and Antoni M. Diehl, Tom R. Hamilton, Irene C. Keeling, and John S. May, "Long-Acting Repository Penicillin in Prophylaxis of Recurrent Rheumatic Fever," *Journal of the American Medical Association* (1954), 155: 1466–1470.

15. Wan Ngo Lim and May G. Wilson, "Comparison of the Recurrence Rate of Rheumatic Carditis among Children Receiving Penicillin by Mouth Prophylactically or on Indication: A Six-Year Study," *New England Journal of Medicine* (1960), 262: 321–325; and Alvan R. Feinstein, Miro Spagnuolo, Saran Jonas, Esther Tursky, Edith K. Stern, and Muriel Levitt, "Prophylaxis of Recurrent Rheumatic Fever: Ineffectiveness of Intermittent 'Therapeutic' Oral Penicillin," *Journal of the American Medical Association* (1965), 191: 451–454.

16. Gene H. Stollerman, "The Prevention of Rheumatic Fever by the Use of Antibiotics," *Bulletin of the New York Academy of Medicine* (1955), 31: 165–180.

17. Ann G. Kuttner and Florence E. Mayer, "Carditis during Second Attacks of Rheumatic Fever: Its Incidence in Patients without Clinical Evidence of Cardiac Involvement in Their Initial Rheumatic Episode," *New England Journal of Medicine* (1963), 268: 1259–1261; for a different opinion, based on observations at Irvington House, see Alvan R. Feinstein and Mario Spagnuolo, "Mimetic Features of Rheumatic-Fever Recurrences," *New England Journal of Medicine* (1960), 262: 533–540.

18. Eloise E. Johnson, Gene H. Stollerman, and Burton J. Grossman, "Rheumatic Recurrences in Patients Not Receiving Continuous Prophylaxis," *Journal of the American Medical Association* (1964), 190: 407–413.

19. American Heart Association, "Prevention of Rheumatic Fever," *Circulation* (1965), 31: 948–952.

20. Joseph M. Miller and Benedict F. Massell, "Studies of Bacterial Throat Flora during Chemoprophylaxis of Rheumatic Fever," *New England Journal of Medicine* (1956), 254: 149–153; Lawrence P. Garrod and Pamela M. Waterworth, "The Risks of Dental Extraction during Penicillin Treatment," *British Heart Journal* (1962), 24: 39–46; and Richard A. Naimon and J. Gordon Barrow, "Penicillin-Resistant Bacteria in the Mouths and Throats of Children Receiving Continuous Prophylaxis against Rheumatic Fever," *Annals of Internal Medicine* (1963), 58: 768–772.

21. Mary Alice Smith, Anton R. Fried, Ernest M. Morris, Lewis C. Robbins, and William J. Zukel, "Rheumatic Fever Prophylaxis: A Community Program through the Private Physician," *Journal of the American Medical Association* (1952), 149: 636–639.

22. William H. Bunn and Hugh N. Bennett, "Community Control of Rheumatic Fever," *Journal of the American Medical Association* (1955), 157: 986–989.

23. Aims C. McGuinness, "The National Attack on Rheumatic Fever," *Public Health Reports* (1959), 74: 870–872.

24. Juanita G. Zagala and Alvan R. Feinstein, "The Preceding Illness of Acute Rheumatic Fever," *Journal of the American Medical Association* (1962), 179: 863–866; and Feinstein, Mario Spagnuolo, Harrison F. Wood, Angelo Taranta, Esther Tursky, and Edith Kleinberg, "Rheumatic Fever in Children and Adolescents: A Long-term Epidemiologic Study of Subsequent Prophylaxis, Streptococcal Infections, and Clinical

Sequelae: VI. Clinical Features of Streptococcal Infections and Rheumatic Occurrences," *Annals of Internal Medicine* (1964), 60: suppl. 5, 68–86.

25. Gabor Czoniczer, Martin Lees, and Benedict F. Massell, "Streptococcal Infection: The Need for Improved Recognition and Treatment for the Prevention of Rheumatic Fever," *New England Journal of Medicine* (1961), 265: 951–952.

26. Burton J. Grossman and Jeremiah Stamler, "Potential Preventability of First Attacks of Acute Rheumatic Fever in Children," *Journal of the American Medical Association* (1963), 183: 985–988; and editorial discussion, "Prevention of Rheumatic Fever," *Journal of the American Medical Association* (1963), 183: 1034.

27. Gabor Czoniczer, Martin Lees, and Benedict F. Massell, "Streptococcal Infection: The Need for Improved Recognition and Treatment for the Prevention of Rheumatic Fever," *New England Journal of Medicine* (1961), 265: 951–952.

28. Bessie L. Lendrum and Charlotte Kobrin, "Prevention of Recurrent Attacks of Rheumatic Fever: Problems Revealed by Long-term Follow-up," *Journal of the American Medical Association* (1956), 162: 13–16.

29. Carl J. Marienfeld, Morton Robins, Roy P. Sandige, and Clare Findlan, "Rheumatic Fever and Rheumatic Heart Disease among U.S. College Freshmen, 1956–60," *Public Health Reports* (1964), 79: 789–811.

30. Basil M. RuDusky, "Heart Murmurs in Youths of Military Age: Evidence of Inadequate Rheumatic Fever Prophylaxis," *Journal of the American Medical Association* (1963), 185: 1004–1007.

31. Benedict F. Massell, Joseph E. Warren, George P. Sturgis, Buford Hall, and Ernest Craige, "The Clinical Response of Rheumatic Fever and Acute Carditis to ACTH," *New England Journal of Medicine* (1950), 242: 641–647, 692–698. For an account of the introduction of cortisone into the practice of rheumatologists, see David Cantor, "Cortisone and the Politics of Drama," *Medical Innovations in Historical Perspective*, ed. J. V. Pickstone (Manchester: University of Manchester, 1992), 165–184, 264–272.

32. Philip S. Hench, Edward C. Kendall, Charles H. Slocumb, and Howard F. Polley, "Effects of Cortisone Acetate and Pituitary ACTH on Rheumatoid Arthritis, Rheumatic Fever, and Certain Other Conditions: A Study in Clinical Physiology," *Archives of Internal Medicine* (1950), 85: 545–666 (section on rheumatic fever, 653–654).

33. Benedict F. Massell, Joseph E. Warren, George P. Sturgis, Buford Hall, and Ernest Craige, "The Clinical Response of Rheumatic Fever and Acute Carditis to ACTH," *New England Journal of Medicine* (1950), 242: 641–647, 692–698.

34. Arlie R. Barnes, Harry L. Smith, Charles H. Slocumb, Howard F. Polley, and Philip S. Hench, "Effect of Cortisone and Corticotropin (ACTH), on the Acute Phase of Rheumatic Fever: Further Observations," *American Journal of Diseases of Children* (1951), 82: 397–425; A. G. Kuttner, J. S. Baldwin, Currier McEwen, J. J. Bunim, Morris Ziff, and D. K. Ford, "Effect of ACTH and Cortisone on Rheumatic Carditis: Observation on Eighteen Cases," *Journal of the American Medical Association* (1952), 148: 628–634; F. Bach, A. Freedman, and L. Bernstock, "Rheumatic Fever: Some Observations on ACTH, Cortisone, and Salicylate Therapy," *British Medical Journal* (1952), 2: 582–587; and Vincent C. Kelley, "Corticotropin (ACTH) Therapy of Initial Attacks of Acute Rheumatic Fever in Children," *American Journal of Diseases of Children* (1952), 84: 151–164.

35. Joseph J. Bunim, Ann G. Kuttner, Janet S. Baldwin, and Currier McEwen, "Cortisone and Corticotropin in Rheumatic Fever and Juvenile Rheumatoid Arthritis," *Journal of the American Medical Association* (1952), 150: 1273–1278; see also Abner

Golden and John Willis Hurst, "Alterations of the Lesions of Acute Rheumatic Myocarditis during Cortisone Therapy," *Circulation* (1953), 7: 218–223.

36. David M. Spain and Daniel Roth, "Effect of Cortisone and ACTH on the Histopathology of Rheumatic Carditis: Report of a Necropsied Case," *American Journal of Medicine* (1951), 11: 128–131; E. N. Chamberlain, John Duncan Hay, and Denis M. Freeman, "Cortisone in Rheumatic Carditis: Some Preliminary Observations," *British Medical Journal* (1952), 1: 1145–1152; Arnold L. Johnson and Charlotte Ferencz, "The Effect of Cortisone Therapy on the Incidence of Rheumatic Heart Disease," *New England Journal of Medicine* (1953), 248: 845–847; and Leo M. Taran, Gaspar A. Gulotta, Nelly Szilagyi, James M. Jablon, and W. Kenneth Lane, "Effect of Cortisone and ACTH on the Protracted Phase of Rheumatic Carditis in Children," *American Journal of Medicine* (1953), 14: 275–283.

37. May G. Wilson, Helen N. Helper, Rose Lubschez, Katharine Hain, and Nathan Epstein, "Effect of Short-Term Administration of Corticotropin in Active Rheumatic Carditis," *American Journal of Diseases of Children* (1953), 86: 131–146; and Wilson and Wan Ngo Lim, "Natural Course of Active Rheumatic Carditis and Evaluation of Hormone Therapy," *Journal of the American Medical Association* (1956), 160: 1457–1460.

38. E. T. Heffer, R. D. Turin, S. R. Slater, and I. G. Kroop, "An Evaluation of Large Doses of Cortisone in First Attacks of Rheumatic Carditis," *Journal of Pediatrics* (1954), 44: 630–639; Nathan M. Greenstein, "Corticotropin in Rheumatic Carditis: Beneficial Effects of High Dosage and Short Duration in Acute Exacerbations of Chronic Rheumatic Carditis," *American Journal of Diseases of Children* (1954), 87: 694–701; and Lawrence Greenman, F. A. Weigand, F. M. Mateer, and T. S. Danowski, "Cortisone Therapy of Initial Attacks of Rheumatic Fever: I. Clinical Data," *American Journal of Diseases of Children* (1955), 89: 426–441.

39. Benedict F. Massell, "ACTH and Cortisone Therapy of Rheumatic Fever and Rheumatic Carditis," *New England Journal of Medicine* (1954), 251: 183–190, 221–228, 263–270.

40. Edward E. Fischel, Charles W. Frank, and Charles Ragan, "Observations on the Treatment of Rheumatic Fever with Salicylate, ACTH, and Cortisone: I. Appraisal of Signs of Systemic and Local Inflammatory Reaction during Treatment, the Rebound Period, and Chronic Activity," *Medicine* (1952), 31: 331–355.

41. Richard D. Rowe, A. D. McKelvey, and John D. Keith, "The Use of ACTH, Cortisone, and Salicylates in the Treatment of Acute Rheumatic Fever," *Canadian Medical Association Journal* (1953), 68: 15–20; R. S. Illingworth, J. Burke, S. A. Doxiadis, J. Lorber, M. G. Philpott, and D. G. H. Stone, "Salicylates in Rheumatic Fever: An Attempt to Assess Their Value," *Quarterly Journal of Medicine* (1954), 23: 177–213; K. S. Holt, "Salicylates in Rheumatic Fever: Difficulties Experienced in Treating Children with Large Doses," *Lancet* (1954), 2: 1197–1199; and Holt, Illingworth, Lorber, and John Rendle-Short, "Cortisone and Salicylates in Rheumatic Fever," *Lancet* (1954), 2: 1144–1148.

42. Benedict F. Massell, "The Medicinal Treatment of Acute Rheumatic Fever," *Medical Clinics of North America* (1953), 37: 1215–1234.

43. *Great Britain*: James Spence, Royal Victoria Infirmary, Newcastle; E.G.L. Bywaters, Canadian Red Cross Memorial Hospital, Taplow (England); Stanley Graham, Royal Hospital for Sick Children, Glasgow; R. S. Illingworth, Children's Hospital, Sheffield; B. E. Schlesinger, Hospital for Sick Children, Great Ormond Street, London; A. G. Watkins, Llandongon Hospital, Cardiff; A. Bradford Hill, statistician.

*USA/Canada*: David Rutstein, American Heart Association; Albert Dorfman, La

Rabida Jackson Park Sanatorium, Chicago; Edward Fischel, Columbia-Presbyterian Hospital, New York; John Keith, Hospital for Sick Children, Toronto; John A. Lichty, University of Colorado; Benedict Massell, House of the Good Samaritan, Boston; Currier McEwen, Bellevue Hospital, New York; Charles Rammelkamp, Jr., Ft. Francis E. Warren, Wyoming (contributed no patients to this study that focused on treatment for children).

44. Medical Research Council of Great Britain and the American Heart Association, "Treatment of Acute Rheumatic Fever in Children: A Co-operative Clinical Trial of ACTH, Cortisone, and Aspirin," *British Medical Journal* (1955), 1: 555–574, also published in *Circulation* (1955), 11: 343–377. For Ft. Francis Warren's participation, see Harold B. Houser, Ernest J. Clark, and Bertrand L. Stolzer, "Comparative Effects of Aspirin, ACTH, and Cortisone on the Acute Course of Rheumatic Fever in Young Adult Males," *American Journal of Medicine* (1954), 16: 168–180.

45. K. S. Holt, "The Rebound Phenomenon in Acute Rheumatic Fever," *Archives of Disease in Childhood* (1956), 31: 444–451; Edward E. Fischel, Charles W. Frank, and Marjorie T. Bellows, "A Study of the Manifestations of Rheumatic Fever Following Cessation of Therapy," *Circulation* (1958), 18: 367–370; and Samuel K. Elster and Elmer Pader, "Studies on Acute Rheumatic Fever in the Adult. II. The Rebound Phenomenon," *Annals of Internal Medicine* (1959), 51: 339–358.

46. Sujoy B. Roy and Benedict F. Massell, "Comparison of Large and Small Doses of Hormones in the Treatment of Acute Rheumatic Carditis," *Circulation* (1956), 14: 44–47; and Roy, George P. Sturgis, and Massell, "Application of the Antistreptolysin-O Titer in the Evaluation of Joint Pain and in the Diagnosis of Rheumatic Fever," *New England Journal of Medicine* (1956), 254: 95–102.

47. J. Lorber, K. S. Holt, John Rendle-Short, and R. S. Illingworth, "Cortisone and Salicylates in Chronic Relapsing Rheumatic Carditis," *Annals of the Rheumatic Diseases* (1957), 16: 481–484.

48. Combined Rheumatic Fever Study Group, "A Comparison of the Effect of Prednisone and Acetylsalicylic Acid on the Incidence of Residual Rheumatic Heart Disease," *New England Journal of Medicine* (1960), 262: 895–902.

49. Medical Research Council and American Heart Association, "The Evolution of Rheumatic Heart Disease in Children: Five-Year Report of a Cooperative Clinical Trial of ACTH, Cortisone, and Aspirin," *Circulation* (1960), 22: 503–515; also published in *British Medical Journal* (1960), 2: 1033–1039.

50. Combined Rheumatic Fever Study Group, "A Comparison of Short-Term, Intensive Prednisone and Acetylsalicylic Acid Therapy in the Treatment of Acute Rheumatic Fever," *New England Journal of Medicine* (1965), 272: 63–70.

51. Medical Research Council of Great Britain and American Heart Association, "The Natural History of Rheumatic Fever and Rheumatic Heart Disease: Ten-Year Report of a Co-Operative Clinical Trial of ACTH, Cortisone, and Aspirin," *Canadian Medical Association Journal* (1965), 93: 519–531; also published in *British Medical Journal* (1965), 2: 607–615; and *Circulation* (1965), 32: 457–476.

52. Albert Dorfman (editorial), "Treatment of Acute Rheumatic Pancarditis," *Circulation* (1964), 29: 811–812; and "Treatment of Rheumatic Fever (editorial)," *New England Journal of Medicine* (1965), 272: 101–102.

53. Dwight E. Harken, Laurence B. Ellis, Paul F. Ware, and Leona R. Norman, "The Surgical Treatment of Mitral Stenosis: I. Valvuloplasty," *New England Journal of Medicine* (1948), 239: 801–809.

54. Robert R. Glover, Charles P. Bailey, and Thomas J. E. O'Neill, "Surgery of Stenotic

Valvular Disease of the Heart," *Journal of the American Medical Association* (1950), 144: 1049–1057; and Charles P. Bailey, Robert P. Glover, and Thomas J. E. O'Neill, "The Surgery of Mitral Stenosis," *Journal of Thoracic Surgery* (1950), 19: 16–49.

55. Charles Baker, R. C. Brock, and Maurice Campbell, "Valvulotomy for Mitral Stenosis: Report of Six Successful Cases," *British Medical Journal* (1950), 1: 1283–1293.

56. Gert H. Brieger, "Mitral Stenosis: A Case Study in the History of Surgery," in A.H.M. Kerkhoff, A. M. Luyendijk-Elshout, and M.J.D. Poulissen, eds., *De Novis Inventis: Essays in the History of Medicine in Honour of Daniel de Moulin on the Occasion of His 65th Birthday* (Amsterdam: APA-Holland University Press, 1984), 27–44. See also Stephen L. Johnson, *The History of Cardiac Surgery, 1896–1955* (Baltimore: Johns Hopkins Press, 1970), 87–99; Harris B. Shumacker, Jr., *The Evolution of Cardiac Surgery* (Bloomington: Indiana University Press, 1992), 31–40, 107–114; R. Heimbecker, T. David, and R. J. Bing, "Valvular Surgery," *Cardiology: The Evolution of the Science and the Art,* ed. Richard J. Bing (Chur, Switzerland: Harward Academic Publishers, 1992), 229–253; Raymond Hurt, *The History of Cardiothoracic Surgery from Early Times* (New York: Parthenon Publishing Group, 1996), 443–460; and W. Bruce Fye, *American Cardiology: The History of a Specialty and Its College* (Baltimore: Johns Hopkins Press, 1996), 115, 168, 170.

57. See Lauder Brunton, "Preliminary Note on the Possibility of Treating Mitral Stenosis by Surgical Methods," *Lancet* (1902), 1: 352; "Surgical Operation for Mitral Stenosis (editorial)," *Lancet* (1902), 1: 461–462; Lauriston E. Shaw, "Surgical Operations for Mitral Stenosis (letter)," *Lancet* (1902), 1: 619; Brunton, "Surgical Operation for Mitral Stenosis (letter)," *Lancet* (1902), 1: 547; Duff S. Allen and Evarts A. Graham, "Intracardiac Surgery—New Method: Preliminary Report," *Journal of the American Medical Association* (1922), 79: 1028–1030; Claude S. Beck, "The Operative Story of the Heart," *Annals of Medical History* (1926), 8: 224–233; Elliott C. Cutler, Samuel A. Levine, and Claude S. Beck, "The Surgical Treatment of Mitral Stenosis: Experimental and Clinical Studies," *Archives of Surgery* (1924), 9: 689–821; Cutler and Levine, "Cardiotomy and Valvulotomy for Mitral Stenosis: Experimental Observations and Clinical Notes Concerning an Operated Case with Recovery," *Boston Medical and Surgical Journal* (1923), 188: 1023–1027; Cutler and Beck, "The Present Status of the Surgical Procedures in Chronic Valvular Disease of the Heart: Final Report of All Surgical Cases," *Archives of Surgery* (1929), 18: 403–416; and H. S. Souttar, "The Surgical Treatment of Mitral Stenosis," *British Medical Journal* (1925), 2: 603–606.

58. Claude S. Beck, "The Technique of Opening the Stenotic Mitral Valve," *Journal of the American Medical Association* (1954), 156: 1400–1401.

59. Robert G. Richardson, *The Surgeon's Heart: A History of Cardiac Surgery* (London: Heinemann Medical Books, 1969), 196–208.

60. Gordon Murray, F. R. Wilkinson, and R. MacKenzie, "Reconstruction of the Valves of the Heart," *Canadian Medical Association Journal* (1938), 38: 317–319.

61. For a discussion of the years just prior to the advent of surgical repair, see Gert H. Brieger, "Mitral Stenosis: A Case Study in the History of Surgery," in *De Novis Inventis: Essays in the History of Medicine in Honour of Daniel de Moulin on the Occasion of His 65th Birthday,* ed. A.H.M. Kerkhoff, A. M. Luyendijk-Elshout, and M.J.D. Poulissen (Amsterdam: APA-Holland University Press, 1984), 27–44.

62. Richard L. Varco and Ivan D. Baronofsky, "The Surgical Problem in Rheumatic Valvular Heart Disease," in *Rheumatic Fever: A Symposium*, ed. Lewis Thomas (Minneapolis: University of Minnesota Press, 1952), 249–264.

63. Dwight E. Harkin, Lewis Dexter, Laurence B. Ellis, Robert E. Farrand, and James F.

Dickson III, "The Surgery of Mitral Stenosis, III. Finger-Fracture Valvuloplasty," *Annals of Surgery* (1951), 134: 722–742; Ralph J. Spiegel, J. Bradley Long, and Lewis Dexter, "Clinical Observations in Patients Undergoing Finger Fracture Mitral Valvuloplasty: I. Auscultatory Changes, II. Electrocardiographic Observations," *American Journal of Medicine* (1952), 12: 626–630 (part I), 631–638 (part II); and Clarence Crafoord and Lars Werkoe, "Surgical Treatment of Rheumatic Heart Disease," *American Journal of Medicine* (1954), 17: 811–825.

64. Thomas J. E. O'Neill, Robert P. Glover, and Charles P. Bailey, "Observations on the Surgical Treatment of Mitral Stenosis by Commissurotomy," *Journal of the American Medical Association* (1951), 147: 1032–1033.

65. O. Henry Janton, Robert P. Glover, and Thomas J. E. O'Neill, "Indications for Commissurotomy in Mitral Stenosis," *American Journal of Medicine* (1952), 12: 621–625.

66. Harry F. Zinnser, Jr., "The Selection of Patients for Mitral Commissurotomy," *American Journal of Medicine* (1954), 17: 804–810.

67. Ibid.; P. F. Angelino, V. Levi, A. Brusca, and A. Actis-Dato, "Mitral Commissurotomy in the Younger Age Group," *American Heart Journal* (1956), 51: 916–925; Albert N. Brest, Joseph Uricchio, and William Likoff, "Valvular Surgery in the Young Patient with Rheumatic Heart Disease," *Journal of the American Medical Association* (1959), 171: 249–251; and Harold A. Collins, Rollin A. Daniel, Jr., H. William Scott, Jr., and Francis A. Puyau, "Surgery for Mitral Valvular Disease during Childhood and Adolescence," *Journal of Thoracic and Cardiovascular Surgery* (1966), 51: 639–648.

68. Gunnar Bieorck, "Rheumatic Heart Disease as a Problem of Preventive Cardiology," *Journal of Chronic Diseases* (1955), 1: 591–600.

69. Marvin Kuschner, Irené Ferrer, Réjane M. Harvey, and Robert Wylie, "Rheumatic Carditis in Surgically Removed Auricular Appendages," *American Heart Journal* (1952), 43: 286–292; David C. Sabiston, Jr., and Richard H. Follis, Jr., "Lesions in Auricular Appendages Removed at Operations for Mitral Stenosis of Presumed Rheumatic Origin," *Bulletin of the Johns Hopkins Hospital* (1952), 91: 178–187; Wilbur A. Thomas, James H. Averill, Benjamin Castleman, and Edward F. Bland, "The Significance of Aschoff Bodies in the Left Atrial Appendage: A Comparison of 40 Biopsies Removed during Mitral Commissurotomy with Autopsy Material from 40 Patients Dying with Fulminating Rheumatic Fever," *New England Journal of Medicine* (1953), 249: 761–765; J. P. Decker, C. Van Z. Hawn, and S. L. Robbins, "Rheumatic 'Activity' as Judged by the Presence of Aschoff Bodies in Auricular Appendages of Patients with Mitral Stenosis: I. Anatomic Aspects," *Circulation* (1953), 8: 161–169; and William F. McNeely, Laurence B. Ellis, and Dwight E. Harkin, "Rheumatic 'Activity' as Judged by the Presence of Aschoff Bodies in Auricular Appendages of Patients with Mitral Stenosis: II. Clinical Aspects," *Circulation* (1953), 8: 337–344.

70. Nicholas P. Christy, "The Effect of Mitral Commissurotomy on the Natural History of Rheumatic Heart Disease," *American Journal of Medicine* (1961), 30: 449–463.

71. Louis A. Soloff, Jacob Zatuchni, O. Henry Janton, Thomas J. E. O'Neill, and Robert P. Glover, "Reactivation of Rheumatic Fever Following Mitral Commissurotomy," *Circulation* (1953), 8: 481–493; and David T. Dresdale, Charles B. Ripstein, Santiago V. Guzman, and Murray A. Greene, "Postcardiotomy Syndrome in Patients with Rheumatic Heart Disease: Cortisone as a Prophylactic and Therapeutic Agent," *American Journal of Medicine* (1956), 21: 57–74.

72. K. Alvin Merendino and Robert A. Bruce, "One Hundred Seventeen Surgically Treated Cases of Valvular Rheumatic Heart Disease: With Preliminary Report of Two Cases of Mitral Regurgitation Treated under Direct Vision with Aid of a Pump-Oxygenator," *Journal of the American Medical Association* (1957), 164: 749–755.

73. T. N. Harris and Sidney Friedman, "Phonocardiographic Differentiation of Vibratory (Functional) Murmurs from Those of Valvular Insufficiency: Further Observations and Application to the Diagnosis of Rheumatic Heart Disease," *American Heart Journal* (1952), 43: 707–712; Crighton Bramwell, "The Diagnosis of Rheumatic Valvular Disease, 1924–1954," *Lancet* (1955), 1: 213–218; Edward M. Kent, William B. Ford, Don L. Fisher, and Theron B. Childs, "The Estimation of the Severity of Mitral Regurgitation: A Correlation of Direct Left Atrial Pressure Recordings with Observations Made during Surgical Palpation of the Valve Area," *Annals of Surgery* (1955), 141: 47–52; Réjane M. Harvey, M. Irené Ferrer, Philip Samet, Richard A. Bader, Mortimer E. Bader, André Cournand, and Dickinson W. Richards, "Mechanical and Myocardial Factors in Rheumatic Heart Disease with Mitral Stenosis," *Circulation* (1955), 11: 531–551; Benjamin G. Musser, James Bougas, and Harry Goldberg, "Left Heart Catheterization: II. With Particular Reference to Mitral and Aortic Valvular Disease," *American Heart Journal* (1956), 52: 567–580; and Jacques B. Wallach, Leslie Lukash, and Alfred A. Angrist, "Mechanisms of Death in Rheumatic Heart Disease in Different Age Periods," *American Journal of Clinical Pathology* (1956), 26: 360–367; and Andrew G. Morrow, "The Surgical Management of Mitral Valve Disease: A Symposium on Diagnostic Methods, Operative Techniques, and Results: Combined Clinical Staff Conference at the National Institutes of Health," *Annals of Internal Medicine* (1964), 60: 1073–1100.

74. Arild E. Hansen, "Importance of Early Diagnosis in Acute Rheumatic Fever," *Journal of the American Medical Association* (1952), 148: 1481–1485.

75. Currier McEwen, "Recent Advances in Diagnosis and Treatment of Rheumatic Fever," *Medical Clinics of North America* (1955), 39: 353–364.

76. Ward Darley, "Denver Rheumatic Fever Diagnostic Service: Purpose and Method of Observation," *Public Health Reports* (1949), 64: 1631–1642; and Frederick J. Lewy, "Diagnostic Problems of Rheumatic Fever and Their Impact on the Management of the Rheumatic Fever Patient," *Annals of Internal Medicine* (1952), 36: 1042–1049.

77. Lindon L. Davis and Marjorie H. Greene, "Rheumatic Fever and Rheumatic Heart Disease in Children as Seen in Clinic Practice," *American Journal of Diseases of Children* (1954), 88: 427–438.

78. Bernice G. Wedum and Paul H. Rhodes, "Differential Diagnosis of Rheumatic Fever in Office Practice," *Journal of the American Medical Association* (1955), 157: 981–986.

79. Committee on Standards and Criteria for Programs of Care, "Jones Criteria (Modified) for Guidance in the Diagnosis of Rheumatic Fever," *Circulation* (1956), 13: 617–620; see also *Public Health Reports* (1956), 71: 672–674.

80. Burton J. Grossman and Balu Athreya, "Sources of Errors in Diagnosis of Acute Rheumatic Fever in Children," *Journal of the American Medical Association* (1962), 182: 830–833.

81. American Heart Association, "Jones Criteria (Revised), for Guidance in the Diagnosis of Rheumatic Fever," *Circulation* (1965), 32: 664–668.

82. Harold C. Anderson and Maclyn McCarty, "Determination of C-Reactive Protein in the Blood as a Measure of the Activity of the Disease Process in Acute Rheumatic Fever," *American Journal of Medicine* (1950), 8: 445–455; Maclyn McCarty, "Present Status of Diagnostic Tests for Rheumatic Fever," *Annals of Internal Medicine* (1952), 37: 1027–1034; Alan G. S. Hill, "C-Reactive Protein in Rheumatic Fever," *Lancet* (1952), 2: 558–560; and Gene H. Stollerman, Samuel Glick, Dali J. Patel, Ilse

Hirschfeld, and Jerome H. Rusoff, "Determination of C-Reactive Protein in Serum as a Guide to the Treatment and Management of Rheumatic Fever," *American Journal of Medicine* (1953), 15: 645–655.

83. Albert J. Simon, Irving Mack, and Philip Rosenblum, "Accelerated Rehabilitation in Rheumatic Fever," *American Journal of Diseases of Children* (1952), 83: 454–462.

84. R. S. Illingworth, "Why Put Him to Bed?," *Clinical Pediatrics* (1963), 2: 108–114.

85. Alvan R. Feinstein, Harry Taube, Ralph Cavalieri, Stanley C. Schultz, and Lawrence Kryle, "Physical Activities and Rheumatic Heart Disease in Asymptomatic Patients," *Journal of the American Medical Association* (1962), 180: 1028–1031.

86. Louis J. Dunman, John H. Githens, and Murray S. Hoffman, "The Role of Bed Rest in Treatment of Rheumatic Fever: Review of Literature and Survey of Current Opinions," *Journal of the American Medical Association* (1957), 164: 1435–1438.

87. Rachel Ash, "Recognition and Management of Rheumatic Fever in Childhood," *Medical Clinics of North America* (1952), 36: 1649–1658; E.G.L. Bywaters, "Treatment of Rheumatic Fever," *Circulation* (1956), 14: 1153–1158; and Bywaters and G. T. Thomas, "Bed Rest, Salicylates, and Steroid in Rheumatic Fever," *British Medical Journal* (1961), 1: 1628–1634.

88. Irving L. Bauer, "Attitudes of Children with Rheumatic Fever," *Journal of Pediatrics* (1952), 40: 796–806.

89. T. Berry Brazelton, Richard Holder, and Beatrice Talbot, "Emotional Aspects of Rheumatic Fever in Children," *Journal of Pediatrics* (1953), 43: 339–358.

90. Ibid., 353.

91. Ibid., 346–347.

92. Ibid., 350.

93. Eugene F. Diamond and Robert Tentler, "The Electroencephalogram in Rheumatic Fever," *Journal of the American Medical Association* (1962), 182: 685–687.

94. Nancy M. Wertheimer, "A Psychiatric Follow-Up of Children with Rheumatic Fever and Other Chronic Diseases," *Journal of Chronic Diseases* (1963), 16: 223–237.

95. Leonore Sacks, Alvan R. Feinstein, and Angelo Taranta, "A Controlled Psychological Study of Sydenham's Chorea," *Journal of Pediatrics* (1962), 61: 714–722.

96. Currier McEwen, "Current Status of Therapy in Rheumatic Fever," *Journal of the American Medical Association* (1959), 170: 1056–1062.

CHAPTER 10    *The Waning of Rheumatic Fever*

1. J. Alison Glover, "The Decline of Mortality from Rheumatic Fever," *Monthly Bulletin of the Ministry of Health and the Emergency Public Health Service* (1946), 5: 222–229 (228).

2. Clifford G. Parsons, "The General Practitioner and the Child with Heart Disease," *British Medical Journal* (1954), 2: 208–212 (209).

3. W. Melville Arnott, "The Changing Aetiology of Heart Disease," *British Medical Journal* (1954), 2: 887–891.

4. Edward F. Bland, "Declining Severity of Rheumatic Fever: A Comparative Study of the Past Four Decades," *New England Journal of Medicine* (1960), 262: 597–599; see also Bland and T. Duckett Jones, "Rheumatic Fever and Rheumatic Heart Disease: A Twenty Year Report on 1000 Patients Followed since Childhood," *Circulation* (1951), 4: 836–843; and Bland and Jones, "The Natural History of Rheumatic Fever: A 20 Year Perspective," *Annals of Internal Medicine* (1952), 37: 1006–1026.

5. Benedict F. Massell, Francisco Amezcua, and Salvatore Pelargonio, "Evolving Picture of Rheumatic Fever: Data from 40 Years at the House of the Good Samaritan," *Journal of the American Medical Association* (1964), 188: 287–294.

6. Ian I. Findlay and Rodney S. Fowler, "The Changing Pattern of Rheumatic Fever in Childhood," *Canadian Medical Association Journal* (1966), 94: 1027–1034.

7. Lawrence Kuskin and Morris Siegel, "The Changing Pattern of Rheumatic Heart Disease: The Experience in New York City Department of Health Cardiac Consultation Clinics, 1943 to 1953," *Journal of Pediatrics* (1956), 49: 574–582.

8. Helen M. Wallace and Herbert Rich, "Changing Status of Rheumatic Fever and Rheumatic Heart Disease in Children and Youth," *American Journal of Diseases of Children* (1955), 89: 7–14.

9. Robert Q. Quinn and Julia P. Quinn, "Decline in Mortality in Acute Rheumatic Fever in New Haven, Connecticut, 1920–1948," *New England Journal of Medicine* (1951), 245: 211–214.

10. Howard A. Joos and Chris P. Katsampes, "A Community Study of Rheumatic Fever," *American Journal of Diseases of Children* (1952), 83: 37–51.

11. Saul J. Robinson, "Incidence of Rheumatic Fever in San Francisco Children: A Ten-Year Study," *Journal of Pediatrics* (1956), 49: 272–279.

12. Samuel L. Lieber and Joe E. Holoubek, "Acute Rheumatic Fever in a Large Southern Hospital over the Five-Year Period 1950 through 1954," *Annals of Internal Medicine* (1956), 45: 118–125.

13. R.A.N. Hitchens, "Decline of Acute Rheumatism," *Annals of the Rheumatic Diseases* (1956), 15: 160–172.

14. S. Rosenbaum and J.D.H. Slater, "An Epidemiological Study of Rheumatic Fever in the Army in 1953," *Journal of the Royal Army Medical Corps* (1957), 103: 109–118.

15. Basil M. RuDusky, "Heart Murmurs in Youths of Military Age: Evidence of Inadequate Rheumatic Fever Prophylaxis," *Journal of the American Medical Association* (1963), 185: 1004–1007.

16. George J. Maresh and John A. Lichty, "Incidence of Heart Disease among Colorado School Children," *Journal of the American Medical Association* (1952), 149: 802–805.

17. George Wolff, "Death Toll from Rheumatic Fever in Childhood," *Journal of the American Medical Association* (1951), 145: 719–724.

18. Joseph Stokes III and Thomas R. Dawber, "Rheumatic Heart Disease in the Framingham Study," *New England Journal of Medicine* (1956), 255: 1228–1233.

19. Carl J. Marienfeld, Morton Robins, Roy P. Sandidge, and Clare Findlan, "Rheumatic Fever and Rheumatic Heart Disease among U.S. College Freshmen, 1956–60," *Public Health Reports* (1964), 79: 789–811.

20. May G. Wilson, Wan Ngo Lim, and Ann McA. Birch, "The Decline of Rheumatic Fever: Recurrence Rates of Rheumatic Fever among 782 Children for Twenty-One Consecutive Calendar Years (1936–1956)," *Journal of Chronic Diseases* (1958), 7: 183–197.

21. R.A.N. Hitchens, "Recurrent Attacks of Acute Rheumatism in School-Children," *Annals of the Rheumatic Diseases* (1958), 17: 293–302.

22. Janet S. Baldwin, Josephine M. Kerr, Ann G. Kuttner, and Eugenie F. Doyle, "Observations on Rheumatic Nodules over a 30–Year Period," *Journal of Pediatrics* (1960), 56: 465–470.

23. Alan M. Aron, John M. Freeman, and Sidney Carter, "The Natural History of

Sydenham's Chorea: Review of the Literature and Long-Term Evaluation with Emphasis on Cardiac Sequelae," *American Journal of Medicine* (1965), 38: 83–95.

24. "Acute Rheumatic Fever: A Changing Disease (editorial)," *Journal of the American Medical Association* (1962), 182: 1035–1036.

25. Edwin P. Maynard, Jr., and Victor Grover, "The Effect of Childbearing on the Course of Rheumatic Heart Disease: A 25-Year Study," *Annals of Internal Medicine* (1960), 52: 163–171.

26. Gene H. Stollerman, Alan C. Siegel, and Eloise E. Johnson, "Variable Epidemiology of Streptococcal Disease and the Changing Pattern of Rheumatic Fever," *Modern Concepts of Cardiovascular Disease* (1965), 34: 45–48.

27. Charles H. Rammelkamp, Lewis W. Wannamaker, and Floyd W. Denny, "The Epidemiology and Prevention of Rheumatic Fever," *Bulletin of the New York Academy of Medicine* (1952), 28: 321–334.

28. John H. Dingle, Charles H. Rammelkamp, Jr., and Lewis W. Wannamaker, "Epidemiology of Streptococcal Infections and Their Non-Suppurative Complications," *Lancet* (1953), 1: 736–738; Floyd W. Denny, Jr., William D. Perry, and Lewis W. Wannamaker, "Type-Specific Streptococcal Antibody," *Journal of Clinical Investigation* (1957), 36: 1092–1100; and Lewis W. Wannamaker and Elia M. Ayoub, "Antibody Titers in Acute Rheumatic Fever," *Circulation* (1960), 21: 598–614. See also Milton Markowitz and Goldie Pelovitz, "Studies on Type-Specific Streptococcal Antibodies as Indicators of Previous Streptococcal Infections in Rheumatic and Nonrheumatic Children," *Journal of Clinical Investigation* (1963), 42: 409–416.

29. Gene H. Stollerman, "Factors That Predispose to Rheumatic Fever," *Medical Clinics of North America* (1960), 44: 17–28; see also Stollerman, Arthur J. Lewis, Irwin Schultz, and Angelo Taranta, "Relationship of Immune Response to Group A Streptococci to the Course of Acute, Chronic, and Recurrent Rheumatic Fever," *American Journal of Medicine* (1956), 20: 163–169.

30. Milton S. Saslaw and Murray M. Streitfield, "Group A Beta Hemolytic Streptococci and Rheumatic Fever in Miami, Fla.," *Public Health Reports* (1954), 69: 877–882; Saslaw, "Case Registry for Rheumatic Fever and Glomerulonephritis," *Journal of the American Medical Association* (1957), 165: 1129–1130; Saslaw and James M. Jablon, "Epidemiology of Group-A B-Hemolytic Streptococci as Related to Acute Rheumatic Fever in Miami, Florida: A Six-Year Study," *Circulation* (1960), 21: 679–683; Saslaw and Morton N. Schwartzman, "Case Registry for Rheumatic Fever in Greater Miami, Florida," *Public Health Reports* (1962), 77: 17–28; and Saslaw, Jablon, and John A. Mazzarella, "Prevention of Initial Attacks of Rheumatic Fever," *Public Health Reports* (1963), 78: 207–221.

31. Alan C. Siegel, Eloise E. Johnson, and Gene H. Stollerman, "Controlled Studies of Streptococcal Pharyngitis in a Pediatric Population: I. Factors Related to the Attack Rate of Rheumatic Fever," *New England Journal of Medicine* (1961), 265: 559–566; and Stollerman, "Factors Determining the Attack Rate of Rheumatic Fever," *Journal of the American Medical Association* (1961), 177: 823–828.

32. Victoria Smallpiece and Hugh Ellis, "Acute Rheumatism and Paediatric Beds," *British Medical Journal* (1960), 1: 1952–1953.

33. Nathan Epstein, "Incidence and Frequency of Infections at Specific Ages in Infancy and Childhood: With Special Reference to Upper Respiratory Infections in Potentially Rheumatic-Susceptible Children," *American Journal of Diseases of Children* (1954), 87: 600–606.

34. Ham Jackson, Jack Cooper, William J. Mellinger, and Arthur R. Olsen, "Streptococcal Pharyngitis in Rural Practice: Rational Medical Management," *Journal of the American Medical Association* (1966), 197: 385–388.

35. Maclyn McCarty, "Maxwell Finland Lecture: An Adventure in the Pathogenic Maze of Rheumatic Fever," *Journal of Infectious Diseases* (1981), 143: 375–385.

36. Maclyn McCarty, "Present State of Knowledge Concerning Pathogenesis and Treatment of Rheumatic Fever," *Bulletin of the New York Academy of Medicine* (1952), 28: 307–320.

37. Rebecca C. Lancefield, "Cellular Constituents of Group A Streptococci Concerned in Antigenicity and Virulence," in *Streptococcal Infections*, ed. Maclyn McCarty (New York: Columbia University Press, 1954), 3–18.

38. L. R. Christensen, "The Streptokinase-Plasminogen System," in *Streptococcal Infections*, ed. Maclyn McCarty (New York: Columbia University Press, 1954), 39–55.

39. Maclyn McCarty, "The Antibody Response to Streptococcal Infections," in *Streptococcal Infections*, ed. Maclyn McCarty (New York: Columbia University Press, 1954), 130–142.

40. Charles H. Rammelkamp, Jr., "Acute Hemorrhagic Glomerulonephritis," in *Streptococcal Infections*, ed. Maclyn McCarty (New York: Columbia University Press, 1954), 197–207.

41. Lowell A. Rantz, Paul J. Boisvert, and Wesley W. Spink, "Hemolytic Streptococcic Sore Throat: The Poststreptococcic State," *Archives of Internal Medicine* (1947), 79: 401–435.

42. Edward E. Fischel, "The Role of Allergy in the Pathogenesis of Rheumatic Fever," *American Journal of Medicine* (1949), 7: 772–793.

43. Joseph M. Miller, Sidney Kibrick, and Benedict F. Massell, "Antibody Response to Non-Streptococcal Antigens as Related to Rheumatic Fever Susceptibility," *Journal of Clinical Investigation* (1953), 32: 691–695.

44. Maclyn McCarty, "Nature of Rheumatic Fever," *Circulation* (1956), 14: 1138–1143; Jerry K. Aikawa, "Hypersensitivity and Rheumatic Fever," *Annals of Internal Medicine* (1954), 41: 576–604; T. N. Harris, "Etiologic Factors in Rheumatic Fever," *Medical Clinics of North America* (1954), 38: 1693–1704; Lloyd Florio, Gertrud Weiss, and Gladys K. Lewis, "Tissue Culture Studies of Cellular Hypersensitivity in Rheumatic Fever: I. The Response of Human White Blood Cells to Streptococci and to Crude Filtrates of Streptococcal Cultures," *Journal of Immunology* (1958), 80: 12–25; and Gertrud Weiss, Florio, and Lewis, "Tissue Culture Studies of Cellular Hypersensitivity in Rheumatic Fever: II. The Response of Fibroblasts from Human Skin and Heart to Disintegrated Streptococci and to Crude Filtrates of Streptococcal Cultures," *Journal of Immunology* (1958), 80: 26–31.

45. George E. Murphy and Homer F. Swift, "The Induction of Rheumatic-like Cardiac Lesions in Rabbits by Repeated Focal Infections with Group A Streptococci," *Journal of Experimental Medicine* (1950), 91: 485–498; L. Kirschner and J. B. Howie, "Rheumatic-like Lesions in the Heart of the Rabbit Experimentally Induced by Repeated Inoculation with Haemolytic Streptococci," *Journal of Pathology and Bacteriology* (1952), 64: 367–377; Otto Saphir, "The Aschoff Nodule," *American Journal of Clinical Pathology* (1959), 31: 534–539; P. S. Tweedy, "The Pathogenesis of Valvular Thickening in Rheumatic Heart Disease," *British Heart Journal* (1956), 18: 173–185; and George E. Murphy, "On Muscle Cells, Aschoff Bodies, and Cardiac Failure in Rheumatic Heart Disease," *Bulletin of the New York Academy of Medicine* (1959), 35: 619–651. For obituaries of Homer Swift, see *Journal of the American Medical*

*Association* (1953), 153: 967; and *Transactions of the Association of American Physicians* (1954), 67: 25–27.

46. Melvin H. Kaplan and Frederick D. Dallenbach, "Immunologic Studies of Heart Tissue: III. Occurrence of Bound Gamma Globulin in Auricular Appendages from Rheumatic Hearts. Relationship to Certain Histopathologic Features of Rheumatic Heart Disease," *Journal of Experimental Medicine* (1961), 113: 1–16.

47. Melvin H. Kaplan, Mary Meyeserian, and Irving Kushner, "Immunological Studies of Heart Tissue: IV. Serologic Reactions with Human Heart Tissue as Revealed by Immunofluorescent Methods: Isoimmune, Wasserman, and Autoimmune Reactions," *Journal of Experimental Medicine* (1961), 113: 17–36.

48. Melvin H. Kaplan and Mary Meyeserian, "An Immunological Cross-Reaction between Group-A Streptococcal Cells and Human Heart Tissue," *Lancet* (1962), 1: 706–710.

49. Melvin H. Kaplan, Robert Bolande, Louis Rakita, and John Blair, "Presence of Bound Immunoglobulins and Complement in the Myocardium in Acute Rheumatic Fever: Association with Cardiac Failure," *New England Journal of Medicine* (1964), 271: 637–645.

50. Evelyn V. Hess, Chester W. Fink, Angelo Taranta, and Morris Ziff, "Heart Muscle Antibodies in Rheumatic Fever and Other Diseases," *Journal of Clinical Investigation* (1964), 43: 886–893.

51. Maclyn McCarty, "Missing Links in the Streptococcal Chain Leading to Rheumatic Fever: The T. Duckett Jones Memorial Lecture," *Circulation* (1964), 29: 488–493; for a similar account but aimed at a larger audience, see Earl H. Freimer and Maclyn McCarty, "Rheumatic Fever," *Scientific American* (December 1965), 213: 66–70.

52. See Edward Klibanoff, Julian Frieden, Mario Spagnuolo, and Alvan R. Feinstein, "'Rheumatic Activity,' A Clinicopathologic Correlation," *Journal of the American Medical Association* (1966), 195: 895–900.

53. For an excellent collection of scientific essays on the state of knowledge about rheumatic fever in the early 1970s, see Lewis W. Wannamaker and John M. Matsen, *Streptococci and Streptococcal Diseases: Recognition, Understanding, and Management* (New York: Academic Press, 1972).

54. Patricia Ferrieri, "Acute Rheumatic Fever: The Come-back of a Disappearing Disease," *American Journal of Diseases of Children* (1987), 141: 725–727; Don M. Hosier, Josepha M. Craenen, Douglas W. Teske, John J. Wheller, "Resurgence of Acute Rheumatic Fever," *American Journal of Diseases of Children* (1987), 141: 730–733; Milton Markowitz and Michael A. Gerber, "Rheumatic Fever: Recent Outbreaks of an Old Disease," *Connecticut Medicine* (1987), 51: 229–233; L. George Veasy, Susan E. Wiedmeier, Garth S. Orsmond, Herbert D. Ruttenberg, Mark M. Boucek, Stephen J. Roth, Vera F. Tait, Joel A. Thopson, Judy A. Daly, Edward L. Kaplan, and Harry R. Hill, "Resurgence of Acute Rheumatic Fever in the Intermountain Area of the United States," *New England Journal of Medicine* (1987), 316: 421–427; Ellen R. Wald, Barry Dashefsky, Cindy Feidt, Darleen Chiponis, Carol Byers, "Acute Rheumatic Fever in Western Pennsylvania and the Tristate Area," *Pediatrics* (1987), 80: 371–374; and Blaise Congeni, Christopher Rizzo, Joseph Congeni, and V. V. Sreenivasan, "Outbreak of Acute Rheumatic Fever in Northeast Ohio," *Journal of Pediatrics* (1987), 111: 176–179.

55. Gene H. Stollerman, "The Nature of Rheumatogenic Streptococci," *Mount Sinai Journal of Medicine* (1996), 63: 144–158; for a similar hypothesis, see Floyd W. Denny, Jr., "A 45–Year Perspective on the Streptococcus and Rheumatic Fever: The Edward H. Kass Lecture in Infectious Disease History," *Clinical Infectious Diseases* (1994),

19: 1110–1122; and Stollerman, "Rheumatogenic Group A Streptococci and the Return of Rheumatic Fever," *Advances in Internal Medicine* (1990), 35: 1–25.

56. Alvin F. Coburn, "Susceptibility to Rheumatic Disease," *Journal of Pediatrics* (1961), 58: 448–451. In the 1960s, Coburn tried to link genetic susceptibility with dietary deficiency, especially the lack of eggs; see Coburn, "The Concept of Egg Yolk as a Dietary Inhibitor to Rheumatic Susceptibility," *Lancet* (1960), 1: 867–870; and Coburn, "The Pathogenesis of Rheumatic Fever—A Concept," *Perspectives in Biology and Medicine* (1963), 6: 493–511.

57. A. C. Stevenson and E. A. Cheeseman, "Heredity and Rheumatic Fever: Some Later Information about Data Collected in 1950–51," *Annals of Human Genetics* (1956), 21: 139–144.

58. May G. Wilson and Morton Schweitzer, "Pattern of Hereditary Susceptibility in Rheumatic Fever," *Circulation* (1954), 10: 699–704.

59. Frieda G. Gray, Robert W. Quinn, and Julia P. Quinn, "A Long-Term Survey of Rheumatic and Non-Rheumatic Families: With Particular Reference to Environment and Heredity," *American Journal of Medicine* (1952), 13: 400–412.

60. A. Michael Davies and Eliahu Lazarov, "Heredity, Infection and Chemoprophylaxis in Rheumatic Carditis: An Epidemiological Study of a Communal Settlement," *Journal of Hygiene* (1960), 58: 263–276.

61. Thomas D. Dublin, A. David Bernanke, Elaine L. Pitt, Benedict F. Massell, Fred H. Allen, Jr., and Francisco Amezcua, "Red Blood Cell Groups and ABH Secretor System as Genetic Indicators of Susceptibility to Rheumatic Fever and Rheumatic Heart Disease," *British Medical Journal* (1964), 2: 775–779; Wan Ngo Lim, A. Kellner, M. D. Schweitzer, D. Smith, and M. G. Wilson, "Association of Secretor Status and Rheumatic Fever in 106 Families," *American Journal of Epidemiology* (1965), 82: 103–111; and A. L. Macafee, "ABO Blood Groups and Rheumatic Heart Disease," *Annals of the Rheumatic Diseases* (1965), 24: 392–393.

62. For a discussion, see Elia M. Ayoub and Salman Ahmed, "Update on Complications of Group A Streptococcal Infections," *Current Problems in Pediatrics* (1997), 27: 90–101.

# GLOSSARY

**ACTH (Adrenocorticotrophic hormone)**—A hormone secreted by the pituitary gland which in turn stimulates the adrenal gland to release steroids, such as cortisol.

**Acute articular rheumatism**—A largely nineteenth-century term for rheumatic fever, used predominantly in Britain.

**Aerobic**—Requiring oxygen for life.

**Alkaline**—A drug or chemical which neutralizes acid, often an oxide or carbonate of metals, such as potash (potassium hydroxide).

**Alpha hemolysis**—Incomplete hemolysis surrounding a colony of bacteria growing on a blood agar plate; its presence serves as an aid in classifying bacteria.

**Anaerobic**—Able to live without oxygen.

**Antibiotic**—An antibacterial agent derived from microorganisms, such as penicillin.

**Antistreptolysin-O (ASO)**—An antibody directed against the Group A beta-hemolytic streptococcus; its presence serves as a diagnostic aid for a preceding streptococcal infection.

**Arthralgia**—Joint pain.

**Arthritis**—Inflammation of joints normally yielding heat, swelling, redness, tenderness, and loss of motion.

**Articular**—Pertaining to joints.

**Aschoff body**—Characteristic inflammmation of the heart muscle found in rheumatic fever.

**Aspirin (acetylsalicylic acid)**—A salicylate drug commonly used to treat rheumatic fever.

**Auscultation**—Listening with a stethoscope to bodily sounds, such as breathing or the heart's beating.

**Bacille d'Achalme**—A rod-shaped bacterium isolated by Pierre Achalme in 1891 from the blood of a patient suffering from rheumatic fever.

**Bacillus (bacilli)**—A rod-shaped bacterium (a).

**Beta hemolysis**—Complete hemolysis, demonstrated by a transparent area surrounding a colony of bacteria growing on a blood agar plate; its presence serves as an aid in classifying bacteria.

**Carditis**—A general term for inflammation of any of the heart's tissues.

**Chorea**—Derived from the Greek word for "dance," a condition characterized by involuntary, repetitive, jerking movements affecting all parts of the body but most noticeable in the limbs, face, and tongue.

**Cinchona**—Genus of evergreen trees whose bark serves as a source of quinine.

**Coccus (cocci)**—Ball-shaped bacterium(a).

**Commissurotomy**—Surgical operation for the correction of mitral stenosis.

**Corticosteroids**—Steroid chemicals secreted by the adrenal glands (and manufactured synthetically) which have many therapeutic uses in medicine; when employed in rheumatic fever, these drugs reduce inflammation.

**Cortisone**—The first corticosteroid used as a drug.

**Cross-reactivity**—A phenomenon in which human antibodies formed to combat streptococcal infections also harm human tissues of similar chemical structure.

**Diplococcus rheumaticus**—Name given to double-balled bacteria, almost certainly *streptococcus viridans,* isolated by Frederick Poynton and Alexander Paine in 1900 from the blood of patients with rheumatic fever.

**Embolus (emboli)**—A mass of material which has traveled from elsewhere through the bloodstream to occlude an artery.

**Endocarditis**—Inflammation of the endocardium, or heart valves.

**Endocardium**—A thin layer of cells that lines the chambers of the heart which help to form the heart valves.

**Erythema marginatum**—A rash commonly associated with rheumatic fever.

**Erythrocyte sedimentation rate (ESR)**—The gradual settling of red blood cells which occurs in an undisturbed sample of whole blood; in rheumatic fever, the rate of sinking is increased; the more active the disease, the higher the rate of fall of red blood cells.

**Group A beta-hemolytic streptococcus (GABS)**—A member of the streptococcus family of bacteria which possesses a specific polysaccharide (A) in the cell wall and which produces beta-hemolysis around colonies on a blood agar plate; infection with GABS precedes rheumatic fever.

**Heart block**—Impaired electrical conduction between the chambers of the heart so that the atria and ventricles beat independently of each other.

**Hemolysis**—Destruction of red blood cells; used as a means of classifying bacteria.

**Hemolytic streptococcus**—A member of the streptococcus family of bacteria that produces clear hemolysis on blood agar plates.

**Hypersensitization**—An allergic overresponse.

**Inflammation**—Local tissue response to injury by bacteria or other agents, which serves a protective function.

**M Protein**—A component of the cell wall of the streptococcus that is responsible for virulence and immunity.

**Mendelian distribution**—Term applied to a law of genetics, enunciated by Johann

Gregor Mendel, that described the expression of dominant and recessive traits in offspring.

**Mitral heart valve**—The valve between the left atrium and left ventricle of the heart.

**Mitral stenosis**—A narrowing of the opening in the mitral valve.

**Myocarditis**—Inflammation of the heart's muscle.

**Myocardium**—Muscular tissue of the heart.

**Nosology**—Classification of diseases.

**Pathognomonic**—Specific and characteristic of a given disease, such as the Aschoff body in rheumatic fever.

**Pericarditis**—Inflammation of the pericardium in which the pericardial sac either adheres to the heart or fills with fluid; in either case, the heart's beating is seriously compromised.

**Pericardium**—A membranous sac surrounding the heart.

**Pleurisy**—Inflammation of the lining of the lungs which can lead to fluid accumulation and to painful and difficult breathing.

**Precordium**—Portion of the chest wall which is anterior to the heart.

**Prednisone**—A synthetic corticosteroid.

**Rheumatism**—An older, generic term for painful joints found in several diseases.

**Salicylate**—A chemical which occurs in several plants or which can be synthesized; salicylate has many medical uses, including the reduction of fever and inflammation. Aspirin is a commonly used derivative.

**Saprophyte**—Germs which usually live upon decaying and dead matter and produce its decomposition.

**Sepsis**—Widespread infection of the blood or other tissues, commonly caused by bacteria.

**Streptococcus**—A large and heterogeneous group of spherical bacteria named for their common tendency to form pairs or chains.

**Streptococcus pyogenes**—An older term for Group A streptococci, which refers to a characteristic of infections with these bacteria to produce pus.

**Streptococcus viridans**—A vague, older term to denote streptococci that produce alpha hemolysis.

**Subcutaneous nodules**—Swellings that occur beneath the skin and are not attached to underlying bone.

**Sulfonamide**—A family of antibacterial drugs.

**Suppuration**—Pus formation, a part of inflammation.

**Valvulotomy**—A surgical operation for the correction of mitral stenosis.

# INDEX

# About the Author

Peter C. English is the Josiah Charles Trent Associate Professor of the History of Medicine at Duke University. He is also a primary care pediatrician. English is the author of *Shock, Physiological Surgery, and George Washington Crile: Medical Innovation in the Progressive Era* and has also written on the history of unwanted children and child abuse, the history of pneumonia and diphtheria, and Abraham Jacobi. He lives in Durham, North Carolina, with his wife, Sarah. They have one son in college.